JB JOSSEY-BASS

QUALITY BY DESIGN

A Clinical Microsystems Approach

Eugene C. Nelson
Paul B. Batalden
Marjorie M. Godfrey
Editors

Foreword by Donald M. Berwick

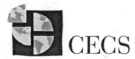

CECS

Center for the Evaluative
Clinical Sciences at Dartmouth

John Wiley & Sons, Inc.

Published by Jossey-Bass
A Wiley Imprint
989 Market Street, San Francisco, CA 94103-1741   www.josseybass.com

Readers should be aware that Internet Web sites offered as citations and/or sources for further
information may have changed or disappeared between the time this was written and when it is read.

Jossey-Bass books and products are available through most bookstores. To contact Jossey-Bass directly
call our Customer Care Department within the U.S. at 800-956-7739, outside the U.S. at 317-572-3986,
or fax 317-572-4002.

Jossey-Bass also publishes its books in a variety of electronic formats. Some content that appears in print
may not be available in electronic books.

Library of Congress Cataloging-in-Publication Data

Quality by design : a clinical microsystems approach / [edited by] Eugene C. Nelson, Paul B. Batalden,
Marjorie M. Godfrey; foreword by Donald M. Berwick.—1st ed.
    p.; cm.
   Includes bibliographical references and index.
   ISBN: 978-0-7879-7898-3 (pbk.)
    1. Medical care—United States—Quality control—Mathematical models.   2. Health services
administration—United States—Mathematical models.   I. Batalden, Paul B.   II. Godfrey, Marjorie
M. III. Nelson, Eugene C.
    [DNLM: 1. Delivery of Health Care—methods.   2. Delivery of Health Care—organization &
administration.   3. Models, Organizational.   4. Quality of Health Care—organization & administration.
W 84.1 Q1535 2007]
   RA399.A3Q343 2007
   362.1068—dc22
                                                  2006036606

FIRST EDITION
PB Printing 10 9 8 7 6 5 4 3

CONTENTS

PART ONE: CASES AND PRINCIPLES   1

TABLES, FIGURES, AND EXHIBITS

Tables

Figures

Exhibits

FOREWORD

Donald M. Berwick

It is remarkable, and sad, that a large proportion of health care professionals today—maybe a majority—would likely describe the environment of their work in terms that bespeak alienation. They might call themselves "battered," "pressured," "hassled," and, deeply, "misunderstood." I do not think they would generally say that about their clinical work; these are not their feelings about their relationships with patients—their experience of trying to help and to heal. These are their feelings about those who set in place the conditions of their work—the rule makers, the paymasters, and to some extent the institutional executives.

It is also remarkable, and sad, that those who shape the environment—the rule makers, the paymasters, and many executives—feel no less pressured than the clinicians do. I believe that many of them feel hassled by their own sense of ineffectiveness. They have hard jobs, involving the navigation of a no-man's-land of goals while also guarding limited resources and pursuing the great ambitions of modern medicine. They are the stewards of possibility, and they seem to me perplexed that the clinical forces so often misunderstand them.

I sat once in a meeting at the highest level in an academic medical center and heard the chief of surgery refer, in public, to the chief finance officer as a "pointy-headed dweeb." The distance between them was vast and the damage to spirit incalculable. This is not at all a one-way problem. How many times have you heard—even laughed at—the unfunny assertion that leading doctors is like "herding cats?" What does the doctor feel who hears that? At least the physicians and nurses have the quiet refuge of the consulting room to retreat to in search of their own meaning. Where does the executive, so abused and so misunderstood, go for renewal?

I sometimes call this the *line-in-the-carpet* problem. I was walking through a multibillion-dollar major medical center once with its powerful CEO. He wanted to introduce me to a clinical leader and brought me to that physician's outpatient clinical office. But the CEO did not walk into the clinical area. At the margin, where the carpet changed color from the deep tan of the waiting area to the lighter tan of the clinical suite, the CEO brought his toes exactly up to the carpet seam, like a racer at the starting line, and leaned awkwardly into the clinical space, asking a passing nurse if Dr. X could be found. He did not set a single foot in the place of patient care. It was as if the CEO of Boeing did not walk into the factory or the CEO of McDonald's avoided the kitchen.

Perhaps it was simply a sign of respect for the flow of work or the confidentiality of patients. But I think not. I think it was a symbol of the torn fabric of health care, deeply divided along the seam between the work of care and the work of shaping the environment of care. Much respected health care management teaching has, I believe, instructed the executives of the future to stay out of the clinical arena—to leave the care to the doctors and nurses—while they, the executives, run the organization that supports the clinicians' work. Elaborate structures involving divided governance, medical staff rituals, hospital bylaws, and even clothing keep the parties on their respective sides of no-man's-land. "Working well" means that neither troubles the other too much and that treaties are fashioned and honored. "Working poorly" leads to open talk of dweebs and cats.

But, even when it produces organizations that are "working well" by these measures, the two-worlds theory of the proper leadership of health care holds the seeds of a disruptive, insulting, dispiriting harvest. When resources are evidently abundant and when patients are generously forgiving, then apparently we can get by. We have so far. In effect we can buy ourselves peace through the allocation of waste. The radiologist gets his (not-truly-needed) new MRI, and the medical staff vote reluctant approval of the hospital's marketing plan. Elaborate medical staff dinners host the visit of the CEO to congratulate retiring physicians and to report on how healthy the organization is. Elaborate executive dinners host the visit of the newly recruited chief of oncology to meet management and tell about the magic of modern chemotherapy in a thirty-minute summary.

But cut the budget, reduce the cash, spend a year or two in red ink, and watch the fabric tear. Misunderstanding takes charge. The clinicians become convinced that the managers could care less about the patients, and the managers become convinced that these "cats" are narcissists who want to have it all.

The authors of this book have spent years now creating a way to heal this rift. Gene Nelson, Paul Batalden, Margie Godfrey, and their colleagues have come to understand that the line-in-the-carpet problem is a deeply embedded cause of the failure of those who give care and those who shape the environment of care to understand themselves, each other, and the mission they share in such a way as to nurture much deeper, authentic respect for all and much more effective action on care itself. What these authors have done is to show us all—clinicians, executives, payers, regulators, and so on—a window through which to understand our shared purpose and our integrated roles. That window is the *clinical microsystem*. The idea seems to me beautifully simple. If our work, at its core, is "to heal and to help" people in distress, then we can get great benefit and guidance for our actions by seeing the work and then figuring out how we can best help *that*. The patient's pain meets the help exactly, and only, at the microsystem—nowhere else. That is in effect the very definition of a clinical microsystem. It is as if all that we do—all that we all do—comes to a point there, and proper judgments about the value of an action or a resource, in the end, can be made only by understanding its effects at that point. Equally, innovations and designs can be judged, in the end, only by tracing them to that point. The microsystem is the exclusive pathway to value. Policy, payment, regulation, clinical training, management training, congressional bills, new drugs, new computers, new architecture, today's meeting, professional ethics, malpractice reforms, the leader's act—all of this can be judged best, improved best, by predicting and tracing its effects on the microsystem where the pain meets the helping.

If clinicians, executives, managers, and others who shape the health care system as a whole can master what this book has to teach, we will have begun a crucial process of reunification of the efforts of many who, in my opinion, at the moment deeply misunderstand each other. We can replace the sadness and insult that come from distance if we will stand together at the window on our work that the microsystem view opens. It is what we are about. Improve microsystems, and we improve everything. Microsystems are where we meet not just the patients we serve but each other as well.

January 2007   *Boston, Massachusetts*

We dedicate this book to

The pioneers—luminaries in the field of improvement, in particular our mentor James Brian Quinn, the "father" of microsystem and macrosystem thinking, and other great thought leaders including W. Edwards Deming, Avedis Donabedian, Parker Palmer, Karl Weick, Donald Schön, and Donald Berwick

All members of the clinical microsystem—all the current and future frontline staff and health care leaders who enjoy the trust of their communities that they will provide the best possible care and caring, as well as all the patients and families who have the potential to benefit from health care done in the right way, in the way they want and need

Our families—all our loved ones who support our passion for excellence in health care, even though it results in peculiar work habits and absences from home

PREFACE

This book is about clinical microsystems—the places where patients and families and careteams meet. It is also about what leaders, at all levels of a health system, need to know and do to create the conditions of excellence in the front lines of care delivery. At the end of the day each patient's care is only as good as the care that is actually delivered by frontline staff. Is the care . . . correct? timely? caring? desired? efficient? The answers pour forth millions of times a day as real patients interact with real providers in real clinical microsystems, the naturally occurring building blocks of every health care system.

In reading this book and in using this book, you will discover many important things about using microsystem thinking and approaches to make lasting improvements in the quality and value of care. Here's a list of distinguishing features of clinical microsystems, the relatively small frontline units of health care. A clinical microsystem is a

- Professional formation locus: the place where people learn how to become competent health care professionals and develop over time
- Living system laboratory: the place to test changes in care delivery and to observe and understand complexity
- Source of workforce motivation or alienation: the place where pride in work flourishes or flounders

- Building block of health care: the place that joins together with other microsystems to make a continuum of care
- Locus of clinical policy in use: the place where clinical care is actually delivered and thereby the place that reflects the authentic clinical policy
- Maker of health care value and safety: the place where costs are incurred and the *sharp end* where reliability and safety succeed or fail
- Maker of patient satisfaction: the place where patients and families interact with staff and experience care as meeting or not meeting their needs

Health professionals, if they are to be effective, should understand these distinguishing features. Here are further illustrative behaviors related to each one:

- *Clinical microsystems are the setting for professional formation.* Professionals *form* themselves over a lifetime. The development and integration of the learning of "the head, the hands, and the heart" that occurs over time and in response to the need to take action linked to values in a particular context is at the heart of the development and formation of the health professional.
- *Clinical microsystems are living, complex systems that have some structure, some patterns of ordered relationships, and some processes; the processes are the means of connecting the patterns and structures to create the output and work.* These microsystems offer opportunities to understand the work of small delivery systems in their natural context. The problems they face are simple, complicated, and complex. Because they are complex, the parts or elements of the systems themselves can change, thereby changing the patterns of interactions and relationships.
- *Clinical microsystems are the locus of control for most of the workforce dissatisfiers and many of the genuine motivators for pride and joy in work.* The *hygiene* factors in work, identified long ago by Herzberg and colleagues, such as work policy and administration, supervision, interpersonal relations, and working conditions, are largely made manifest in the microsystems (Herzberg, 1987). So too, the *motivating factors,* such as the work itself, responsibility, recognition, and a sense of achievement, are found—or not—in the microsystems.
- *Clinical microsystems are the basic building blocks of health care.* In primary, secondary, and tertiary care settings these small systems connect the core competencies of health professionals to the needs of patients, families, and communities. In personal care settings and in public health settings these small systems must operate well if the knowledge, skills, and values of sophisticated professionals are to be applied. In both relatively economically advantaged and relatively economically disadvantaged settings the small frontline system can work well or poorly as a system. In isolation or in concert with other microsystems the clinical microsystem makes it easy or difficult to do the *right* thing. Microsystems

exist—not because we have installed them—but because today we have noticed them and we have noticed that they are the way real health care work gets done. The idea that patients and providers are *members* of the same system is not new. In the 1930s the famed physiological biochemist L. J. Henderson noted that patients and their caregivers were best thought of as members of the same system (Henderson, 1935).

- *Clinical microsystems are the units of clinical policy-in-use.* Much has been made of formal guidance for caregivers, from the aphorisms of Hippocrates to today's guidelines, protocols, pathways, and evidence syntheses. Often, however, this formal guidance is the guidance we *espouse* but do not *practice.* Clinical microsystems have policies-in-use about access, about the use of information and telecommunication technologies to offer care, about the daily use of science and evidence, about staffing and the continuing development of people, and more. Sometimes a policy-in-use is written, sometimes not. Debates often rage about the espoused policies, whereas the policies-in-use often remain misunderstood and unexamined.

- *Clinical microsystems are where good value and safe care are made.* Clinical microsystems, like other systems, can function to make it *easy to do the right thing* in the work of clinical care, or not. If added energy and work are required to be sure that the right care is offered for the right patient at the right time, the inherent value of that clinical microsystem is less than the value of the microsystem that does not require that added investment to do the right thing. Microsystems that work as high-reliability organizations, similar to those described by Weick and colleagues, are "mindful" of their interdependent interactions (Weick, 2002; Weick & Sutcliffe, 2001).

- *Clinical microsystems are the locus of control for many, if not most, of the variables that account for patient satisfaction with health care.* Ensuring that patients get access when they want and need it is, or is not, a goal of the scheduling processes of the microsystem. Making needed information readily available is, or is not, a priority of the microsystem. A culture that reflects genuine respect for the patient and careful listening to what patients have to say results in *social learning* for the microsystem; a less responsive culture results in something else. The patterns of staff behavior that the patients perceive and interpret as meeting their special needs, or not, are generated at the level of the microsystem (Schein, 1999).

Because microsystems are so critically important to patients, families, health care professionals, and the communities they serve, and because they have heretofore been for the most part, overlooked or invisible, we felt it was imperative to write this book. In doing so we hope that the reality and the power of health systems thinking in general—and clinical microsystem thinking in particular—can be unleashed and popularized so that outcomes and value can be improved continuously (from the inside out and from the bottom up) and that health professionals at all organization levels may have a better chance of having their everyday work be in sync with their core values and their strong desire to do the right thing well.

December 2006   Eugene C. Nelson
                                                         Lebanon, New Hampshire
                                                         Paul B. Batalden
                                                         Hanover, New Hampshire
                                                         Marjorie M. Godfrey
                                                         Hanover, New Hampshire

References

Henderson, L. J. (1935). Physician and patient as a social system. *New England Journal of Medicine, 212*, 819–823.

Herzberg, F. (1987, September/October). One more time: How do you motivate employees? *Harvard Business Review*, pp. 109–120.

Schein, E. H. (1999). *The corporate culture survival guide: Sense and nonsense about culture change.* San Francisco: Jossey-Bass.

Weick, K. E. (2002). The reduction of medical errors through mindful interdependence. In M. M. Rosenthal & K. M. Sutcliffe (Eds.), *Medical error: What do we know? What do we do?* (pp. 177–199). San Francisco: Jossey-Bass.

Weick, K. E., & Sutcliffe, K. M. (2001). *Managing the unexpected: Assuring high performance in an age of complexity.* San Francisco: Jossey-Bass.

ACKNOWLEDGMENTS

We are indebted to many wonderful people and outstanding organizations that helped make this book possible. Although it is impossible to recognize everyone who contributed to this endeavor, we would like to make mention of some individuals and organizations that merit special attention, and we ask forgiveness from those that we should have mentioned but somehow overlooked.

This book was inspired by the groundbreaking scholarship of James Brian Quinn, professor emeritus at Dartmouth's Tuck School of Business Administration. He is a friend and colleague and a never ending source of ideas and insights about what it takes to make great organizations great. In a similar vein we wish to acknowledge the encouragement of and the ideas developed by Donald Berwick, Maureen Bisognano, Thomas Nolan, and Pat Rutherford and their colleagues at the Institute for Healthcare Improvement who are working to transform health systems in North America and throughout the world. We also benefited from the insights about planning care in clinical microsystems that were provided by Edward Wagner and Connie Davis.

We wish to thank all the staff in the twenty clinical microsystems that we studied, who taught us so much about what can be done to innovate and provide superior care to patients and community residents. These wonderful clinical programs were Bon Secours Wound Care Team (St. Petersburg, Florida); Center for Orthopedic Oncology and Musculoskeletal Research (Washington, D.C.); Dartmouth-Hitchcock Spine Center (Lebanon, New Hampshire); Gentiva Rehab

Without Walls (Lansing, Michigan); Grace Hill Community Health Center (St. Louis, Missouri); Henry Ford Neonatal Intensive Care Unit (Detroit, Michigan); Hospice of North Iowa (Mason City, Iowa); Interim Pediatrics (Pittsburgh, Pennsylvania); Intermountain Shock/Trauma/Respiratory Intensive Care Unit (Salt Lake City, Utah); Iowa Veterans Home, M4C Team (Marshalltown, Iowa); Massachusetts General Hospital Downtown Associates Primary Care (Boston, Massachusetts); Mayo Health System, Midelfort Behavioral Health (Eau Claire, Wisconsin); Norumbega Medical, Evergreen Woods Office (Bangor, Maine); On Lok SeniorHealth Rose Team (San Francisco, California); Intermountain Healthcare, Orthopedic Specialty Practice (Boise, Idaho); Over-look Hospital, Emergency Department (Summit, New Jersey); Sharp Diabetes Self Management Training Center (La Mesa, California); Shouldice Hernia Repair Centre (Thornhill, Ontario, Canada); ThedaCare Physicians, Kimberly Office Family Medicine (Kimberly, Wisconsin); and Visiting Nurse Service of New York, Congregate Care, Queens Team 11s (New York City).

Moreover, hundreds of practices in the United States, Canada, England, Sweden, Norway, Italy, Kosovo, and elsewhere have cheerfully tested and provided feedback on the principles, tools, worksheets, and methods that we have created, and for this we are most grateful. We particularly appreciate the advanced use of microsystem strategies in the Geisinger Health System, Danville, Pennsylvania; the Cincinnati Children's Hospital Medical Center, Exempla Health System, Denver, Colorado; the Cystic Fibrosis Foundation, Bethesda, Maryland; the Vermont Oxford Network, Burlington, Vermont; and the Jönköping County Council Health System in Sweden.

Many of the health care leaders and staff in the clinical microsystems in which we conducted the original research went above and beyond our expectations in providing assistance to our research team. In this respect we wish to thank Craig Melin, the CEO of Cooley Dickinson Hospital (Northampton, Massachusetts), for his help in developing a case study and his insights as an outstanding senior leader; Robert Stark and his associates in the primary care practice at Massachusetts General Hospital Downtown (MGHD) for their generous sharing of their work experiences; and Charles Burger and his staff at the Evergreen Woods Office of Norumbega Medical (Bangor, Maine), for their gracious hospitality and continued collaborative learning. We also wish to thank the staff at the Dartmouth-Hitchcock Medical Center (DHMC) PainFree program for providing a remarkable case study, James Weinstein and his staff at the innovative Dartmouth-Hitchcock Spine Center, and William Edwards and the exemplary Intensive Care Nursery team. Finally, Carol Kerrigan, Barbara Rieseberg, and the Plastic Surgery Section at DHMC and Edward Catherwood, Jean Ten Haken, and the ICCU team at DHMC have been masterfully applying microsystem techniques; their work is represented in the case examples in Part Two of this book. We appreciate their extraordinary leadership and their permission to display some of their work.

Further, we wish to express our appreciation for the extensive contributions made by our research team—Thomas Huber, John H. Wasson, Kerri Ashling, Tina Foster, Richard Brandenburg, Curtis Campbell, Linda Headrick, Julie Johnson, David Rudolf, and Valerie Stender—including their rigorous and extraordinary work on qualitative and quantitative analyses, medical record reviews, financial performance assessments, and operational assessments. We have special appreciation for the graphic designs developed by Coua Early and initial manuscript preparation and research by Elizabeth Koelsch, Joy McAvoy, Alyssa Cretarola, and Gerald Collins. Linda Billings is accorded special mention and accolades for her editorial and graphic assistance; she worked on the manuscript for months on end, always with an eye to accuracy and clarity.

We deeply appreciate the editorial skills and long-time support from Steven Berman, who edits the *Joint Commission Journal on Quality and Patient Safety;* many chapters in this book were first published as articles in that journal. Moreover, we are deeply grateful to Andrew Pasternack, our editor at Jossey-Bass, who encouraged us to write this book and assisted us in important and tangible ways.

Finally, we are exceedingly grateful to the Robert Wood Johnson Foundation for its generous support of the Clinical Microsystem Research Program, RWJ Grant Number 036103, and to our project officer and colleague at the foundation, Susan Hassmiller, who has always been deeply interested in supporting and promoting this body of work.

INTRODUCTION

The health care system needs to work well for patients, each time a patient needs help and every time a patient needs help. The health care system needs to work for the professionals and other people who take care of patients, every day of their working life, so they can be proud of the services they provide to patients. In short we need a health care system that works right—for patients, families, and staff. Not only this, we need a health care system that is capable of getting better all the time, because the scientific community is making new discoveries that can benefit patients and because people are presenting new health needs that must be met. If you are the patient, you want to receive high-quality care that meets your special needs. If you are there to take care of the patient, you want to provide high-quality health care that gives you a sense of accomplishment. Patients and families, clinicians and staff, are all part of the same system, and they want the same thing. They want the system to work the way it needs to work 100 percent of the time.

We all know that sometimes the system works perfectly and lives are saved; we celebrate these events and are thankful. We also recognize that sometimes the system fails and errors are made and at times lives are lost; we deplore these events and are remorseful. The question is what can health care professionals and staff do to improve care, to transform the system, and to work toward perfect care?

Need

The health care system is seriously flawed. In the words of the Institute of Medicine (U.S.), Committee on Quality of Health Care in America (2001), "the chassis is broken." Lives are sometimes lost that could have been saved. Patients and families often experience both the best of care and the worst of care in a single illness episode. There are many problems both large and small. Sometimes the system does too much (overuse), sometimes too little (underuse); sometimes the system does it wrong (misuse). The health care system must be transformed to be safe, timely, effective, efficient, equitable, and most important, patient centered. The need for change is clear, but the pathway to affordable, durable, attractive system change often lies hidden.

Purpose

This book aims to improve the health care system by making clear a new pathway—for improving care *from the inside out*. It is a microsystem approach, and it is both complex and simple. It is complex because it involves a deep understanding of patients and professionals and the changing environments that they work in. It is simple because, at the end of the day, the goal is just this—to achieve the best patient outcomes by developing reliable, efficient, and responsive systems that have the capability of meeting the individual needs of "this" patient and continually improving care for the "next" patient.

We believe there is a need to transform health care and that it is possible to make this change from the inside out by focusing full attention on the *front lines* of care, the small clinical units where quality and value and safety are made. Although our main focus is on changing care where it is made—at the front lines of care—we recognize that this change will not take place absent excellent senior and midlevel leadership to promote the change *from the outside in*. The microsystem approach invites senior and midlevel leaders to align policy—mission, vision, and values—with strategy, operations, and people and to create what Quinn (1992) has referred to as an "intelligent enterprise," that is to say, an organization that is smart and is able to get smarter (see also Bossidy, Charan, & Burck, 2004; Liker, 2004). This organization's intelligent activity results in

- Doing and improving: realizing the synergy between proactive work to improve care—at all levels of the system and the business of providing care to patients and families when they need care
- Refining operations and learning: blending a constant drive for operational excellence with organizational learning, by relentless reflection on actual

performance compared to the patients' needs and by never-ending trials of new ways to improve performance to meet patients' needs, with conscious learning from each attempt.

Scope and Treatment

The scope of this book is broad. It presents ideas and methods for all levels of health care leadership—senior, midlevel, and frontline. It offers research results on high-performing clinical microsystems, case studies featuring individual clinical programs, guiding principles with wide application, and very specific tools, techniques, and methods that can be adapted to diverse clinical practices and clinical teams. Of necessity, it has not only wide scope but considerable depth. In short this book aims to provide a comprehensive and detailed understanding of what it will take for health care professionals to transform the health care systems that they are part of.

Health care is the concern of small units and large health systems, of microsystems and macroorganizations. Our primary focus is on the *sharp end* of care—the places where care is actually delivered in the real world. We call these small frontline systems of care *clinical microsystems.* They are, literally, the places where patients and families and careteams meet. Microsystems form around patients and families in times of illness or injury or other health need; whether we recognize it or not, clinical microsystems (for example, medical practices, emergency response teams, emergency departments, open-heart surgery teams, intensive care units, inpatient care units, nursing home units, home health teams, and palliative care teams) are the basic building blocks of all health care systems. Therefore the quality of care of any health care system can be summarized by this equation:

$$Q_{HS} = Q_{m1} + Q_{m2} + Q_{m3} + Q_{mn.}$$

That is to say, the quality of the health care system (Q_{HS}) for any individual patient (or any group of patients) is a function of the quality of care provided to that patient in each of the microsystems (Qm)—the first through the nth—where he or she receives care, *plus* the quality of the *interactions* of all the microsystems providing care to that patient (interactions between microsystems involve the handoff of patients, of information about patients, and of supporting services needed to provide care for patients). This is what we mean when we use the term the *sharp end* of care—the point at which services are delivered and do good or do harm or do nothing at all except consume resources and add cost.

Although care is *made* in the frontline units (the clinical microsystems), most of these small systems are not freestanding, rather they are usually part of a larger organization. Therefore it is essential to draw out the relationships between the small frontline systems that actually provide care and the macroorganizations—such as hospitals, group practices, integrated health systems, extended care facilities, and home health agencies—that exist to deliver care. A top-performing health system will successfully knit together mission, vision, strategy, and operations, from the top to the bottom of the organization, in a way that makes sense, that gives the organization the capability of providing high-quality and high-value care, of improving care, and of competing under challenging market conditions.

Overview of the Contents

This book is divided into two parts. The chapters in Part One explore the many facets of microsystem thinking. Part One provides frameworks, case studies, principles, and practical examples. Here is a brief preview of what we cover in Part One.

- Chapter One presents background information, including a description of clinical microsystems, and summarizes recent research on the factors that blend together to generate high performance.
- Chapter Two describes the developmental journey that microsystems can take to attain peak performance.
- Chapter Three explores the essence of leadership within clinical microsystems, focusing on three essential facets of leading—gathering knowledge, taking action, and reflecting on the current condition and the gap between that condition and the desired state.
- Chapter Four shifts attention from frontline leaders to senior and midlevel leaders and explores what they can do to create the conditions that enable peak performance at the front lines of care.
- Chapter Five turns the spotlight on the growth and development of staff—the greatest asset of all clinical microsystems.
- Chapters Six and Seven deal with the design and redesign of core services and the planning of care to match the needs of individual patients with the services offered by the health system.
- Chapter Eight delves into the issue of safety—a fundamental property of all clinical microsystems as they attempt to do the right things in the right way, performing each and every time in a perfectly safe and reliable manner.

- Chapter Nine describes the vital role that data play in creating a rich and positive information environment that supports care delivery in real time and systemic improvement over time.

   Part Two of this book aims to propel organization-wide transformation by increasing the capability of frontline units to improve themselves from the inside out *and* to respond with intelligence and energy to strategic change initiatives that come from higher levels of the organization. Chapter Ten is an introduction to the next fourteen chapters, as follows:

M3 Matrix

   Chapter Ten provides an overview of the path forward to making durable improvements in a health system, and it offers the M3 Matrix. This matrix suggests actions that should be taken by leaders at three levels of the health system (the top, or macrosystem, level; the middle, or mesosystem, level; and the frontline, or microsystem, level) to begin the transformation journey.

Dartmouth Microsystem Improvement Curriculum (DMIC)

   Chapters Eleven through Twenty-Four provide a core curriculum that can be used over time with frontline microsystems to build their capability to provide excellent care, to promote a positive work environment, and to contribute to the larger organization in essential ways. This curriculum sketches out an *action-learning* program that can be adapted for use in many different ways and in virtually any health care delivery setting. The topics covered sequentially in this action-learning program are

- An introduction to microsystem thinking (Chapter Eleven)
- Using effective meeting skills (part one) (Chapter Twelve)
- Assessing your microsystem by using the 5Ps (Chapter Thirteen)
- Using the PDSA↔SDSA model for improvement (Chapter Fourteen)
- Selecting themes for improvement (Chapter Fifteen)
- Writing a global aim statement to guide improvement (Chapter Sixteen)
- Performing process mapping (Chapter Seventeen)
- Specific aim (Chapter Eighteen)
- Using cause and effect diagrams (Chapter Nineteen)
- Using effective meeting skills (part two): brainstorming and multi-voting (Chapter Twenty)
- Understanding change concepts (Chapter Twenty-One)

- Measuring and monitoring (Chapter Twenty-Two)
- Using action plans and Gantt charts (Chapter Twenty-Three)
- Following up on improvement with storyboards, data walls, and playbooks (Chapter Twenty-Four)

Chapter Twenty-Five recaps the main ideas presented in this book and suggests ways to continue on the path to excellence.

The Outpatient Primary Care Practice "Assess, Diagnose and Treat" Workbook is in the appendix to support your efforts to gather and analyze data and information about your clinical microsystem. These worksheets are easily adaptable to any health care setting across the continuum of care—we offer this version because it was the first version we customized and contains the most worksheets for use in a variety of settings. Additional customized workbooks can be found at www.clinicalmicrosystem.org.

The scientific approach to improvement requires data and information supplemented by intuitive knowledge of your microsystem to enable the best decision making for improvement. The collection of worksheets complement the work in Part Two of this book and are necessary to gain deep insight into information and data not commonly explored by all members of the clinical microsystem. Increasingly, health care systems have the capability of providing some of the data and information suggested to collect in the workbook. If your organization does have the data and information easily available and it is current, you do not need to use the worksheets. If you cannot find *current* information and data, the worksheets are helpful tools to aid your collection of data and information to inform your improvement selection and decision making.

For more information related to the material in Part Two and the DMIC action-learning program, as well as information on what organizations are doing with these techniques, visit our microsystem Web site: http://www.clinicalmicrosystem.org.

How to Use This Book

The book is designed to provide you with powerful theoretical frameworks and principles, valuable tools and techniques, and an action-learning program. It can be used in several ways. Part One features cases and principles; it provides a comprehensive understanding of microsystem thinking, principles, and approaches. It should be read by anyone who wishes to gain wide and deep understanding of microsystem thinking. Part Two offers suggestions for leaders at all levels of the organization about practical actions they can take to build effective performance capability. It features the M3 Matrix and an action-learning program complete with tools, methods, and techniques; it offers very specific information that can be used to assess, diagnose, and improve health care, medical practices, and clinical units of many types. The chapters in Part Two should be read and put into practice by anyone who wishes to improve health care and to lead large and small systems to achieve peak performance in their frontline microsystems—the places where patients and families and careteams meet.

References

Bossidy, L., Charan, R., & Burck, C. (2004). *Confronting reality: Doing what matters to get things right*. New York: Crown Business.

Institute of Medicine (U.S.), Committee on Quality of Health Care in America. (2001). *Crossing the quality chasm: A new health system for the 21st century.* Washington, DC: National Academies Press.

Liker, J. K. (2004). *The Toyota way: 14 management principles from the world's greatest manufacturer.* New York: McGraw-Hill.

Quinn, J. B. (1992). *Intelligent enterprise: A knowledge and service based paradigm for industry.* New York: Free Press.

THE EDITORS

Eugene C. Nelson is director of Quality Administration for the Dartmouth-Hitchcock Medical Center (DHMC) and professor of Community and Family Medicine at Dartmouth Medical School. He is a national leader in health care improvement and the development and application of measures of system performance, health outcomes, and customer satisfaction. He is the recipient of the Joint Commission on Accreditation of Healthcare Organizations' Ernest A. Codman lifetime achievement award for his work on outcomes measurement in health care.

For over twenty years, Nelson has been one of the nation's leaders in developing and using measures of health care delivery system performance for the improvement of care. His success in developing the *clinical value compass* and *instrument panels* to measure health care system performance has made him one of the premier quality and value measurement experts in the country.

During this same time period, Nelson was doing pioneering work in bringing modern quality improvement thinking into the mainstream of health care. Working with friends and colleagues—Paul Batalden, Donald Berwick, James Roberts, and others—he helped launch the Institute for Healthcare Improvement and served as a founding board member. In the early 1990s, Nelson and his colleagues at Dartmouth began to develop clinical microsystem thinking, and he started to use these ideas in his work as a professor (in Dartmouth Medical School's graduate program in the Center for Clinical and Evaluative Sciences), as a health system leader at DHMC, and as an adviser to innovative health care systems in North America and Europe.

Although based at Dartmouth, Nelson works with many organizations in the United States and abroad and is the author of more than one hundred articles, books, and monographs.

He received his AB degree from Dartmouth College, his MPH degree from Yale Medical School, and his DSc degree from the Harvard School of Public Health. He is married to Sandra Nelson, who practices law, and has three children—Lucas, Alexis, and Zach.

Paul B. Batalden is professor, Pediatrics and Community and Family Medicine, and director of Health Care Improvement Leadership Development in the Center for the Evaluative Clinical Sciences at Dartmouth Medical School.

He is a national leader in health care improvement and health professional development. Over the past three decades he has developed theory, practical approaches, and health professional education policy and educational programs for improving care.

He developed the VA National Quality Scholar Program and the Dartmouth-Hitchcock Leadership Preventive Medicine combined residency program—offering training in leading microsystem change for the improvement of health care quality, safety, and value—which he currently directs. He chaired the Accreditation Council for Graduate Medical Education's National Advisory Committee on Outcomes, which helped to develop the "general competencies for graduate medical education," and the American Association of Medical College's committee to define the desired content and outcomes of medical student learning about "quality" of health care.

Since the early 1990s, he has focused on the work and vitality of the clinical microsystem. This research, teaching, mentoring, and advising of health professionals has involved individuals from several countries and representing all levels of organizational responsibility, every stage of professional development, and several health professional disciplines.

Batalden was the founding board chairman of the Institute for Healthcare Improvement and he has been a member and chair of the U.S. National Quality Council, an examiner for the Malcolm Baldrige National Quality Award, and a judge for the VA's Kizer Quality Award. His health care roles have included clinical practitioner, assistant surgeon general, United States Public Health Service (USPHS), clinical researcher, clinical scholar program developer, and governing board member for hospitals and health systems. He has written many articles, books, and monographs and has made videotapes about the improvement of health care quality.

He has received several awards for his work: the Ernest A. Codman lifetime achievement award for quality improvement and measurement, the Alfred I. duPont Award for Excellence in Children's Health Care, the American Hospital Association's Award of Honor for his health care quality improvement work, and the Founder's Award of the American College of Medical Quality. He is a member of the Institute of Medicine of the National Academy of Sciences.

Batalden received his BA degree from Augsburg College, his MD degree from University of Minnesota Medical School, and his pediatric specialty training from the University of Minnesota.

Marjorie M. Godfrey has a rich background in health care improvement, covering her thirty years of clinical leadership experience.

At the Center for the Evaluative Clinical Sciences at Dartmouth, she is an adjunct instructor in Community and Family Medicine and director, Clinical Microsystem Resource Group. She is the senior program advisor and faculty for major professional organizations including the National Cystic Fibrosis Foundation, the Vermont Oxford Network, Traumatic Brain Injury Foundation, Quality Improvement Organizations (QIOs) Cincinnati Children's Hospital Medical Center, Exempla Health System, University California, Davis, and the Geisinger Health System.

She is a faculty member and technical advisor to the Idealized Design of Clinical Office Practices initiative at the Institute for Healthcare Improvement. For twelve years, she was the director of Clinical Practice Improvement at Dartmouth-Hitchcock Medical Center leading and teaching improvement science throughout the complex health care system. Prior to that role she was the director of the Post Anesthesia Care Unit and Radiology Nursing; and previous to that she was a staff nurse in cardiology and postanesthesia care.

Godfrey coaches and supports many health care organizations across the United States and throughout Europe, including the National Primary Care Development Team for the National Health Service of England and Jönköping County Council Qulturum Leadership in Sweden.

Since 1994 she has focused on the practical application of clinical microsystem concepts and theories. She is the lead author of the *Dartmouth Clinical Microsystem Workbook* series and the lead developer of teaching materials and action learning curriculum endorsed by the IHI and the American Hospital Association.

She has collaborated with the Cystic Fibrosis Foundation (CFF) to design, develop, and distribute the CFF toolkit, including a CF-specific action guide and video. She is the originator and lead editor of www.clinicalmicrosystem.org, a Web site created to serve as a vehicle for information sharing and networking for the community of microsystem thinkers and designers. She speaks regularly at national and international meetings to share practical application stories and to provide instruction on microsystem concepts and theories. She is also an author of numerous articles published in peer-reviewed journals.

Godfrey is passionate about strategies for improving the vitality of microsystems. She is leading many improvement initiatives that are testing various collaborative models and adapting them to local settings. She codevelops improvement strategies with senior leaders to ensure engagement and development of frontline clinical teams that include patients and families, and she is a strong advocate for young professionals and students in health care, identifying opportunities to support their professional development and their integration into health care systems.

Godfrey has an MS degree in outcomes, health policy, and health care improvement from the Center for the Evaluative Clinical Sciences at Dartmouth, a BSN degree from Vermont College at Norwich University, and a nursing diploma from Concord Hospital School of Nursing.

THE CONTRIBUTORS

Kerri Ashling, MD, MS, medical director, Correctional Health and Rehabilitation Services, Seattle and King County Department of Public Health, Seattle, Washington.

Paul Barach, MD, MPH, associate professor, University of South Florida College of Medicine Miami, Florida

George T. Blike, MD, professor in Anesthesiology and Community and Family Medicine, Dartmouth Medical School, Medical Director for Office of Patient Safety, Dartmouth-Hitchcock Medical Center, Lebanon, New Hampshire.

Christine Campbell, BA, research assistant Robert Wood Johnson Foundation Grant, Dartmouth Medical School, Hanover, New Hampshire.

Joseph P. Cravero, MD, medical director, CHAD PainFree Program, Dartmouth-Hitchcock Medical Center, Lebanon, New Hampshire.

William H. Edwards, MD, professor and vice chair of Pediatrics, Neonatology Division chief, section chief, Neonatal Intensive Care Unit, Children's Hospital at Dartmouth, Lebanon, New Hampshire.

Paul Gardent, MBA, executive vice president, Dartmouth-Hitchcock Medical Center, Lebanon, New Hampshire.

Linda A. Headrick, MD, MS, senior associate dean for Education and Faculty Development, School of Medicine, University of Missouri-Columbia, Missouri.

Karen Homa, PhD, improvement specialist, Dartmouth-Hitchcock Leadership Preventive Medicine Residency Program, Lebanon, New Hampshire.

Thomas P. Huber, MS, ECS, Thomas Patrick Consulting Co., San Francisco, California.

Julie K. Johnson, MSPH, PhD, assistant professor of medicine, University of Chicago, Illinois; director of research, American Board of Medical Specialties, Evanston, Illinois.

Linda Kosnik, RN, MSN, CS, chief nursing officer, Overlook Hospital, Summit, New Jersey.

John H. Wasson, MD, research director, the Dartmouth/Northern New England COOP Project; Herman O. West Professor of Geriatrics; director, Center for Aging; professor in Community and Family Medicine, Dartmouth Medical School, Hanover, New Hampshire.

QUALITY BY DESIGN

PART ONE

CASES AND PRINCIPLES

CHAPTER ONE

SUCCESS CHARACTERISTICS OF HIGH-PERFORMING MICROSYSTEMS

Learning from the Best

Eugene C. Nelson, Paul B. Batalden, Thomas P. Huber, Julie K. Johnson, Marjorie M. Godfrey, Linda A. Headrick, John H. Wasson

Chapter Summary

Background. Clinical microsystems are the small, functional frontline units that provide most health care to most people. They are the essential building blocks of larger organizations and of the health system. They are the place where patients, families, and careteams meet. The quality and value of care produced by a large health system can be no better than the services generated by the small systems of which it is composed.

Methods. A wide net was cast to identify and study a sampling of the best-quality, best-value small clinical units in North America. Twenty microsystems, representing a variety of the component parts of a health system, were examined from December 2000 through June 2001, using qualitative methods supplemented by medical record and finance reviews.

Results. The study of these twenty high-performing sites generated many best-practice ideas (processes and methods) that microsystems use to accomplish their goals. Their success characteristics were related to high performance and include leadership, macrosystem support of microsystems, patient focus, community and market focus, staff focus, education and training, interdependence of care team, information and information technology, process improvement, and performance results. These ten

3

success factors were interrelated and together contributed to the microsystem's ability to provide superior, cost-effective care and at the same time create a positive and attractive working environment.

Conclusions. A seamless, patient-centered, high-quality, safe, and efficient health system cannot be realized without transformation of the essential building blocks that combine to form the care continuum.

The health care system in the United States can, under certain conditions, deliver magnificent and sensitive state-of-the-art care. It can snatch life from the jaws of death and produce medical miracles. The case of Ken Bladyka, presented later in this chapter, is one positive example of the health care system's performance. Yet the system is often severely flawed and dysfunctional. The Institute of Medicine (IOM) report *Crossing the Quality Chasm: A New Health System for the 21st Century* (Institute of Medicine [U.S.], Committee on Quality of Health Care in America, 2001), makes the point of system failure clear:

- "Health care today harms too frequently and routinely fails to deliver its potential benefits"(p. 1).
- "Tens of thousands of Americans die each year from errors in their care, and hundreds of thousands suffer or barely escape from nonfatal injuries that a truly high quality care system would largely prevent" (p. 2).
- "During the last decade alone, more than 70 publications in leading peer-reviewed clinical journals have documented serious quality shortcomings" (p. 3).
- "The current system cannot do the job. Trying harder will not work. Changing systems of care will" (p. 4).

This chapter introduces the concept of the clinical microsystem, summarizes recent research on twenty high-performing microsystems sampled from the care continuum, and stresses the strategic and practical importance of focusing health system improvement work specifically on the design and redesign of small, functional clinical units.

Qualitative research methods were used to analyze 250 hours of conversations with microsystem personnel; these conversations were augmented by chart reviews and financial data. Principles, processes, and examples were gleaned from the interviews to describe what these exemplary microsystems are doing to achieve superior performance.

So, what *is* the true nature of our health system? Sometimes it works well, but all too often it fails to deliver what is needed.

True Structure of the System, Embedded Systems, and Need to Transform Frontline Systems

The true structure of the health system the patient experiences varies widely. Patients in need of care may find

- Clinical staff working together—or against each other
- Smooth-running frontline health care units—or units in tangles
- Information readily available, flowing easily, and in a timely fashion—or not
- Health care units that are embedded in helpful larger organizations—or cruel, Byzantine bureaucracies
- Health care units that are seamlessly linked together—or totally disjointed
- High-quality, sensitive, efficient services—or care that is wasteful, expensive, and at times harmful or even lethal

In brief it can be said that the true structure of the health system is composed of a few basic parts—frontline clinical microsystems, mesosystems, and overarching macrosystems. These systems have a clinical aim and are composed of patients, staff, work patterns, information, and technology, and they exist in a context. These elements are interrelated to meet the needs of patient subpopulations needing care. As the Bladyka case will illustrate, "it is easy to view the entire health care continuum as an elaborate network of microsystems that work together (more or less) to reduce the burden of illness for populations of people" (Nelson et al., 2000, p. 669).

Here are three fundamental assumptions about the structure of the health system:

1. Bigger systems (*macrosystems*) are made of smaller systems.
2. These smaller systems (*microsystems*) produce quality, safety, and cost outcomes at the front line of care.
3. Ultimately, the outcomes of a macrosystem can be no better than the outcomes of the microsystems of which it is composed.

The concept of clinical microsystems is spreading and has been used in many national and international programs: the IOM's *Crossing the Quality Chasm* report, the Institute for Healthcare Improvement's Idealized Design of Clinical Office Practice program and also its Pursuing Perfection program (Kabcenell, 2002) and Transforming Care at the Bedside program (Rutherford, Lee, & Greiner, 2004), the Cystic Fibrosis Foundation's Accelerating Improvement in CF CareCollaborative, the Vermont Oxford Network of Neonatal Intensive Care Units ("Your Ideal NICU") program, the United Kingdom's health system renewal program, and so on.

FIGURE 1.1. CHAIN OF EFFECT IN IMPROVING HEALTH CARE QUALITY.

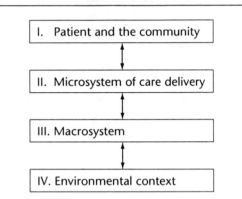

Source: Donald M. Berwick. Used with permission.

Donald Berwick's "chain of effect in improving health care quality" (Berwick, 2001) (see Figure 1.1) shows the major elements that need to work well and work together well for high-quality care to be delivered, and highlights the pivotal role played by the microsystems of care delivery. Clinical microsystems are the places where patients and families and health care teams meet, and consequently they are positioned at the *sharp end* of the health care delivery system, where care is delivered, medical miracles happen, and tragic mistakes are made. Our approach in this book is focused primarily on this microsystem level, where frontline clinical teams interact with patients and produce outcomes.

To bring about fundamental change of the magnitude required in the health system, our country needs a systematic transformation *at all levels* of the system. This requires a *system-based* approach, one that recognizes the reality and functional integrity of human systems. Although many attempts have been made to change the health system—by focusing on the individual patients, the individual physicians serving these patients, the larger provider organizations, the payment system, and other aspects of health care policy—there have been very few efforts to understand and change the frontline clinical units that actually deliver the care. To move toward a *perfected* macrosystem of care, the performance of each individual microsystem must be optimized within that system's context and the linkages between all the various clinical microsystems must be seamless, timely, efficient, and thoroughly reliable. Although change is required at all levels of the system, the powerful new idea here is that the microsystem concept offers an opportunity to transform health care at the front line of service delivery.

Describing Clinical Microsystems

Microsystems involve people in varying roles, such as patients and clinicians; they also involve processes and recurring patterns—cultural patterns, information flow patterns, and results patterns. This book defines microsystems in health care in the following way:

> A clinical microsystem is a small group of people who work together on a regular basis to provide care to discrete subpopulations of patients. It has clinical and business aims, linked processes, and a shared information environment, and it produces performance outcomes. Microsystems evolve over time and are often embedded in larger organizations. They are complex adaptive systems, and as such they must do the primary work associated with core aims, meet the needs of their members, and maintain themselves over time as clinical units.

Microsystems, the essential building blocks of the health system, can be found everywhere and vary widely in terms of quality, safety outcomes, and cost performance. A microsystem is the local milieu in which patients, providers, support staff, information, and processes converge for the purpose of providing care to individual people to meet their health needs. If a person were to explore his or her local health system, he or she would discover myriad clinical microsystems, including a family practice, a renal dialysis team, an orthopedic practice, an in vitro fertilization center, a cardiac surgery team, a neonatal intensive care unit, a home health care delivery team, an emergency department, an inpatient maternity unit, a rapid response team, and an extended care facility. Clinical microsystems are living units that change over time and *always* have a patient (a person with a health need) at their center. They come together to meet patients' needs—and they may disperse once a need is met (for example, a rapid response team, or a *fast* squad, forms quickly, comes together around the patient for a short period of time, and disperses after the patient has been stabilized or transported).

As described in the Bladyka case in the following box and illustrated in Figure 1.2, these individual microsystems are tightly or loosely connected with one another and perform better or worse under different operating conditions. Our ability to see them as functional, interdependent systems is challenged by our conventions of compartmentalizing and departmentalizing, considering separately, for example, human resources, accounting, and information technology. Our commitment to professional disciplines and specialties as a prime organizing principle often creates barriers that impede the daily work of clinical microsystems.

The Bladyka Case

Ken Bladyka is a thirty-nine-year-old resident of New Hampshire who has a wife, two children, and a sixth degree black belt. He has earned several national and international karate championships. Last summer, while attending the Amateur Athletic Union National Karate Championships to watch his son compete, he noticed bruises on his arm. When he got home he noticed more bruises and petechiae on his legs, and Paige, Ken's wife, was horrified when she saw severe bruises on his back as well. This happened on the Fourth of July, and the following sequence of activities transpired over the next three months:

- 7/4: Ken calls his family physician, his primary care provider, to report findings.
- Family physician sees Ken and Paige that same day.
- Family physician refers Ken to Dartmouth-Hitchcock Medical Center (DHMC) hematology department in Lebanon, New Hampshire.
- Doctor on call sees Ken and orders labs.
- Ken starts his own medical record.
- Ken admitted to DHMC with diagnosis of aplastic anemia complicated by auto-immune disease.
- Inpatient care—daily labs and transfusions—provided under direction of hematologist.
- Ken discharged to home, receives outpatient daily labs and transfusions as needed, and readmitted to DHMC hematology service as needed.
- Ken's four siblings tested for bone marrow matches at DHMC, and at health care facilities in Hartford, Connecticut, and San Francisco, California.
- One sibling, his sister Mary, has a positive match.
- Ken begins a search for "best place with best outcomes in world" and selects Fred Hutchinson Cancer Research Center (FHCRC) in Seattle, Washington.
- 8/23: Ken, Paige, and Mary fly to Seattle, and on 8/24 Ken is admitted to FHCRC.
- 9/3: Chemotherapy is begun at FHCRC.
- 9/10: Bone marrow transplant procedure done at FHCRC.
- 9/12: Ken celebrates his fortieth birthday while an inpatient at FHCRC.
- 9/27: Ken transferred to Paul Gross Housing unit for 100 days of follow-up care.
- 10/3: Testing at FHCRC reveals that bone marrow transplant has started to produce positive results.
- Ken continues to recover and recuperate while residing at Paul Gross Housing unit and anxiously awaiting his return to home and family and work. . . .

Figure 1.2 uses a flowchart to depict Ken's health system journey. It shows the frontline clinical units, the different small groups of people who worked directly with Ken at each step of his care, such as the office of his primary care provider (PCP), the DHMC hematology inpatient unit, and the bone marrow testing units. These small, frontline clinical units are what this book calls *clinical microsystems*. Figure 1.2 also

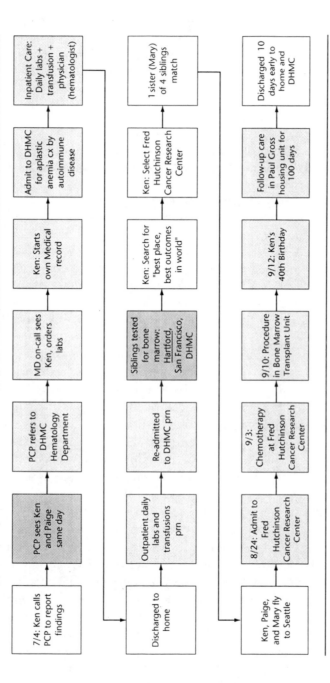

FIGURE 1.2. FLOWCHART OF KEN BLADYKA'S JOURNEY THROUGH THE HEALTH SYSTEM.

shows the larger umbrella organizations, or *macrosystems*—the Dartmouth-Hitchcock Medical Center, and the Fred Hutchinson Cancer Research Center—that played a part in Ken Bladyka's care. This case study provides a glimpse of the true structure of the health system. Before examining this structure further it is important to emphasize some facts that arise from the Bladyka case:

- This could happen to you.
- This could happen to your family and friends.
- Ken needed high-quality, safe, and affordable care.
- Ken found frontline health systems that met his special needs, but these pockets of gold were spread across the country.
- We need a solid-gold system—meaning a high-quality, high-value, high-reliability system—throughout the nation to serve all Americans.

Another way to describe clinical microsystems is with a high-level diagram that portrays a typical microsystem's *anatomy*—the set of elements that come together, like biological structures that work together toward a common goal, to form the microsystem organism. Figure 1.3 illustrates the anatomy of a typical internal medicine practice. This clinical microsystem, like all others, has a mission, or core *purpose*—in this case, to achieve the best possible outcomes for patients—and is composed of *patients* who form different subpopulations (such as healthy, chronic, and high risk). The patients interact with *professionals*, including clinicians and support staff, who perform distinct roles, such as physician, nurse, nurse practitioner, medical assistant, and so on. The patients and staff work to meet patients' needs by engaging in direct care *processes*, such as accessing systems, assessing needs, diagnosing problems, establishing treatment plans, and following up over time. These direct care processes are assisted by supporting processes that involve distinct tools and resources, such as medical records, scheduling, diagnostic tests, medications, and billing. The results of the interactions between patients and staff and clinical and support processes can be used to produce *patterns* of critical results, such as biological and safety outcomes, functional status and risk outcomes, patient perceptions of goodness of care, and cost outcomes, that combine to represent the value of care. The patterns of results also include the elements of practice culture, what it *feels like* to work in the clinical unit, as well as elements important to business success, such as direct costs, operating revenues, and productivity.

Another important feature of the clinical unit is that it has a semipermeable boundary that mediates relationships with patients and families and with many support services and other microsystems. Furthermore it is embedded in, influences, and is influenced by a larger organization that itself is embedded in a particular environment—a payment environment; a regulatory environment; or

FIGURE 1.3. ANATOMY OF A CLINICAL MICROSYSTEM.

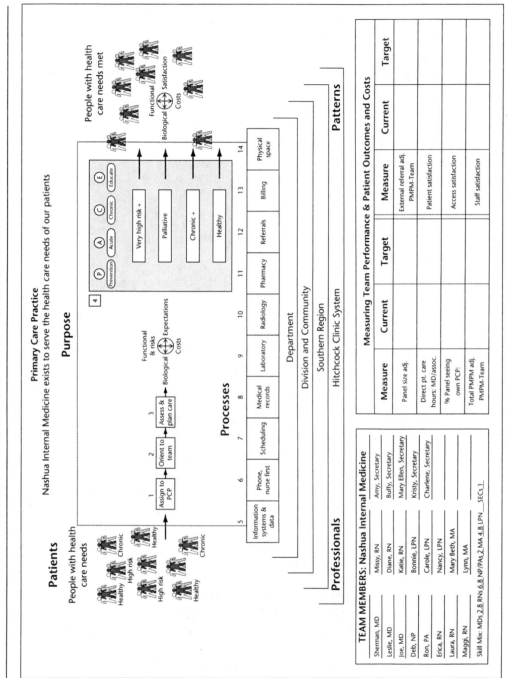

Source: Nelson, E. C., & Batalden, P. B., unpublished document, 1998.

a cultural, social, and political environment. Thus the clinical microsystem, although a comparatively simple concept, is still in fact a complex, adaptive system that evolves over time.

Complex adaptive systems are found in nature and in human groups. They can be contrasted with mechanical systems, which tend to be more predictable and not subject to emergent behavior. Fritof Capra, a noted physicist and author, suggests that a useful way to analyze complex adaptive systems arising in nature is to use a framework that addresses structure, process, and patterns (Capra, 1996; Nelson et al., 1998). Patterns are the consistent behaviors, sentiments, and results that emerge from the relationships of the parts involved in a complex adaptive system (Zimmerman, Lindberg, & Plsek, 1999).

Previous Research on Microsystems, Organizational Performance, and Quality

The clinical microsystem work described in this chapter represents an extension of the authors' earlier work on improvement in health care. For example, in 1996 the authors wrote a four-part series on clinical improvement that was published in the *Joint Commission Journal on Quality Improvement* (Nelson, Mohr, Batalden, & Plume, 1996; Nelson, Batalden, Plume, & Mohr, 1996; Mohr, Mahoney, Nelson, Batalden, & Plume, 1996; Batalden, Mohr, Nelson, & Plume, 1996). That series described concepts and methods for improving the quality and value of care provided for specific subpopulations of patients.

The microsystem work described herein amplifies this earlier work by taking into account the structural units—that is, clinical microsystems—responsible for delivering care to specific patient populations, and the manner in which these microsystems function, which involves the interplay of patients, professionals, processes, and patterns within and between microsystems. The primary emphasis of the authors' former work was on the clinical process that generates outcomes—quality and costs—for patients served by clinical systems. This new body of work retains a strong emphasis on clinical processes and patient-based outcomes but expands the frame to include

- An explicit focus on the local context—that is, the naturally occurring clinical units that form the front line of health care delivery
- Consideration of the information environment that supports or undermines care delivery
- The interactions and relationships among people within microsystems and the interactions between clinical microsystems that work together to provide comprehensive care

- The relationships between clinical microsystems and the larger systems in which they are embedded—for example, the mesosystems, macrosystem, and larger community

The research on microsystems described in this chapter generally builds on ideas developed by Deming (1986), Senge (1990), Wheatley (1992), and others who have applied systems thinking to organizational development, leadership, and improvement. The emerging fields of chaos theory, complexity science, and complex adaptive systems have also influenced our thinking (Arrow, McGrath, & Berdahl, 2000; Hock, 2005; Kelly, 1994; Peters, 1987; Wheatley, 1992).

The seminal idea for the microsystem in health care stems from work of James Brian Quinn that he summarized in *Intelligent Enterprise* (Quinn, 1992). In this book he reports on primary research conducted on the world's best-of-the-best service organizations, such as FedEx, Mary Kay Inc., McDonald's, Intel, SAS, and Nordstrom. His aim was to determine what these extraordinary organizations were doing to enjoy such explosive growth, high margins, and wonderful reputations with customers. He found that these service sector leaders organized around, and continually engineered, the frontline interface that connected the organization's core competency with the needs of the individual customer. Quinn called this frontline activity the *smallest replicable unit*, or the minimum replicable unit, that embedded the service delivery process. The smallest replicable unit idea—or the microsystem idea, as we call it—has critical implications for strategy, information technology, and other key aspects of creating intelligent enterprise. Two excerpts from Quinn's book convey the power and scope of this organizing principle and the need for senior leaders to focus their attention on creating the conditions to continually improve the performance of frontline delivery units.

- On core strategy: "Critical to relevant effective system design is conceptualizing the smallest replicable unit and its potential use in strategy as early as possible in the design process" (p. 104).
- On informatics and improvement: "Through careful work design and iterative learning processes, they both reengineered their processes to use this knowledge and developed databases and feedback systems to capture and update needed information at the micro levels desired" (p. 105).

Donaldson and Mohr (2000) investigated high-performing clinical microsystems; this research provided important background material for the IOM's Committee on Quality of Health Care in America in writing *Crossing the Quality Chasm*. Donaldson and Mohr's work was based on a national search for the highest-quality clinical microsystems. Forty-three clinical units were identified, and leaders of those units participated in extensive interviews conducted by the report authors. The results of the interviews were analyzed to determine the characteristics that seemed to be most responsible for enabling these high-quality microsystems to be successful. The results suggested that eight dimensions were associated with high quality:

- Constancy of purpose
- Investment in improvement
- Alignment of role and training for efficiency and staff satisfaction
- Interdependence of care team to meet patient needs
- Integration of information and technology into work flows
- Ongoing measurement of outcomes
- Supportiveness of the larger organization
- Connection to the community to enhance care delivery and extend influence

Our study of clinical microsystems has built directly on Mohr and Donaldson's work.

Study of Clinical Microsystems

The aim of our research study, which we conducted from June 2000 through June 2002, was to identify the success characteristics—the principles, processes, and methods—that high-performing clinical microsystems use to provide care that is characterized by both high quality and cost efficiency. Our method was to identify twenty high-performing clinical microsystems representing different parts of the care continuum and to study their performance through site visits, detailed personal interviews, direct observations, and reviews of medical record and financial information. The research was sponsored by the Robert Wood Johnson Foundation and was conducted by a research team based at Dartmouth Medical School's Center for the Evaluative Clinical Sciences. The research methods are described in more detail in the following section.

Research Design

The research design was an observational study that for the most part used qualitative methods, such as personal interviews and direct observations, with a limited review of medical records and analysis of financial data. Figure 1.4 displays an overview of the research design.

FIGURE 1.4. RESEARCH DESIGN FOR STUDY OF TWENTY CLINICAL MICROSYSTEMS.

Sampling

Selecting high-performing clinical microsystems via a multitiered search pattern

1. Award winners and measured high performance
2. Literature citations
3. Prior research and field experience
4. Expert opinion
5. Best within best

Choosing 20 clinical microsystems for study

1. Assess outcomes of search pattern
2. Create table of sites by search pattern
3. Conduct survey and telephone interview
4. Choosing and inviting sites to participate

Data Collection

Two data collection instruments

Self-administered microsystem survey
Self-assessment of performance based on key characteristics

Telephone interview
Examination of delivery processes, the quality of care and services, and cost efficiency and waste reduction

Two-day site visit for interviews and direct observation

In-depth interviews
   Microsystem staff and larger organization staff

Medical chart review
   Assessment of technical clinical quality of care

Finance review
   Assessment of operational performance and cost efficiency

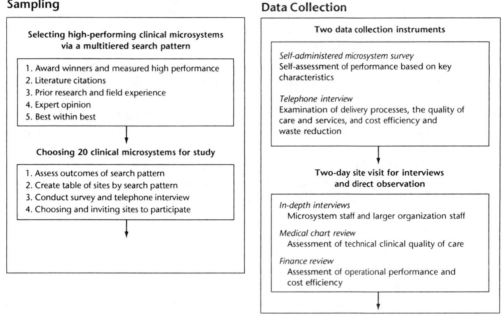

Data Analysis

Assessment of screening interviews and face-to-face depth interviews

1. Entered and analyzed via QSR NUD*IST
2. Major success characteristics determined from cross-case analysis

Assessment of chart review and financial performance

Medical chart review
1. Specific and aggregate quality indicators assessed
2. Scoring, rating, and ranking completed for each site

Finance review
1. Aggregate financial information reviewed
2. Each site rated on a rank-order, cost-efficiency success scale

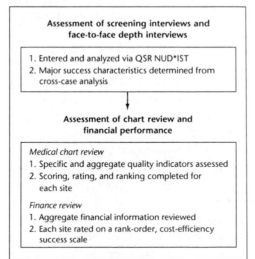

Sampling

The objective was to select a total of twenty high-performing clinical microsystems (that is, small groups of people who work together regularly to provide care to discrete subpopulations of patients) that represented a number of different components of the care continuum: primary care, specialty care, inpatient care, nursing home care, and home health care.

First, to begin the process of identifying twenty of the best performers across North America, we employed five complementary search patterns:

- Award winners and measured high performance. We searched for clinical units that had won national or regional awards or had the best quality and cost measures in established databases.
- Literature citations. We searched, using resources such as Dow Jones Interactive, LexisNexis, Tablebase, and ProQuest, for clinical units prominently mentioned in the professional literature.
- Prior research and field experience. We used the lists of top-performing clinical units from prior research conducted by the Institute of Medicine (Donaldson & Mohr, 2000), and we used the field experience from the Institute for Healthcare Improvement's Breakthrough Series on the performance of the best-known clinical units.
- Expert opinion. We interviewed national health care leaders and quality-of-care experts to request their nominations for best-performing microsystems in North America.
- Best within best. We interviewed leaders of exemplary large organizations, such as the Mayo Clinic, Massachusetts General Hospital, Henry Ford Health System, and Scripps Clinic, and requested nominations for the best-performing small clinical units within their organizations.

Second, we entered the names of the identified clinical units into a table that enabled the research team to identify those microsystems that had garnered the most mentions across the five different search patterns and to review the strength of each clinical unit with respect to exemplary performance (120 sites identified). We then selected the most promising microsystems within each category (primary care, specialty care, inpatient care, nursing home care, and home health care) and invited these sites, using a mailed invitation and personal phone calls, to take part in an interview (75 sites invited).

Third, we conducted structured screening interviews over the telephone with potential sites and asked their leaders to complete a brief questionnaire that gathered further background information on each site and its quality-cost performance (60 sites completed a screening interview).

Fourth, we selected the final 20 sites on the basis of the results of the screening interview, questionnaire, and willingness to participate.

Data Collection

We used several methods to collect data for the project. To screen sites for possible inclusion in the study, we used two data collection instruments:

Self-administered microsystem survey. This fifteen-item survey was mailed to potential sites for self-completion and was used for self-assessment of performance based on key characteristics identified in Donaldson and Mohr's IOM study in 2000.

Telephone interview. A thirty-minute telephone survey was conducted with potential sites. Lead field researchers used a semistructured interview guide to gather data on the nature of the microsystem and its delivery processes, the quality of care and services, cost efficiency, and waste reduction.

After sites had been selected for inclusion in the study, a two-day site visit was held to conduct in-depth interviews and to provide an opportunity for direct observation. As part of this site visit, information was gathered using these methods:

In-depth interviews. An interview guide was used to conduct detailed, face-to-face interviews with staff in each microsystem. These interviews ranged in length from approximately twenty to ninety minutes, with most lasting either thirty or sixty minutes. Interviews were conducted with a mix of staff in each microsystem, to gain perspectives from all types of staff—the clinical leader, administrative leader, physicians, nurses, clinical technicians, clinical support staff, and clerical staff. In addition, interviews were held with selected staff (for example, the senior leader, financial officer, and information officer) of the larger organization of which the clinical microsystem was a part.

Medical chart review. A medical record expert who was part of the research team coordinated a review of medical records in each of the microsystems. A detailed protocol was used to select the medical records of 100 relevant patients of each clinical microsystem. These records represented cases involving typical services provided and medical problems commonly treated by the unit. Structured data collection forms were used to gather specific information on the technical quality of care provided in each clinical unit.

Finance review. Information related to the financial performance of each microsystem was collected from available data and reports, such as annual reports, quarterly reports, and productivity data reflecting operating revenues, operating costs, waste reduction efforts, and operational efficiency.

For each microsystem site, complete data included the screening survey; screening interview; personal, in-depth interviews; and medical and financial records. The interviews were documented by the study's lead field researcher (T.P.H.), using a tape recorder or taking detailed notes (or doing both). The only data set with partial information related to finance. With some notable exceptions most of the microsystems studied did not have sufficient accurate, detailed information to provide a sound basis for determining actual costs, revenues, and savings accrued over time. Financial information tended to reflect classic accounting system assumptions that focus detailed data collection on individual practitioners and standard departments rather than on the functional unit, the actual microsystem. Consequently, it was not possible to assess accurately each site's financial performance and productivity.

Data Analysis

The verbatim information from the screening interviews and the face-to-face, in-depth interviews was transcribed and entered into a content analysis program called QSR NUD*IST. The interview information was then analyzed, with the assistance of the content analysis software, using the method known as cross-case analysis (Miles & Huberman, 1994). This is a standard, qualitative research method that involves deconstructing all the meaningful utterances (interview segments) into individual text units and then placing the text units into affinity groups and reconstructing the information for the purpose of identifying common themes—in this case major success characteristics. Some text units had content that could be coded into two or more affinity groups, and the classification system we used allowed us to assign a text unit to one or more categories.

Major success characteristics can be described as the primary factors that these high-performing microsystems appeared to have in common and that appeared to be associated with high-quality and high-efficiency patterns of performance. Two members of the research team (T.P.H. and J.J.M.) independently analyzed all the verbatim content and placed the content into affinity groups (coding categories). Using conventional content analysis methods enabled these categories to evolve as case material was processed. The coding results from the two analysts were compared, and discrepancies between the two were discussed, and consensus was reached to resolve differences. The data were aggregated for each site to determine what proportion of the coded verbatim text units fell within each of the primary success characteristics.

The screening process was designed to identify high-quality, high-efficiency sites. The subsequent site visits provided strong confirmation that the site selection process was successful at identifying high performers. All twenty sites were exemplary in many ways. Nevertheless each site was to some extent unique and had its own set of particular strengths and further improvement opportunities with respect to quality and efficiency.

Results of the medical record reviews and financial analyses were used primarily to help us identify sites that might be especially promising for best-of-best processes and methods.

Analysis of the medical charts was based on a review of 100 randomly selected records, which were coded for five features of care:

- A problem list
- A medication list
- An allergy list
- Evidence of patient teaching
- A site-specific clinical measure of process or outcome quality (for example, glycosolated hemoglobin level or mortality rate) that was relevant for the patient subpopulation treated by the clinical unit

After all the data were in, some sites displayed evidence of superior performance across the board. That is to say, internal trend data on technical quality, health outcomes, costs, and revenues, in addition to the results from the site interviews and the medical record reviews, provided extremely strong evidence of stellar, summa cum laude performance. We used these sites somewhat more heavily in identifying best-of-best processes and methods within the set of twenty high-performing clinical units. We relied especially on several clinical microsystems that had extraordinary results. The members of this select group shared many common methods and processes, even though they were in different regions of the country and had little knowledge of one another. For example, all these units made extensive use of daily interdisciplinary huddles; monthly performance review sessions; data displays showing results over time; home-grown, real-time informatics solutions; and annual, all-staff retreats for establishing improvement themes and monitoring performance in mission-critical areas.

Results

The twenty clinical microsystems selected for study represented sixteen states and Canadian provinces (see Appendix 1.1 at the end of this chapter for a complete listing). There were four primary care practices, five medical specialty practices, four inpatient care units, four home health care units, and three nursing home and hospice facilities. Many of these clinical microsystems were parts of larger, well-known systems, such as the Mayo Clinic, Massachusetts General Hospital, and Intermountain Health Care. Others, however, were parts of smaller, lesser-known organizations, such as Norumbega (Maine), ThedaCare (Wisconsin), and Intermountain Orthopedics (Idaho).

Success Characteristics of High-Performing Sites

Analysis of the results suggests that each of the twenty high-performing clinical units is indeed a complex, dynamic system, with interacting elements that come together to produce superior performance. No single feature or success characteristic can stand alone to produce high-quality, high-value systemic results. That being said, these microsystems shared a set of primary success characteristics, and these characteristics interacted with one another to produce highly favorable systemic outcomes:

- Leadership of microsystem
- Macrosystem support of microsystem
- Patient focus
- Staff focus
- Interdependence of care team
- Information and information technology
- Process improvement
- Performance results

These primary success characteristics fall into five main groups and interact dynamically with one another. Figure 1.5 displays these groupings. It also shows two additional success characteristics that involve health professional education and training and the external environment (including the financial, regulatory, policy, and market environments) in which the microsystem is embedded. These themes were often mentioned in our research, although not as frequently as the primary ones we identified. A third additional theme, patient safety, was also identified, but again in a less frequent pattern so it was not included in the final success characteristics.

Content analysis of the interview text showed that seven of the eight primary success characteristics were mentioned frequently. For example, process improvement methods were mentioned in 13.5 percent of all text units coded, and staff focus was mentioned in 9.4 percent. Organizational support of microsystem (3.2 percent) was important but less frequently mentioned.

FIGURE 1.5. SUCCESS CHARACTERISTICS OF HIGH-PERFORMING CLINICAL MICROSYSTEMS.

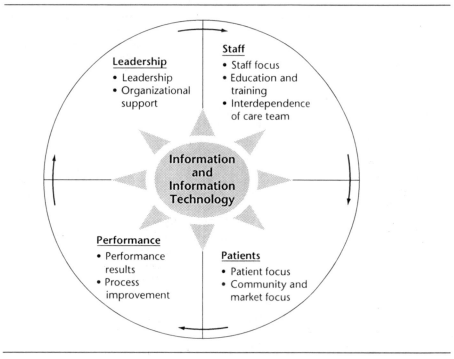

There was substantial variation in the prominence of the primary success characteristics across sites. For example, leadership, which accounted for 7.7 percent of the coded comments on average, ranged from a high of 13.2 percent in a nursing home to a low of 3.1 percent in a home health site. Similarly, staff focus, which accounted for 9.4 percent of coded comments on average, ranged across sites from a high of 20.9 percent in a home health unit to 1.6 percent in a specialty medicine unit. This variation suggests that different clinical units in different contexts serving different types of patients may possess these success characteristics in greater or lesser degrees.

Principles Associated with the Success Characteristics

Each of the primary success characteristics reflects a broad range of features and also reflects underlying principles. Table 1.1 provides more information on the nature of the success characteristics and the illustrative principles that underlie them. For example, patient focus reflects a primary concern with meeting all patient

TABLE 1.1. SCOPE OF PRIMARY SUCCESS CHARACTERISTICS AND ILLUSTRATIVE UNDERLYING PRINCIPLES.

Scope of Success Characteristic	Illustrative Underlying Principle
Leadership. The role of leadership for the microsystem is to maintain constancy of purpose, establish clear goals and expectations, foster positive culture, and advocate for the microsystem in the larger organization. There may be several types of leaders in the microsystem, including *formal* leaders, *informal* leaders, and *on-the-spot* leaders.	The leader balances setting and reaching collective goals with empowering individual autonomy and accountability.
Organizational support. The larger organization provides recognition, information, and resources to enhance and legitimize the work of the microsystem.	The larger organization looks for ways to connect to and facilitate the work of the microsystem. The larger organization facilitates coordination and handoffs between microsystems.
Patient focus. The primary concern is to meet all patient needs—caring, listening, educating, responding to special requests, innovating in light of needs, providing a smooth service flow, and establishing a relationship with community and other resources.	We are all here for the same reason—the patient.
Staff focus. The microsystem does selective hiring of the right kind of people, integrates new staff into culture and work roles, and aligns daily work roles with training competencies. Staff have high expectations for performance, continuing education, professional growth, and networking.	A *human resource value chain* links the microsystem's vision with real people on the specifics of staff hiring, orienting, and retaining and of providing continuing education and incentives for staff.
Education and training. Expectations are high regarding performance, continuing education, professional growth, and networking.	Intentional training and development of all staff is key to professional formation and optimal contributions to the microsystem.
Interdependence of care team. The interaction of staff is characterized by trust, collaboration, willingness to help each other, appreciation of complementary roles, and recognition that all contribute individually to a shared purpose.	A multidisciplinary team provides care. Every staff person is respected for the vital role he or she plays in achieving the mission.

(continued)

TABLE 1.1. (*Continued*)

Scope of Success Characteristic	Illustrative Underlying Principle
Information and information technology. Information is essential; technology smoothes the linkages between information and patient care by providing access to the rich information environment. Technology facilitates effective communication, and multiple formal and informal channels are used to keep everyone informed all the time, help everyone listen to everyone else's ideas, and ensure that everyone is connected on important topics.	Information is *the* connector—staff to patients, staff to staff, needs with actions to meet needs. The information environment is designed to support the work of the clinical microsystem. Everyone gets the right information at the right time to do his or her work.
Process improvement. An atmosphere for learning and redesign is supported by the continuous monitoring of care, the use of benchmarking, frequent tests of change, and a staff empowered to innovate.	Studying, measuring, and improving care is an essential part of our daily work.
Performance results. Performance focuses on patient outcomes, avoidable costs, streamlining delivery, using data feedback, promoting positive competition, and frank discussions about performance.	Outcomes are routinely measured, data is fed back to the microsystem, and changes are made based on the data.

needs—caring, listening, educating, responding to special requests, innovating in light of needs, providing a smooth service flow, and establishing a relationship with community and other resources—and can be encapsulated with a simple principle: we are all here for the same reason—the patient.

Specific Examples of Success Characteristics

The site interviews provide many varied and rich examples of the ways that the primary success characteristics manifest themselves in these clinical microsystems. Table 1.2 provides some examples from the original interview notes for each of the primary success characteristics. For example, here is a typical statement revealing patient focus: "At first you think you would miss the big cases that you had at a general hospital, and you do at first, but then after a while you realize they were just cases. Here you get to interact with the patient and the patient is not just a case but instead is a person."

TABLE 1.2. SPECIFIC EXAMPLES OF THE PRIMARY
SUCCESS CHARACTERISTICS.

Success Characteristic	Specific Example
Leadership	"Leadership here is fantastic, they outline the picture for us and provide a frame, then hand us the paint brushes to paint the picture."
	"I have been here for 25 years and it has allowed me to create a system that allows me the freedom to interact and manage the staff like human beings. I get to interact with them as real people and being highly organized allows that flexibility."
Organizational support	"We are not one of the top priorities so we have been left alone; I think that's been one of the advantages. We have a good reputation, and when we need something we get it. The larger organization is very supportive in that we get what we want, mostly in terms of resources."
	"One of the things that we do fight quite often is the ability to create the protocols that fit our unit, the larger organization protocols don't work. We need to tweak them—and so we do."
Patient focus	"At first you think you would miss the big cases that you had at a general hospital, and you do at first, but then after a while you realize they were just cases. Here you get to interact with the patient and the patient is not just a case but instead is a person."
	"I think medicine had really come away from listening to the patient. People can come in here for a heart disease appointment and all of a sudden they will start to cry. You think, okay, let's see what else is going on. I'd like to think our clinical team is real sensitive to that. . . . 'My wife left me, I don't see my kids anymore, my job is going down hill.' Jeez and you're feeling tired? I wonder why. . . . Our purpose is to set an example to those who have forgotten about what it means to be in medicine, which is to help people. It's not about what is the most expensive test you can order."
	"We created the unit for patients first. For instance, when we designed the new [unit], we didn't give up family room space."
Staff focus	"We have high expectations about skills and how we hire new staff. . . . When we hire new staff we look for interpersonal skills, and a good mesh with values and the mission. We can teach skills but we need them to have the right attitude."
Education and training	"I like molding people into positions. . . . I would rather take someone with no experience and mold them than take someone who thinks they already know everything. We have a way of doing things here for a reason, because it works, so we want people to work here that can grasp this and be part of the organization."

(continued)

TABLE 1.2. (*Continued*)

Success Characteristic	Specific Example
	"They allow you here to spread your wings and fly. There are great safety nets as well. You can pursue initiatives. There are always opportunities. They encourage autonomy and responsibility."
Interdependence of care team	"Together, the team works. When you take any part away, things fall apart. It's really the team that makes this a great place to work."
	"We decided as a team that our patients needed flu vaccinations, so we all volunteered on a Saturday, opened the practice and had several hundred patients come through. We ended up doing quite a bit more than flu shots including lab work, diabetic foot checks and basic checkups."
	"Here it's a real team atmosphere. Nobody gets an attitude that is disruptive. People get past the point of acting as individuals and instead work as a real team. It seems that people respect each other. For instance, when I get a new prescription, I go to the residents first. I don't try to bypass them by going to other staff alone. I will sometimes ask the residents to come with me to talk to other staff to make sure we are doing the right thing for the patient."
Information and information technology	"We use face-to-face, e-mail, and telephone. All of us try to get to the five different clinics. We have about 250 people in our staff. I know all of them, and [the executive director] and [the director of disease care] know most of them. It's about staying in touch. . . . And there is good documentation."
	"We have a system of electronic discharge. The computer is great. The physician anywhere in a satellite clinic has instantaneous access."
	"We have good information systems on labs, outpatient notes, immunization, pharmacy. . . . For instance, the immunization record here is linked to the state database. So they can get that information directly."
Process improvement	"It goes back to our processes. When we talk about how we do something in our office, we create a flow sheet. We get out the yellow stickies and we talk about every step in the process. And as a group we come up with this. Then we step back and we look at all this extra work that we make for ourselves, and then we streamline it."
	"Buried treasure. We are constantly on the lookout for tiny things that will improve care for our patients or our own lives, whether it's financial, a system component that needs improvement, or a process change."
	"I can tell you when I was practicing by myself it was painful at times, to say, 'Here you've got to do this,' and you know we're going to shut down the practice for half a day to get people really up to speed in these principles. But I would say, if you look at industry, they've learned that . . . you have to do that. The Toyota plant out in Fremont,

(*continued*)

TABLE 1.2. SPECIFIC EXAMPLES OF THE PRIMARY SUCCESS CHARACTERISTICS. (*Continued*)

Success Characteristic	Specific Example
	California, being one of the more prominent examples. The GM executives asked just exactly that. 'How can you afford to shut down the production line?' and they say, 'Well how can you afford *not* to shut down the production line?'"
Performance results	"It takes a little over a minute for us to turn around an operating room. Since we do the same surgery and we know how many cases there will be in each room, we have shelves with operating packs that after a surgery can be replaced very fast with all the appropriate tools."
	"We have a very low disposable cost per case, around $17–$18, compared to an average hospital that has $250–$500 for a similar case."
	"We have the lowest accounts receivable in the entire system. We are very proud of this. What we did was basically look at every category of expense and worked through each detail to get to the most efficient care, for instance, scheduled drugs via the pharmacy."

Best Practices: Processes and Methods Associated with High Performance

The study of the high-performing sites generated many *best practice* ideas (processes and methods) that microsystems use to accomplish their goals. Some of these noteworthy practices are discussed in *The Clinical Microsystem Action Guide* (Godfrey et al., 2002). Although a complete list of all these noteworthy practices is beyond the scope of this chapter, Table 1.3 provides a sampling of them across the major themes. For example, one process used in many sites to ensure that the patient focus was correct was to hold a daily case conference to discuss the status of each patient and to develop an optimal treatment plan that best matched the patient's changing needs.

Discussion

The results showed that the top-performing clinical units were vibrant, vital, dynamic, self-aware, and interdependent small-scale clinical organizations led with intelligence and staffed by skilled, caring, self-critical staff. Although each clinical unit was extraordinary and unique in many respects, each nevertheless shared ten success characteristics that interacted with each other dynamically and over time to produce superior, efficient care and services.

The success characteristics were generally consistent with the findings of the IOM's 2001 report *Crossing the Quality Chasm*, but there was one important

TABLE 1.3. ILLUSTRATIVE BEST PRACTICES USED BY HIGH-PERFORMING CLINICAL MICROSYSTEMS.

Best Practice Category	Description of Noteworthy Practice
Leading organizations	• Annual retreat to promote mission, vision, planning, and deployment throughout microsystem • Open-door policy among microsystem leaders • Shared leadership within the microsystem (for example, among physician, nurse, and manager) • Use of storytelling to highlight improvements needed and improvements made • Promotion of culture to value reflective practice and learning • Intentional discussions related to mission, vision, values
Staff	• Daily huddles to enhance communication among staff • Daily case conferences to focus on patient status and treatment plans • Monthly all staff (*town hall*) meetings • Continuing education *designed into* staff plans for professional growth • Screening of potential hires for attitude, values, and skill alignment • Training and orientation of new staff into work of microsystem
Information and information technology	• Tracking of data over time at microsystem level • Use of *feed forward* data to match care plan with changing patient needs • Information systems linked to care processes • Inclusion of information technology (IT) staff on microsystem team
Performance and improvement	• Use of benchmarking information on processes and outcomes • Use of *data walls* and displays of key measures for staff to view and use to assess microsystem performance • Extensive use of protocols and guidelines for core processes • Encouragement of innovative thinking and tests of change

difference. This was the emergence of leadership as a key success factor at the microsystem level. Careful review of the IOM findings and discussion with the report's lead investigator (J. J. Mohr, telephone conversations with E. C. Nelson, November 2001), however, reveal that leadership was threaded through many of the eight dimensions discussed in that report and was strongly present in the

high-performing microsystems that were studied. Thus some of the difference between our findings and the IOM findings arises from the use of different systems of classification when examining study results.

The results from our study differ from Quinn's findings reported in *Intelligent Enterprise* (Quinn, 1992), which were derived from study of world-class service
organizations outside the health care sector. The senior leaders Quinn studied
had a laserlike strategic and tactical focus on the smallest replicable units within
their organizations. They viewed those units as the microengines that generated
quality and value for their customers, as the vital organs that linked customers
with the organization's core competency through the actions taken by frontline
service providers at what we are calling the sharp end. Given the importance that
Quinn's leaders placed on these units, they iteratively designed, improved, provided incentives for, monitored, and replicated units throughout the organization.
In contrast, the senior leaders of the larger delivery systems in which our twenty
high-performing health care microsystems were embedded were for the most part
not focused on supporting excellence in the frontline clinical units. These health
system leaders showed some recognition of outstanding performance and some
degree of special assistance for outstanding units, but they lacked a strategic focus
on creating the conditions that would generate excellent interdependent performance in all the microsystems that constituted their health system. In short they
did not make the attainment of microsystem excellence a basic pillar of their management strategy.

Finally, our microsystem study has some important limitations, briefly summarized in the following list:

> *Reality and reductionism.* The reality of clinical microsystems and the health
> systems in which they are embedded is immensely complex. To study it
> and learn about it, we inevitably had to reduce, enormously, the actual
> reality to a relatively small number of features, dimensions, and interac-
> tions. Much is lost in this reduction. By focusing down on *this* we tend to
> ignore all of *that*.
>
> *Methods.* The case study approach adopted for this study gave us scope
> and depth of analysis but also tended to produce bias in several ways.
> For example, in case studies the point of view of the investigators will
> create insights in some areas and cause blind spots in others. Some of
> the staff interviewed may be inclined to place their organization in a
> somewhat more favorable light than warranted by actual conditions and
> may direct the investigators to learn more about its strengths than its
> weaknesses.

Sample. The observations are based on a small sample of just twenty microsystems that were drawn purposefully from a universe of microsystems that numbers in the tens of thousands.

Data. The data used in the study were primarily subjective and qualitative. Only limited amounts of objective data were gathered and used in the research.

Analysis. The method of content analysis, although it is a conventional and time-honored research tool, requires classification of the raw data—in this case the text units from the interviews—by the researchers. A different research team analyzing the same raw interview content might arrive at different conclusions.

Time-limited findings. The observations are cross-sectional and time limited. Although the microsystems themselves are likely to be changing in small and large ways over time and although each has its own development history and staging, the study "sliced" into the world of each microsystem and "biopsied" its structure, content, processes, outcomes, and patterns at a single point in time.

In sum the methods that were used to learn about clinical microsystems were conventional and useful, but they are clearly imperfect and restricted in diverse, important ways. Much remains to be done to quantitatively validate these findings and to make them predictive for health system and clinical microsystem leaders.

Practical Implications

This opening chapter introduced the new idea—of microsystem thinking—and summarized important research on what makes some microsystems so very good. There are grounds for excitement and hope for the health care system if we can put these ideas to work in the real world of health care delivery. Of course, as Robert Galvin, the director of Global Healthcare for General Electric, has written: "there is a reason to be cautious. New ideas in health care have a tendency to over-simplify and overpromise. Whether it be managed care, continuous quality improvement, or defined contribution, proponents seem to subscribe to the 'domino theory' of health policy: that is if only this one new idea could be applied appropriately, the great stack of complicated issues in health care would fall into place one by one" (Galvin, 2001, p. 57).

As discussed at the outset of this chapter, the health system is immense, complex, and able to deliver delightful and dreadful care. Change must contend with a linked chain of effect that connects individual patients, communities, and clinicians with small, naturally occurring frontline units and these units with countless large and small host organizations, all of which exist in a modulating policy, legal, social, financial, and regulatory environment. Oversimplification of the health system is as common as it is foolhardy.

Yet with this caution in mind, we believe that the critical role of these naturally occurring, small clinical units, which represent a vital link in the larger health care chain of effect, has been largely ignored. For the most part, fundamental changes in the health system have been directed elsewhere—at clinicians, consumers, purchasers, large managed care organizations, reimbursement policymakers, and so on—and have for the most part ignored targeting the system's essential building blocks.

The domino effect cannot ripple through the system if some of the dominoes are absent. Clinical microsystem thinking has been absent in health system reform. Once again we are reminded of Quinn's observation, "Critical to relevant effective system design is conceptualizing the smallest replicable unit and its potential use in strategy as early as possible in the design process" (Quinn, 1992, p. 104).

We hope that the remaining chapters in this book on clinical microsystems will provide useful theories and models, practical ideas, and helpful tools that readers can use to

- Plan individual patient care and efficient services
- Create rich information environments
- Promote the strategic spread of high-performing clinical microsystems that excel at meeting patients' needs and are stimulating work environments

Conclusion

Clinical microsystems are the smallest replicable units in the health system. Health system redesign can succeed only with leaders who take action to transform these small clinical units in order to optimize performance to meet and exceed patient needs and expectations and to perfect the linkages between the units. A seamless, patient-centered, high-quality, safe, and efficient health care system cannot be realized without the transformation of the essential building blocks that combine to form the care continuum.

APPENDIX 1.1. THE TWENTY SITES EXAMINED
IN THE CLINICAL MICROSYSTEM STUDY.

Name of Microsystem	Location	Name of Macrosystem
Home Health Care		
Gentiva Rehab Without Walls	Lansing, MI	Gentiva Health Services
Interim Pediatrics	Pittsburgh, PA	Interim HealthCare of Pittsburgh
On Lok SeniorHealth Rose Team	San Francisco, CA	On Lok SeniorHealth
Visiting Nursing Service Congregate Care Program, Queens Team 11S	New York, NY	Visiting Nursing Service of New York
Inpatient Care		
Henry Ford Neonatal Intensive Care Unit	Detroit, MI	Henry Ford Hospital, Henry Ford Health System
Intermountain Shock/Trauma/Respiratory Intensive Care Unit	Salt Lake City, UT	Latter-Day Saints Hospital, Intermountain Healthcare
Center for Orthopedic Oncology and Musculoskeletal Research	Washington, DC	Washington Cancer Institute, Washington Hospital Center, MedStar Health
Shouldice Hernia Repair Centre	Thornhill, Canada	Shouldice Hospital
Nursing Home Care		
Bon Secours Wound Care Team	St. Petersburg, FL	Bon Secours Maria Manor Nursing and Rehabilitation Center
Hospice of North Iowa	Mason City, IA	Mercy Medical Center North Iowa, Mercy Health Network
Iowa Veterans Home, M4C Team	Marshalltown, IA	Iowa Veterans Home, Veterans Commission
Primary Care		
Grace Hill Community Health Center	St. Louis, MO	Grace Hill Neighborhood Health Centers, Inc.
Massachusetts General Hospital Downtown Associates Primary Care	Boston, MA	Massachusetts General Hospital, Partners Healthcare
Evergreen Woods Office	Bangor, ME	Norumbega Medical, Eastern Maine Healthcare
ThedaCare Kimberly Office Family Medicine	Kimberly, WI	ThedaCare Physicians

(continued)

APPENDIX 1.1. THE TWENTY SITES EXAMINED
IN THE CLINICAL MICROSYSTEM STUDY (*Continued*).

Name of Microsystem	Location	Name of Macrosystem
Specialty Care		
Dartmouth-Hitchcock Spine Center	Lebanon, NH	Dartmouth-Hitchcock Medical Center
Midelfort Behavioral Health	Eau Claire, WI	Midelfort Clinic at Luther Campus, Mayo Health System
Orthopedic Specialty Practice	Boise, ID	Intermountain Healthcare
Overlook Hospital Emergency Department	Summit, NJ	Overlook Hospital, Atlantic Health System
Sharp Diabetes Self Management Training Center	La Mesa, CA	Grossmont Hospital, Sharp HealthCare

References

Arrow, H., McGrath, J., & Berdahl, J. (2000). *Small groups as complex systems.* Thousand Oaks, CA: Sage.

Batalden, P. B., Mohr, J. J., Nelson, E. C., & Plume, S. K. (1996). Improving health care: Part 4. Concepts for improving any clinical process. *Joint Commission Journal on Quality Improvement, 22*(10), 651–659.

Berwick, D. (2001). Which hat is on? Plenary Address at the Institute for Healthcare Improvement's 12th Annual National Forum, Orlando, FL.

Capra, F. (1996). *The web of life: A new scientific understanding of living systems.* New York: Anchor Books.

Deming, W. E. (1986). *Out of the crisis.* Cambridge, MA: MIT Center for Advanced Engineering Study.

Donaldson, M., & Mohr, J. (2000). *Exploring innovation and quality improvement in health care microsystems: A cross-case analysis.* Technical Report for the Institute of Medicine Committee on Quality of Health Care in America. Washington, DC: Institute of Medicine.

Galvin, R. (2001). The business case for quality. *Health Affairs, 20*(6), 57–58.

Godfrey, M. M., Batalden, P. B., Wasson, J. H., & Nelson, E. C. (2002). *Clinical microsystem action guide* (Version 2.1). Hanover, NH: Dartmouth Medical School.

Hock, D. (2005). *One from many.* San Francisco: Berrett-Koehler.

Institute of Medicine (U.S.), Committee on Quality of Health Care in America. (2001). *Crossing the quality chasm: A new health system for the 21st century.* Washington, DC: National Academies Press.

Kabcenell, A. (2002). Pursuing perfection: An interview with Don Berwick and Michael Rothman. *Joint Commission Journal on Quality Improvement, 28*, 268–278.

Kelly, K. (1994). *Out of control: The rise of neo-biological civilization.* Reading, MA: Addison-Wesley.

Miles, M., & Huberman, A. (1994). *An expanded sourcebook: Qualitative data analysis.* Thousand Oaks, CA: Sage.

Mohr, J. J., Mahoney, C. C., Nelson, E. C., Batalden, P. B., & Plume, S. K. (1996). Improving health care: Part 3. Clinical benchmarking for best patient care. *Joint Commission Journal on Quality Improvement, 22*(9), 599–616.

Nelson, E. C., Batalden, P. B., Mohr, J. J., & Plume, S. K. (1998). Building a quality future. *Frontiers of Health Service Management, 15*(1), 3–32.

Nelson, E. C., Batalden, P. B., Plume, S. K., & Mohr, J. J. (1996). Improving health care: Part 2: A clinical improvement worksheet and users' manual. *Joint Commission Journal on Quality Improvement, 22*(8), 531–547.

Nelson, E. C., Mohr, J. J., Batalden, P. B., & Plume, S. K. (1996). Improving health care: Part 1. The clinical value compass. *Joint Commission Journal on Quality Improvement, 22*(4), 243–258.

Nelson, E. C., Splaine, M. E., Godfrey, M. M., Kahn, V., Hess, A., Batalden, P., et al. (2000). Using data to improve medical practice by measuring processes and outcomes of care. *Joint Commission Journal on Quality Improvement, 26*(12), 667–685.

Peters, T. J. (1987). *Thriving on chaos: Handbook for a management revolution.* New York: Knopf.

Quinn, J. B. (1992). *Intelligent enterprise: A knowledge and service based paradigm for industry.* New York: Free Press.

Rutherford, P., Lee, B., & Greiner, A. (2004). *Transforming care at the bedside.* Retrieved June 20, 2006, from http://www.ihi.org/IHI/Results/WhitePapers/TransformingCareattheBedsideWhitePaper.htm.

Senge, P. M. (1990). *The fifth discipline: The art and practice of the learning organization.* New York: Doubleday.

Wheatley, M. J. (1992). *Leadership and the new science: Learning about organization from an orderly universe.* San Francisco: Berrett-Koehler.

Zimmerman, B., Lindberg, C., & Plsek, P. (1999). *Edgeware: Insights from complexity science for health care leaders.* Irving, TX: VHA.

CHAPTER TWO

DEVELOPING HIGH-PERFORMING MICROSYSTEMS

Eugene C. Nelson, Paul B. Batalden, William H. Edwards, Marjorie M. Godfrey, Julie K. Johnson

Chapter Summary

Background. This chapter focuses on what it takes, in the short term and the long term, for clinical microsystems— the small, functional frontline units that provide most health care to most people—to attain peak performance.

Case study. A case study featuring the intensive care nursery at Dartmouth-Hitchcock Medical Center illustrates the ten-year evolution of one particular clinical microsystem. Related evolutionary principles begin with the intention to excel, involve all the players, focus on values that matter, keep both discipline and rhythm, use measurement and feedback, and create a learning system.

Discussion. A microsystem's typical developmental journey toward excellence entails five stages of growth—

awareness of being an interdependent group with the capacity to make changes, connecting routine daily work to the high purpose of benefiting patients, responding successfully to strategic challenges, measuring the microsystem's performance as a system, and juggling improvements while taking care of patients.

A model curriculum. Health system leaders can sponsor an action-learning program to catalyze development of clinical microsystems. The Dartmouth Microsystem Improvement Curriculum (DMIC) can help clinical staff members acquire the fundamental knowledge and skills they will need to master if they are to increase their capacity to attain higher levels of performance. It uses action-learning theory and sound educational principles to provide staff with the opportunity to learn, test, and gain some degree of mastery; it involves people in the challenging real work of improving the care that they provide. It represents improvement from the inside out, because it begins with the professionals inside the system working together to get better results for the patients they serve while simultaneously finding ways to improve worklife.

This chapter focuses on what it takes, in the short term and long term, for clinical microsystems—the small functional, frontline units that provide most health care to most people—to realize their potential and to attain peak performance. Attention is placed on both long-run issues and short-term actions related to attaining high levels of performance that both benefit patients and energize staff. To achieve long-term gains, it may be important to have a sense of how actual clinical microsystems can grow, learn, adapt, and improve over extended periods of time. We provide a case study to highlight one microsystem's ten-year journey toward excellence and to offer a framework that reflects a microsystem's developmental journey toward high performance. This case study, like other case studies presented in this book, contributes to the evolution of clinical microsystem theory.

To make swift progress in the short term, it may be wise for the leaders of health systems to sponsor an action-learning program to catalyze proactive development of clinical microsystems. We describe the Dartmouth Microsystem Improvement Curriculum (DMIC), which addresses microsystem fundamentals and which can be used to initiate forward progress and to begin to anchor strategic and operational microsystem thinking in the local culture. This chapter concludes with a summary of important points, including what leaders can do to foster effective progress toward best performance.

Case Study: A Decade of Progress for an Intensive Care Nursery

This case draws on a decade of experience, planned change, and growth in the intensive care nursery (ICN) at Dartmouth-Hitchcock Medical Center (DHMC). The ICN serves a mostly rural region of New Hampshire and Vermont, with a total population of approximately 750,000 people. The ICN was started in 1972 and currently has thirty-one beds.

Initial Stimulus and First Project: Quiet Pleases, 1992

In 1992, Gene Nelson and Bill Edwards, the latter a neonatologist and the ICN's medical director, were in conversation about the ICN. When asked about his vision for the ICN, Edwards said he would like to see it become the best in the world— not to claim bragging rights but rather to make it possible for infants and their families to have the best chance possible for successful outcomes. He asked, rhetorically, "Would any family want anything less?"

This conversation was in effect a tipping point (Gladwell, 2000). It set in motion events that accelerated and provided structure for a long and continuing quest for excellence in this ICN. With this vision in mind, Edwards and Nelson, who had recently joined DHMC, decided to start explicitly working toward the goal of achieving best possible outcomes. A brief synopsis of the early activity follows.

Edwards invited an interdisciplinary team of about seven ICN staff to embark with him on an action-learning activity, or *studio course*, based on the principles that Donald Schön presents in his 1990 book, *Educating the Reflective Practitioner*. For approximately six months this ICN team met weekly or biweekly for sixty minutes at a time. The first thing the team members did was to talk about the team's mission and aim. Team members used clinical *value compass* thinking to do the following:

- Sharpen the team's aim, which became— "to optimize the outcome of <1500-gram babies, to decrease the incidence of major morbidity and mortality, and to do this at a lower cost"
- Clarify critical outcomes of care for key beneficiaries (the infants, their families, and community providers)

The ICN value compass that was developed in 1992 (Figure 2.1), and is still used today, summarizes the team's outcomes model. The team then identified high-leverage areas that might be improved to realize better outcomes. This led to the selection of an initial, novel improvement theme that centered on noise reduction. This topic was selected because research had suggested that high noise levels could disturb the delicate physiology of low birth weight infants and had the potential to cause serious adverse events. Assessment of the current sound levels in the ICN revealed that frequent loud noises occurred and that all staff members could be involved in noise reduction. The next steps involved assessing the sources of loud noises (people and equipment), gathering baseline data on noise levels, and planning tests of change using the scientific method. This effort used the plan-do-study-act (PDSA) approach (Nelson, Batalden, & Ryer, 1998).

FIGURE 2.1. VALUE COMPASS FOR THE DHMC INTENSIVE CARE NURSERY.

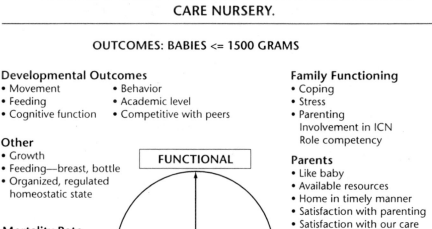

OUTCOMES: BABIES <= 1500 GRAMS

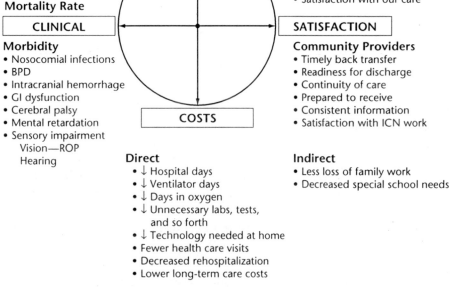

Developmental Outcomes
- Movement
- Feeding
- Cognitive function
- Behavior
- Academic level
- Competitive with peers

Other
- Growth
- Feeding—breast, bottle
- Organized, regulated homeostatic state

Family Functioning
- Coping
- Stress
- Parenting
  Involvement in ICN
  Role competency

Parents
- Like baby
- Available resources
- Home in timely manner
- Satisfaction with parenting
- Satisfaction with our care

FUNCTIONAL

Mortality Rate

CLINICAL

SATISFACTION

Morbidity
- Nosocomial infections
- BPD
- Intracranial hemorrhage
- GI dysfunction
- Cerebral palsy
- Mental retardation
- Sensory impairment
  Vision—ROP
  Hearing

Community Providers
- Timely back transfer
- Readiness for discharge
- Continuity of care
- Prepared to receive
- Consistent information
- Satisfaction with ICN work

COSTS

Direct
- ↓ Hospital days
- ↓ Ventilator days
- ↓ Days in oxygen
- ↓ Unnecessary labs, tests, and so forth
- ↓ Technology needed at home
- Fewer health care visits
- Decreased rehospitalization
- Lower long-term care costs

Indirect
- Less loss of family work
- Decreased special school needs

The first set of changes focused on noise produced by staff, family, and visitors and was signified by the theme—prominently displayed—of *Quiet Pleases*. The second set of changes targeted equipment noise produced by myriad alarms—"buzzers, bells, and whistles"—that were constantly erupting to signal possible danger. After all these changes were initiated, noise levels decreased in the intermediate care area within the ICN (Figure 2.2).

Beyond the impact on noise reduction (which was real yet modest), this initial improvement work gave all the ICN staff disciplines—physicians, nurses, nursing

FIGURE 2.2. NOISE LEVELS IN THE ICN INTERMEDIATE CARE UNIT BEFORE AND AFTER QUIET PLEASES.

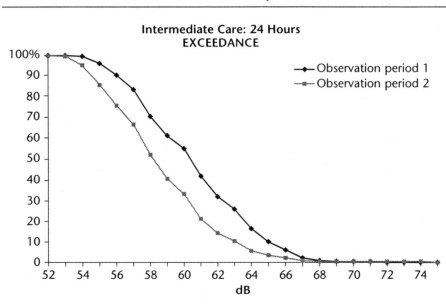

Note: The exceedance is the percentage of time the noise level exceeded each decibel level (C-weighted scale) during a twenty-four-hour period.

assistants, administrative staff—an opportunity to work together to learn principles and methods that could be used in the future. It gave them a sense that they could change their work, and it generated a visible, short-term *win*, promoted local improvement knowledge, created a guiding coalition, used the scientific method (which was revered in the local culture), and fostered respectful interdependence and shared leadership patterns, all of which built a solid foundation for continuing on the path toward excellence and transformation (Kotter, 1996; Schein, 1999; Weick, 1995).

System Cost-Cutting Imperatives and Adaptive Responses, 1994 to 1997

In 1994, the DHMC health system faced significant financial challenges; all the clinical units were challenged to reduce costs. The ICN embarked on a length of stay (LOS) reduction program to reduce costs while maintaining or improving quality. Members of the interdisciplinary team focused on three high-leverage processes—discharge planning and case management, management of apnea and

FIGURE 2.3. ICN MEDIAN COST PER INFANT ADMITTED IN 1996–1997 INTENSIVE CARE NURSERY.

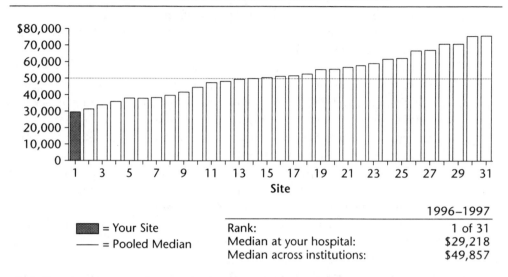

	1996–1997
▓ = Your Site	
— = Pooled Median	
Rank:	1 of 31
Median at your hospital:	$29,218
Median across institutions:	$49,857

Note: The geographical adjustment adjusts for area differences in input prices: that is, cost for each hospital is measured as though that hospital faced average U.S. input prices.

related discharge criteria, and management of infants' transitions to oral feeding. These and other subsequent changes (for example, reducing unnecessary diagnostic tests, decreasing total parenteral nutrition costs, and changing antibiotic prescribing patterns) led to recurring savings (estimated at $1.3 million per year) and measurable decreases in LOS. The ICN was subsequently able to achieve the lowest geographically adjusted, median cost per infant admitted in 1996–1997 compared with the cost at thirty other hospitals participating in the Vermont Oxford Network (VON) quality improvement collaborative described in the following section (Figure 2.3).

Collaborative Work with VON: 1995 to 2003

Another important factor in the DHMC ICN's quest for best possible care has been the ICN's participation in the Vermont Oxford Network. In 1994, VON initiated a focus on collaborative, multidisciplinary quality improvement, with the DHMC ICN as a charter member (Horbar et al., 2001; Rogowski et al., 2001). Approximately 100 ICNs worked together, either directly or via teleconferencing, to improve the quality of neonatal care.

By working with VON the ICN at DHMC was able to

- Reduce its nosocomial infection rate by approximately 70 percent in three years, from an annual rate of 39 percent to 13 percent among infants with birth weights ranging from 501 to 1500 grams.
- Help plan and colead an international, multicenter, randomized controlled trial on the effectiveness of prophylactic skin care with an emollient on nosocomial infection rates and skin integrity in extremely low birth weight infants (501 to 1,000 grams) (Edwards, Conner, & Soll, 2001, 2004).
- Improve use of nasal continuous positive airway pressure (CPAP) by benchmarking the best-known practices and best-observed outcomes and applying these practices and outcome measures. This activity led to large measurable improvements—for example, a substantial decline in the mean number of days that infants used mechanical ventilation (see Figure 2.4).
- Colead and participate with ten other centers in a program to increase family involvement in each child's care, which involved including parents, as members

FIGURE 2.4. LONGITUDINAL TRENDS IN NUMBER OF DAYS ICN INFANTS SPEND ON MECHANICAL VENTILATION.

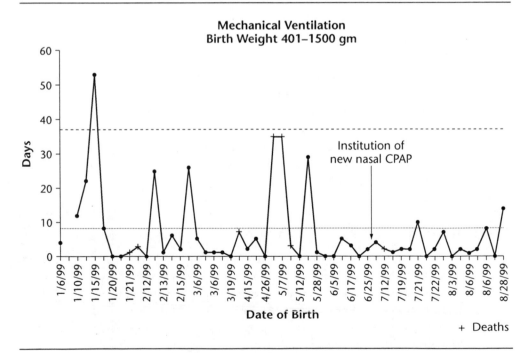

of the care team, in daily rounds (Cisneros-Moore, Coker, DuBuisson, Swett, & Edwards, 2003; Saunders, Abraham, Crosby, Thomas, & Edwards, 2003).

- Experience the power and attractiveness of learning from and with others in a *community of practice* (Wenger, 1999).

Evolutionary Principles: Transformation of Improvement Patterns

The DHMC ICN case study reveals a clinical unit that is on the move and headed toward something better. It always had the intention to achieve superior results, but it lacked a method for doing so. This case study embodies the following principles, which may be helpful in guiding other microsystems' progress toward the best possible performance.

Begin with the Intention to Excel. The improvement process is initiated and sustained with the intention to achieve the best possible results. This aim is motivated not so much by the desire to capture the high ground or to bask in the limelight but by the desire to do what is best for the patients and families that have the potential to benefit from care.

Involve All the Players. The leaders who are successful will, over time, find a variety of opportunities and ways to involve all the microsystem players—interdisciplinary staff and patients and families—in the action of analyzing and improving processes and outcomes.

Focus on Values That Matter. The leadership activity that will sustain a virtuous cycle of improvement in performance connects change to core values that matter to patients, families, and staff.

Keep Both Discipline and Rhythm. Improvement work can be sustained over time and become part of a clinical microsystem's culture when leaders inculcate new habits and new patterns that produce an internal discipline and reliable rhythm. *Discipline* relates to such things as use of the scientific method and open, respectful inquiry into authentic causes and full effects. *Rhythm* relates to devoting some time to improving patient care even as large amounts of time are spent on providing patient care.

Use Measurement and Feedback. Both the discipline and the rhythm—the pattern essential for fostering learning systems—are aided and abetted by the use of measurement and feedback to assess the gap between current results and the desired state.

Create a Learning System. A statement often attributed to Galileo holds that "you cannot teach anyone anything, you can only help him find it within himself." People learn in many ways—by being confronted with a worthy challenge, by taking action and reflecting on the results, by using the scientific method, by becoming keen participant observers of their own work processes and the related outcomes, by exchanging ideas and methods about what works and what fails, and so on. It is important to create a learning system and thereby the conditions under which staff members can learn and discover, test out new ideas, realize their own potential, and attempt to innovate.

A Model of Development and a Curriculum to Catalyze Microsystem Growth

In this section we first provide a general model that portrays a clinical microsystem's developmental journey toward best possible performance. We then introduce a curriculum that can be used to jump-start clinical microsystems to embark on their own paths toward peak performance.

A Microsystem's Developmental Journey

To complement the previous case study, which provides some details of one particular microsystem's developmental journey, Figure 2.5 provides a general model for the journey. The model is based on work with and observations of hundreds of clinical microsystems during the past two decades. It calls attention to the following five stages of growth over time.

Stage 1: Create **Awareness of Our Clinical Unit as an Interdependent Group of People with the Capacity to Make Changes.** Often it is the invitation to describe the work of a clinical microsystem in a diagram that initiates that microsystem's enhanced self-awareness. Members of the clinical microsystem will often note routines, habits, or processes that do not work very well or that do not make sense when they look at the system's functioning as a whole, and they may decide to change them. The experience of working on what some describe as the *foolishness* of work—the things no one wants to admit to, much less brag about (such as confusion and rework in patient flow)—can lead to staff members' realization that change as a unit is possible. The sense that "we" can take action on "our" unit begins a journey of empowerment for the microsystem.

FIGURE 2.5. A MODEL FOR A MICROSYSTEM'S DEVELOPMENTAL JOURNEY.

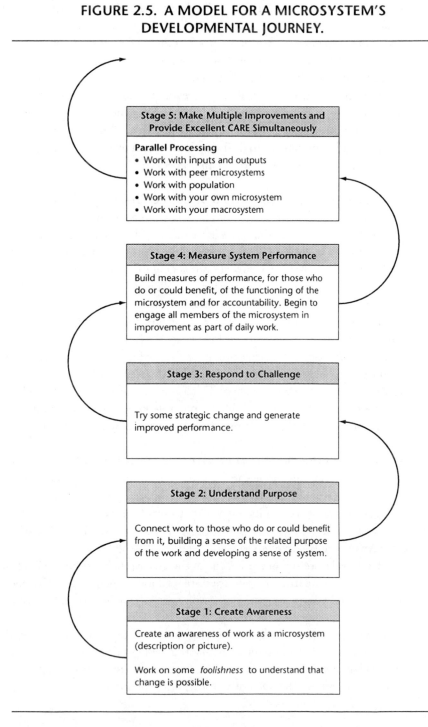

Stage 5: Make Multiple Improvements and Provide Excellent CARE Simultaneously

Parallel Processing
- Work with inputs and outputs
- Work with peer microsystems
- Work with population
- Work with your own microsystem
- Work with your macrosystem

Stage 4: Measure System Performance

Build measures of performance, for those who do or could benefit, of the functioning of the microsystem and for accountability. Begin to engage all members of the microsystem in improvement as part of daily work.

Stage 3: Respond to Challenge

Try some strategic change and generate improved performance.

Stage 2: Understand Purpose

Connect work to those who do or could benefit from it, building a sense of the related purpose of the work and developing a sense of system.

Stage 1: Create Awareness

Create an awareness of work as a microsystem (description or picture).

Work on some *foolishness* to understand that change is possible.

*Stage 2: Connect Our Routine Daily Work to the High **Purpose** of Benefiting Patients; See Ourselves as a **System.*** Once its members have a sense of *agency* ("we can take action on our own work"), a team is often able to come to a deeper realization than it had before; it sees that it exists for a purpose: the benefit of patients and families. With this clarification of an aim—to benefit a defined population of patients—it is easier for everyone to see the providers, processes, and patterns as a system (Godfrey, Nelson, Wasson, Mohr, & Batalden, 2003; Wasson, Godfrey, Nelson, Mohr, & Batalden, 2003). This step of relating the needs of a population of patients to the hurly-burly world of everyday work is a challenge clinical microsystems have often skipped over.

*Stage 3: Respond Successfully to a **Strategic** **Challenge.*** When a microsystem that has a sense of itself as a system faces a strategic challenge, such as "eliminate waiting for access to appointments in primary and specialty care," or, "cut costs by reducing LOS in the ICN," it can successfully change its processes and make things work better. However, for a clinical unit lacking this self-awareness, responding to a challenge such as this is often a matter of "following the recipe" or "looking like we are moving forward and attending to the issue when we are really walking in place." The results usually show up later as a slow decline in the changed performance to the previous unsatisfactory level (recipe following) or as no measurable improvement after all (walking in place but looking attentive). Recipe followers often worry about "holding the gains," whereas walkers in place often demand valid measures that will reveal how good the performance really is. Clinical microsystems that have well-developed identities as systems are better able to integrate large and small changes into their regular operations—their identity—and as a result they sustain them over time.

*Stage 4: **Measure** the Performance of Our System as a System.* The clinical microsystem that has made some changes, that has developed an explicit sense of itself as a system, and that is producing many important outcomes tends to be curious about its results—it wants to track its performance after making changes. Visual reminders of performance in the form of *data walls* (large, detailed displays of results) are often present (Nelson et al., 2003).

Data walls are designated areas in the clinical microsystem where data over time specific to the microsystem are displayed for all members of the microsystem to review and take action on. Data walls typically include data over time from

- The larger organization-strategic measures that might be collected by the larger organization, such as patient satisfaction, staff satisfaction
- Service line data, such as time to catheterization laboratory for a cardiac microsystem or infections rates for a surgical service

- Clinical microsystem data that reflect current performance data, such as cycle time from the time a patient enters the microsystem until they leave in an ambulatory practice, length of stay in an inpatient unit, or number of days from last infection to other improvement cycle data specific to current improvement activities

Measurement becomes a friend of forward progress and of the microsystem's enhanced sense of itself. The microsystem often begins to track important indicators of its process for providing services and its outcomes to gain a better understanding of what is happening and to put itself in a better position to manage and improve care. The leaders of the microsystem begin to engage all the staff in the work of improving and innovating.

Stage 5: Successfully Juggle **Multiple** **Improvements** *While Taking Excellent Care of Patients, . . . as We Continue to Develop an Enhanced Sense of Ourselves as a System.* With self-understanding, the ability to change, and the ability to track and reflect on its performance, the clinical microsystem is able to engage its context—the macrosystem in which it works and the other microsystems with which it regularly interacts. It is now in a better position to

- Analyze, modify, and standardize its own operations, such as the internal flows (from input to output).
- Reach out and involve all members of the clinical microsystem, including those who are only marginally connected to this newfound identity.
- Focus renewed energy on finding ways to meet the needs of each individual patient, one by one, and the needs of the population of patients the microsystem serves.

The clinical microsystem finds it is now possible to engage many people in many ways in taking actions to provide and improve care, to run multiple tests of change simultaneously, and to create a work environment that recognizes good work and promotes personal and professional growth (Huber et al., 2003). It finds ways to foster a *virtuous* cycle, or positive, upward, evolutionary spiral.

A microsystem's developmental journey does not always work this way. "All models are wrong, some are useful," as Box (1978, p. 202) reminds us. The model is depicted in a stagewise, linear fashion. However, the microsystem's developmental journey does not necessarily occur in this sequence; it has interactions and feedback loops. Although the model seems to imply an *entity*—that is, *the* clinical microsystem—many clinical microsystems more often resemble a loosely coupled group than a tightly linked interdependent crew (Scott, 1981; Weick, 2001). These caveats notwithstanding, this developmental model has proven helpful for members and leaders of clinical microsystems who are eager to reflect on their work and on their efforts to attain the highest levels of quality, safety, service, and efficiency. A developmental journey is not an overnight occurrence, and leadership that seeks knowledge, takes action, and reviews and reflects can help keep everyone's focus on the journey (Batalden et al., 2003).

A Model Curriculum for the Developmental Journey

Researchers can sometimes identify clinical units and clinical programs that are extraordinary. Most health systems have many exemplary clinical units. However, most health systems also recognize that what they need is not a *few pockets of gold* but a total system that is *solid gold*.

The question is, How do we begin the evolution toward a solid-gold health system—one that is composed of many small systems that are excellent in what they do? Recall that the patient's health care journey often requires him or her to interact with many small clinical units that come together into a health system (care continuum) that addresses the patient's changing health needs (Nelson et al., 2002).

There are many answers to this fundamental and challenging question, How might we embark successfully on improving the health system by improving the small systems of which it is composed? One very good answer is offered in Chapter Four of this book. That chapter demonstrates the powerful strategic value of applying microsystem thinking to the problem of organization-wide improvement in a large, complex health system.

Another complementary (and partial) answer to this question of organization-wide transformation is to provide each and every clinical microsystem (and the clinical support units such as human resources, information services, billing, and purchasing) with a basic learning program that will enable each individual microsystem to gain the skill and knowledge needed to start and sustain its own self-improvement from the inside out. Part Two of this book introduces the Dartmouth Microsystem Improvement Curriculum, which is based on more than ten years of direct experience in working with clinical units as they redesign their work or design completely new health care programs. (Table 10.1, in Chapter Ten, provides an overview of this curriculum.)

This curriculum performs the following functions:

- Helps clinical staff acquire the fundamental knowledge and skills that they will need to master if they are to increase their capacity to attain higher levels of performance

- Uses action-learning theory and sound educational principles to provide people with the opportunity to learn, test, and gain some degree of mastery
- Involves people in the challenging real work of improving—assessing, diagnosing, treating—the small systems in which they work, in ways that will matter

This curriculum has been applied to diverse clinical units—such as primary care practices, specialty medical practices, inpatient clinical units, home health teams, and clinical support units, such as pharmacy, radiology, and pathology—in the United States and in many settings throughout Europe—and has been offered in various formats (for example, one day per month for six months, one day per week for ten weeks, and an accelerated workshop running for five consecutive half days).

Two points about the Dartmouth Microsystem Improvement Curriculum learning model merit special emphasis.

Studio Course Principles. Donald Schön uses the architectural studio course as a model for effective learning to emphasize creating the conditions under which people can learn rather than focusing mostly on direct teaching or skills training (Schön, 1983). We base the microsystem improvement curriculum on Schön's studio-course model and capitalize on the power of these strategies:

- Giving people a meaningful challenge to work on (for example, improve access, reduce errors, delight patients)
- Offering longitudinal learning—a by-product of working on the challenge
- Evoking the magic of interactive learning, which involves peer-to-peer exchanges, teacher-to-student dialogues, microsystem-to-microsystem discussions, and microsystem-to-macrosystem conversations
- Learning from concrete experience and reflecting on the experience
- Drawing on other life experiences and knowledge bases and applying them to the challenge at hand

Many health care professionals do not regularly take the time to reflect on their practice. Once they have *protected time* to do this, self-awareness grows.

Three-Thread Tactic. The aim of the Dartmouth Microsystem Improvement Curriculum is to intertwine three vital threads and to develop them in the learners over time. These three threads are

1. Finding ways to better meet each patient's special needs
2. Making the work experience for staff meaningful and joyous through their learning to work in an interdisciplinary manner to design and provide patient-centered care

3. Increasing each staff person's capability to improve his or her work and to contribute to the betterment of the system as a whole

Several years ago Donald Wolfe called attention to the needed competence within microsystems and macrosystems for work in the "applied behavioral sciences." He noted that *competence* always has a context (the microsystem work life), is rooted in a knowledge base and in analytical skills (clinical knowledge and improvement knowledge), and is inevitably interdependent with values and involves the whole person (unity of organizational mission with personal values) (Wolfe, 1980). The Dartmouth Microsystem Improvement Curriculum and the style of teaching that accompanies it are designed to reflect these themes.

Conclusion

The challenge for all of us, leaders of health systems and people who work in those systems, is to provide high-quality care that is patient centered, safe, effective, timely, equitable, and efficient (Institute of Medicine [U.S.], Committee on Quality of Health Care in America, 2001). This cannot be done today, but it could be done tomorrow if, and only if, we can redesign our systems. We need system-based improvement methods to make lasting improvements in the health care system.

A successful redesign requires creating the conditions for learning, improvement, and accountability at multiple levels—the large-system level (populated by macroorganizations that exist in reimbursement, legal, policy, and regulatory milieus), the mesosystem level (which represents the middle layers of large organizations and links the front office with the front line), and the small-system level (characterized by clinical microsystems such as outpatient clinics, inpatient units, and other frontline delivery teams and clinical support groups). We must pay close attention to the large-system issues; if we fail to do so, our progress will be limited. However, we must also pay close attention to the small-system realities if we are to meet the quality challenge. There are many reasons why this is so. As noted earlier in this book, a small system can be described as a

- Basic building block of health care
- Unit of clinical policy-in-use
- Place where good value and safe care are *made.*
- Locus of control for most of the variables that account for patient satisfaction
- Setting for interdisciplinary professional formation
- Locus of control of most of the worklife *dissatisfiers* and many of the *genuine motivators* for health professionals' pride and joy in work

For us, the joy of these insights is that they allow us to see the familiar with "new eyes," as Marcel Proust observed about the discovery process. The challenge comes from using our new eyes to see and asking ourselves questions such as these:

1. What will it take for the processes of health professional education and development to recognize the cooperative and interdependent work of professionals from different disciplines and prepare these professionals accordingly?
2. What will help health system leaders recognize the opportunity they have to actively foster the development of clinical microsystems, on which their macrosystem depends, and what will help those macrosystem leaders hold their microsystems accountable for the quality, value, and safety of patient care?
3. What *structures* of organization and work will enable clinical microsystems to regularly improve value by facilitating the never-ending removal of waste and cost?
4. What practices and disciplines in clinical microsystems will hold and honor the vitality of the paradox of the health care of the individual and the health of populations (that doing what seems best for the health of the individual and doing what seems best for the health of the population may seem to or may actually conflict).

We hope that this book, by focusing attention on clinical microsystems—the places where patients and care teams meet—will contribute to lasting improvements in patient care as well as betterment of the working lives of those who provide the care.

References

Batalden, P. B., Nelson, E. C., Mohr, J. J., Godfrey, M. M., Huber, T. P., Kosnik, L., et al. (2003). Microsystems in health care: Part 5. How leaders are leading. *Joint Commission Journal on Quality and Safety, 29*(6), 297–308.

Box, G. (1978). *Statistics for experimenters: An introduction to design, data analysis, and model building.* Hoboken, NJ: Wiley-Interscience.

Cisneros-Moore, K. A., Coker, K., DuBuisson, A. B., Swett, B., & Edwards, W. H. (2003). Implementing potentially better practices for improving family-centered care in neonatal intensive care units: Successes and challenges. *Pediatrics, 111*(4, Pt. 2), 450–460.

Edwards, W. H., Conner, J. M., & Soll, R. F., for the Vermont Oxford Network. (2001). The effect of Aquaphor® original emollient ointment on nosocomial sepsis rates and skin integrity in infants of birth weight 501 to 1000 grams. *Pediatric Research, 49*(4, Pt. 2), 388A.

Edwards, W. H., Conner, J. M., & Soll, R. F., for the Vermont Oxford Network Neonatal Skin Care Study Group. (2004). The effect of prophylactic ointment therapy on nosocomial sepsis rates and skin integrity in infants of birth weight 501–1000 grams. *Pediatrics, 113*(5), 1195–1203.

Gladwell, M. (2000). *The tipping point: How little things can make a big difference.* Boston: Little, Brown.

Godfrey, M. M., Nelson, E. C., Wasson, J. H., Mohr, J. J., & Batalden, P. B. (2003). Microsystems in health care: Part 3. Planning patient-centered services. *Joint Commission Journal on Quality and Safety, 29*(4), 159–170.

Horbar, J. D., Rogowski, J., Plsek, P. E., Delmore, P., Edwards, W. H., Hocker, J., et al. (2001). Collaborative quality improvement for neonatal intensive care. NIC/Q Project Investigators of the Vermont Oxford Network. *Pediatrics, 107*(1), 14–22.

Huber, T. P., Godfrey, M. M., Nelson, E. C., Mohr, J. J., Campbell, C., & Batalden, P. B. (2003). Microsystems in health care: Part 8. Developing people and improving work life: What front-line staff told us. *Joint Commission Journal on Quality and Safety, 29*(10), 512–522.

Institute of Medicine (U.S.), Committee on Quality of Health Care in America. (2001). *Crossing the quality chasm: A new health system for the 21st century.* Washington, DC: National Academies Press.

Kotter, J. P. (1996). *Leading change.* Boston: Harvard Business School Press.

Nelson, E. C., Batalden, P. B., Homa, K., Godfrey, M. M., Campbell, C., Headrick, L. A., et al. (2003). Microsystems in health care: Part 2. Creating a rich information environment. *Joint Commission Journal on Quality and Safety, 29*(1), 5–15.

Nelson, E. C., Batalden, P. B., Huber, T. P., Mohr, J. J., Godfrey, M. M., Headrick, L. A., et al. (2002). Microsystems in health care: Part 1. Learning from high-performing front-line clinical units. *Joint Commission Journal on Quality Improvement, 28*(9), 472–493.

Nelson, E. C., Batalden, P. B., & Ryer, J. C. (Eds.). (1998). *Clinical improvement action guide.* Oakbrook Terrace, IL: Joint Commission on Accreditation of Healthcare Organizations.

Rogowski, J., Horbar, J. D., Plsek, P. E., Baker, L. S., Deterding, J., Edwards, W. H., et al. (2001). Economic implications of neonatal intensive care unit collaborative quality improvement. *Pediatrics, 107*(1), 23–29.

Saunders, R. P., Abraham, M. R., Crosby, M. J., Thomas, K., & Edwards, W. H. (2003). Evaluation and development of potentially better practices for improving family-centered care in neonatal intensive care units. *Pediatrics, 111*(4, Pt. 2), 437–449.

Schein, E. H. (1999). *The corporate culture survival guide: Sense and nonsense about culture change.* San Francisco: Jossey-Bass.

Schön, D. A. (1983). *The reflective practitioner: How professionals think in action.* New York: Basic Books.

Schön, D. A. (1990). *Educating the reflective practitioner: Toward a new design for teaching and learning in the professions.* San Francisco: Jossey-Bass.

Scott, W. R. (1981). *Organizations: Rational, natural and open systems.* Upper Saddle River, NJ: Prentice Hall.

Wasson, J. H., Godfrey, M. M., Nelson, E. C., Mohr, J. J., & Batalden, P. B. (2003). Microsystems in health care: Part 4. Planning patient-centered care. *Joint Commission Journal on Quality and Safety, 29*(5), 227–237.

Weick, K. E. (1995). *Sensemaking in organizations.* Thousand Oaks, CA: Sage.

Weick, K. E. (2001). *Making sense of the organization.* Malden, MA: Blackwell.

Wenger, E. (1999). *Communities of practice: Learning, meaning, and identity.* New York: Cambridge University Press.

Wolfe, D. M. (1980). Developing professional competence in the applied behavioral sciences. In E. Byrne & D. E. Wolfe (Eds.), *Developing experiential learning programs for professional education.* New Directions in Experiential Learning, No. 8. San Francisco: Jossey Bass.

CHAPTER THREE

LEADING MICROSYSTEMS

Paul B. Batalden, Eugene C. Nelson, Julie K. Johnson, Marjorie M. Godfrey, Thomas P. Huber, Linda Kosnik, Kerri Ashling

Chapter Summary

Background. Leading and leadership by formal and informal leaders goes on at all levels of microsystems—the essential building blocks of all health systems. Leading goes on between microsystems and at all levels of the systems in health care. This chapter on high-performing clinical microsystems is based on interviews and site visits to twenty clinical microsystems in North America. It describes how leaders contribute to the performance of those microsystems.

Analysis of interviews. Interviews of leaders and staff members offer a rich understanding of the three core processes of leading. First, *building knowledge* requires many behaviors of leaders and has many manifestations as leaders seek to build knowledge about the structure, processes, and patterns of work in their clinical microsystems. Second, *taking action* covers many different behaviors that involve making things happen, executing plans, and making good on intentions. It focuses action on the way people are hired and developed and involves the way the work gets done. Third, *reviewing* and *reflecting* provides insights into the ways the microsystem's patterns, processes, and structure enable the desired work to get done; into what *success* looks like; and into what will be next after that success is created.

Conclusion. This focus on the processes of leading is intended to enable more people to develop into leaders and more people to share the roles of leading.

Much is written about leading health care systems today, but little is written about leading health care at the level of the microsystems of care that work at the place where patients and careteams meet. Many times what is written about leading small health care systems leaves out the voices of those staffing the front lines of care delivery. Even less is heard about the perspectives of those engaged in the daily work of the best of the small systems. This chapter is about the active process of leading that we observed in our research on high-performing microsystems, the things these microsystems' leaders and staff told us about leading and leaders, and the ideas and practices we have come to think of as being helpful to the daily work of a clinical microsystem.

Leader, Leadership, Leading

It is tempting to think of *leading* as what a person—the leader—does. But what if you consider the three commonly used words *leader, leadership,* and *leading* as all arising from the same ancient root words *laitho* and *laithan,* meaning "way" or "journey" and "to travel" (Ayto, 1991; Barnhart, 2000)?

Leader is a word that we use to label a person who is guiding or leading. *Leadership* is a word that we use to describe the phenomenon of leading. *Leading* describes the active process. What we learned from the twenty high-performing clinical microsystems we studied is that they used all three words in describing their *journeying,* but it was the active process of leading that they described as being helpful to their work.

Leading and leadership by formal and informal leaders goes on at all levels of an organization. Leading goes on within microsystems and between them. It goes on between microsystems and other levels of the health care system. It goes on at the level of the larger organizations in which these smaller clinical units function.

The information in this chapter is based on our qualitative research (summarized in the box titled "Recap of Methods"). It focuses on the ways that leadership contributes to high performance across the twenty clinical microsystems studied.

Our research methods ultimately generated the results summarized in Tables 3.1, 3.2, and 3.3. These tables contain the actual comments made by microsystem leaders and staff about leading; some of the behaviors illustrated in their words are also noted in these tables (Denzin & Lincoln, 2000; Patton, 1990). The members of a clinical microsystem can be described as the small team of people who work together on a regular basis—or as needed—to provide care and the individuals who receive that care (who can also be recognized as members of a discrete subpopulation of patients). Herbert Simon, the Nobel economist, has noted that in the information age the resource in short supply is attention

(Kelly, 1998). Ronald Heifetz (1994) has proposed that the gift of attention is essential to the process of leading. Karl Weick (2002) has observed that systems cannot become more reliable or safer until the performance of the factors preventing failure is noticed. People then need to make sense of what has been noticed, and after making sense of what has been noticed, they need to be prepared to take action. Attending to and noticing prepares them for leading. But for this type of leading to be possible, some space must be created in a life of over-stimulation, a life that suffers from too much input. Schön (1983) invited all of us to become reflective practitioners and to constantly intermingle the practice of our profession with reflection on what is being done and what the antecedents and consequences of action are. What happens? Why does it happen? What results are intended, anticipated and desired? What outcomes are unintended, unanticipated, and undesired? Heifetz suggests that the good leader needs to be both "on the dance floor" in the middle of the action and "up in the balcony" seeing the larger pattern of what is happening and knowing when and how to intervene in a way that promotes progress on difficult problems (Parks, 2005).

Recap of Methods

The Dartmouth microsystem research project sponsored by the Robert Wood Johnson Foundation was conducted from June 2000 through June 2002. First, the research team used multiple search patterns to identify high-performing clinical microsystems in the United States and Canada. Second, the most promising sites were screened, using brief survey instruments and telephone interviews with key contacts at the sites. Third, the team selected twenty of the most exemplary sites from across the health care continuum for in-depth study. Fourth, the team conducted two-day site visits during which in-depth, semistructured individual interviews and group interviews were conducted with diverse staff representing the major work roles in each microsystem. In addition, the team observed care processes, interviewed some senior leaders in the microsystem's larger organization, and gathered clinical data via chart review and financial data from administrative sources. Fifth, to analyze the information collected, the team entered verbatim data transcribed from the staff interviews into a computer and used a software program to perform a content analysis on those data. The data were placed into affinity groups to identify themes that contributed to high performance and that appeared across the twenty microsystems. One of the affinity groups of verbatim comments was labeled leadership. Sixth, focusing on the leadership affinity group of verbatim comments, the team used induction to develop a framework for the data reflected in the verbatim comments and other aspects of the site visit. Seventh, the team classified the comments on leading into three categories: building knowledge, taking action, and reviewing and reflecting. (Refer to Chapter One for more information on research methods.)

Three Fundamental Processes of Leading: What Clinical Microsystem Team Members Observe and Report

Through observing and listening to leaders at work, three fundamental processes of leading can be recognized: (1) building knowledge, (2) taking action, and (3) reviewing and reflecting (Batalden & Splaine, 2002). As described in this chapter, employing helpful tools, such as those found in the second section and the Appendix of this book (and at http://www.clinicalmicrosystem.org), can increase a leader's knowledge of a microsystem in an organized fashion.

The comments of the individuals we interviewed reflect these three themes, and for convenience, we have grouped them by these themes in Tables 3.1, 3.2, and 3.3. These tables provide the actual words of the people who were interviewed in our microsystem study. They offer a rich understanding of the three core processes of leading.

Building Knowledge

Building knowledge occurred in many ways, required many behaviors, and had many manifestations as leaders acted on their curiosity to build knowledge about the structure, processes, and patterns of work in their clinical microsystems.

As Table 3.1 reveals, leading involves building knowledge of the basic structural characteristics of the microsystem: its organization and language, its physical arrangements and technology to promote flow of patient care, its intended—and its practiced—policy about patient care and about work, the constraints impeding daily good work, and the current skills and knowledge base of those who work in it.

Leading involves building knowledge of the processes of work, the sources of unwanted variation in those processes, and the methods associated with better practice performance, including ways of measuring and monitoring processes (as covered in Chapter Nine). Leading includes building knowledge of the patterns, habits, and traditions that support learning and creativity and that help everyone focus on the patient. Leadership helps people notice the work processes and patterns of interactions and relationships that need to be changed. Leadership involves inviting *questions* by creating opportunities for asking staff questions and by learning from their responses (Revans, 1966, pp. 91–99).

Taking Action

Taking action covers many different behaviors—making things happen, executing plans, and making good on intentions. It focuses action on the way people are hired and developed, involves the way work gets done, and fosters accountability.

TABLE 3.1. BUILDING KNOWLEDGE IN CLINICAL MICROSYSTEMS: VIEWS ON LEADING QUOTED FROM OUR INTERVIEWS.

Observation and Comments	Behaviors Illustrated
"In 1994, the facility had a pressure ulcer rate of 33% among its residents. They hired . . . a very dedicated nurse to start a wound care team. In 1995 the team really took off when Dr. _____ joined and began to go to the nursing home and round weekly on the patients with wounds. By observing the patients in their natural environment he was able to recognize factors that contributed to wounds, such as nutrition, positioning and bedding. As the floor nurses realized that he would be around reliably and [Nurse] _____ would pursue the treatment orders throughout the week, they became more interested in wound care. Dr. _____ took the opportunity to educate them about different types of wounds and treatments in a nonaccusatory manner. He took the heat off the nurses by talking to the patients and families about the wounds himself. As the question changed from 'What did I do wrong?' to 'What is going on with this patient?' all the staff became more proactive in looking for and treating wounds early. Wound recognition and treatment decisions improved as the team learned and worked together. [Nurse] _____ took the lead in creating protocols for wound assessment and treatment. Together, Dr. _____ and [Nurse] _____ brought the pressure ulcer rate down to less than 2%, where they have kept it since 1996." *—Director*	• Observe actual context of work. • Have a predictable presence. • Be interested in follow-up. • Lead learning as needed. • Focus on *what*, not *who*. • Encourage proactive thinking.
"The _____ Center brought together twenty different disciplines to care for patients with . . . disorders. One of the challenges facing . . . the medical director was that the neurosurgeon, the chiropractor, the physical therapist, the nurse, the physiatrist, the orthopedic surgeon, the family practitioner, the internist, the psychologist, and others each had their own language for discussing . . . care. How could they all understand each other to collaborate in the care of their mutual patients?" *—Medical director*	• Foster a common language for the common work.
"If the health center finds that a needed service is not provided in the community, their practice is to find the funding and develop the capacity to provide it themselves." *—Staff member*	• Determine the need for new services, based on community availability.
"At _____ they are asked to collect data that demonstrates the problem and pinpoints where the flaw is. As [the] nurse practitioner in . . . clinic explains, 'If we want change, we track our data. So when I looked at 20 people and found out it was taking me 45 seconds to	• Use data to characterize problems, foster change.

(continued)

TABLE 3.1. BUILDING KNOWLEDGE IN CLINICAL MICROSYSTEMS: VIEWS ON LEADING QUOTED FROM OUR INTERVIEWS. (*Continued*)

Observation and Comments	Behaviors Illustrated
open and close a normal mammogram report, this is not a good use of my time. So then I had the data and I got [a faster] computer. So you can't just whine.'" *—Staff nurse*	
"[The medical director] does a 'state of the office' presentation each year for his employees, in which he shares the financial details of the practice, including his own salary, as well as his goals for himself and the practice for the upcoming year. And it's all shared. We all know that. It's not just like the managers and the supervisors know that and we know there is something going on, but we don't know what it is." *—Staff nurse*	• Create widespread information about operational performance.
"I get more questions where they want me to do research to come up with the latest data. . . . [They] utilize that information and seek information in a way that's different than perhaps what we're accustomed to in other areas." *—Pharmacist*	• Seek information from every helpful source.
"This is the first place that I've ever worked where I could come to work and use my imagination in coming up with how to do something. Other places that I've worked, you have ideas, but . . . there's no point to bring it up because nobody's going to listen. And so it's exciting even though you think of primary care as being the same old thing, it really is not the same old thing at _____." *—Staff member*	• Encourage use of imagination and ideas by listening to them and using them.
"The unit leaders kicked off their patient safety project by presenting their systems-focused philosophy toward medical errors to their entire staff. Next, they streamlined the process for reporting errors and established a categorization system. Lastly, they set a contest to motivate their staff—whoever reports the most errors over the coming year gets two free dinners at the nicest restaurant in [the city], paid for by the unit medical director. Thus far, error reporting has increased dramatically and they are getting much better data." *—Director*	• Share your own theories, assumptions. • Make it easy to do the right thing. • Recognize the desired behaviors.
"I would say empowerment is really important. It starts with [the medical director]; he feels that you can do anything you want to do. He has certainly helped me in that respect. He has a way in instilling self-confidence. He has enabled me and empowered me to be able to do what I wanted to learn how to do and to do it well." *—Staff member*	• Instill confidence.

TABLE 3.1. (*Continued*)

Observation and Comments	Behaviors Illustrated
"[The leader] has to have a passion for whatever that program is going to be. Um. But you also have to be able to push all of your information down." *—Staff member*	• Have a *passion* for the future. • Move information everywhere.
"It is not telling someone to do, but [it] is showing what is right to do." *—Nurse director*	• *Show,* don't *tell.*
"I speak the language of the people I work with and the different languages of the people I work with. I answer the telephone at the . . . center sometimes, at the reception desk, to understand what the patients are asking. I will try to do a job that is not ever my job to understand the system and when I do that it provides me the incredible ability to communicate with all parts of the system." *—Medical director*	• Directly experience the work of others in order to better understand the systems.
. . ."[Here] the issues are dealt with." *—Staff member*	• Build knowledge of how issues are *dealt with.*
"The group gets to [have] discussions on where we're going to go in the future." *—Staff member*	• Encourage conversations about the future.
"If your primary language is English, and you were born in this country, that is a stumbling block. It was for me, certainly, in the beginning. But I worked on that . . . over time. And actually, it adds richness to the team. That's how I see it now. Things get reduced to nouns and adjectives and not a whole lot of other verbiage." *—Director*	• Work on a common language.
"Meeting as a microsystem can have a great efficiency if you have one day that you just meet massively and we do. So when people call with complaints, compliments, concerns, whatever, we give them times inside this microsystem management day and we literally have people from [everywhere; it seems like] the whole world comes to us during that day." *—Medical director*	• Create predictable *space* for communication in the midst of busyness.
"I started the breakfast club where people came in to eat if they wanted to from 7:30–9:00 unpaid; we start here around 9 for pay. Since folks were not getting paid they figure it would be OK to voice their opinions. The way we started was simply to sit down together and invite whomever wanted to come and have a relaxed breakfast, sometimes we talked about issues, other times we talked about personal family stuff. There was no agenda, no leader, everyone came into the room as	• Find ways to learn informally, even from personal and family issues.

(*continued*)

TABLE 3.1. BUILDING KNOWLEDGE IN CLINICAL MICROSYSTEMS: VIEWS ON LEADING QUOTED FROM OUR INTERVIEWS. (*Continued*)

Observation and Comments	Behaviors Illustrated
equals until 9:00 A.M. when once again I was the boss and they were employees." —*Director*	
"I'm just an aide. They don't care. I don't know anything. They don't care. All I know how to do is clean poop or wipe the floor up, and in shock trauma the nurses will teach you anything you want to know. Anything you ask them, if they're not—things aren't coming out of their ears, or something. . . . You can learn anything." —*Aide*	• Foster inquiry—by everyone.

As a review of Table 3.2 reveals, leading means taking action on the structure to create and modify formal reporting relationships, to have clearly identified *go to* people for the multitude of different microsystem processes, and to change the physical arrangements for work when they stand in the way of an optimal work flow. It means championing the integration of information technology into the care processes. It means hiring people who share the values of the clinical microsystem and bringing the right people together. It means noticing what needs to be done and having the courage to initiate action while also inviting others to join in the detailed specification of work processes.

Leading by taking action means having specific processes for making things happen. It involves having careful, authentic respect for all the people who staff the clinical microsystem. It means being vigilant about ways that the current processes might fail or are failing. It usually involves active engagement of the leader in the daily workings of the microsystem and in the actions to be taken. It means involving the patients and families as full members in the care that the microsystem creates and gives. It means using process knowledge to cross-train members of the microsystem in order to increase the system's process capabilities.

Leading involves taking action on the patterns of work in order to promote the cooperative functioning of all microsystem members and to recognize their interdependence. It means caring for one another. It means celebrating in the midst of the work. It involves fostering trust and respect in caring for patients. It involves the daily practice of respect and trust among microsystem members. It means paying attention to the ways that differences and conflicts are addressed.

TABLE 3.2. TAKING ACTION IN CLINICAL MICROSYSTEMS: VIEWS ON LEADING QUOTED FROM OUR INTERVIEWS.

Observations and Comments	Behaviors Illustrated
"If you have a group of people and you know there has to be a change, you *have* to change. I mean, you can't just wait for it to run into the ground." —*Director*	• Take timely action.
"I think the first step [for our management team] was the three of them realizing that they were a team, that each one in one area wasn't totally responsible for the entire unit, that all three represent nursing, medicine, with a team approach, and I think they've instilled in all the rest of us that you don't ever say something can't be done without looking at it, assessing it, proposing a change, implementing it, and then evaluating it." —*Clinician*	• Act together to encourage ideas and suggestions.
"When hiring new employees, the leadership team at the _____ Center looks for individuals whose values closely match the mission and values of the clinic." —*Staff member*	• Hire for shared values.
"Patients become more compliant when [this doctor] gives them a copy of their office visit record and relevant self-management flow sheets, thus empowering them to better understand and manage their health issues." —*Nurse*	• Share information in a format that connects to taking action.
"The cross-training is facilitated by extensive process flow-charting, which clearly defines the work to be done. With the work clearly defined, competency-based training protocols can more easily be created." —*Staff nurse*	• Foster process literacy as an adjunct to clarity of work definition.
"[Here] the issues are dealt with.". . . —*Staff member*	• Take action on *issues* of concern.
"_____ RN, the practice manager at . . . , uses 'I statements' to build trust and deal with conflict among her staff." —*Observer*	• Deal openly and directly with conflicting points of view.
"[Our leaders] don't feel like they're up here and you're down there. And as long as you come with the attitude of wanting to do something positive, they'll stand with you on that. I don't have any master's degree or anything. These people have master's degrees and they don't act like they have to stand out because they have them. They just treat you right. . . . They meet you where you're at. And then they help you to grow." —*Staff member*	• Accept coworkers as colleagues, and promote their individual development.

(continued)

TABLE 3.2. TAKING ACTION IN CLINICAL MICROSYSTEMS: VIEWS ON LEADING QUOTED FROM OUR INTERVIEWS. (*Continued*)

Observations and Comments	Behaviors Illustrated
"The leader has to have credibility. And credibility, I learned, is different than competence. You can be a very competent physician and still not have credibility. Credibility has to do with supporting others, walking the talk, doing what you say you're going to do, being reliable, and being accountable; all of those things are very important in leadership. Being the person that the front line respects and knows that they can turn to. Once you have that relationship then the ability to involve the front line in the process and teach them how to do it rather than doing it for them, I think, is very important." —*Medical director*	• Support others. • Minimize the gap between what you say and what you do. • Follow through, connecting your voice and your actions. • Take the actions you say you are going to take—predictably. • Recognize the others who depend on you. • Maintain the respect of others by the actions you take.
"I find one of the most incredible things is how empowered we feel as employees to make various decisions. Combined with all the computer programs that we are using, when a patient calls, we can right then and there know whether to get them in, to get a medication into them, to tell them to take some hot chicken soup, or to go to the ER." —*Staff member*	• Enable others to act. • Provide the technology needed to do a good job.
"One of the goals for the corporation, that I talked about last night a little bit, was their desire to liberate the potential of people. I love that. I mean that I think that is one of the best phrases or slogans, or whatever you want to call it. . . . Liberate the potential of the people is an awesome concept. And what that says to me—there is so much potential out there that the quiet employee is as valuable as the extrovert. And if you tap into people and find out what drives them and what moves them, there are a lot of opportunities." —*Staff member*	• Recognize the potential of people, and take steps to enable it.
"We have an administrator who is terrific. . . . I wouldn't describe him as religious, but I would describe him as a human being who has such a tremendous value system that it guides his life." —*Staff member*	• Demonstrate your values.
". . . The eight values that are on the wall . . . they are not just on the wall, they are what we do." —*Staff member*	• Make daily work and values congruous.
"[The key is] people who are cognizant of the philosophy of how the process is running." —*Nurse director*	• Build process knowledge, including the underlying rationale for the process.

TABLE 3.2. (*Continued*)

Observation and Comments	Behaviors Illustrated
"We're all treated as valued employees and not just an employee." —*Staff member*	• Treat people so they feel respected.
"[R]espect and . . . trust [are] critical. . . . And you know that is something that is earned all the time." —*Medical director*	• Work to earn respect and trust.
"You always have to have someone to go to." —*Staff member*	• Be reliably available and accessible.
"[The patient] was so glad she got to die of a terminal illness and be in hospice because she had waited all of her life to feel loved and accepted and to be treated with dignity and respect, and she finally got it those last few months before she died because she was [under our care], and she . . . got what she had wanted all of her life." —*Staff member*	• Foster an environment of respect and love for patients.
"And if it's not working from my perspective, I'm going to get back to them, say, 'You know, it's not working. We need to fix it.' But I'm not going to come up with the solution. I'm not going to come up with the details of, you know, fixing it. I'm going to let them decide. I'll tell what the problem is and then [they can] work [it] out." —*Director*	• Tell the truth about what isn't working well. • Offer *room* for others to solve the problem.
"We start from the assumption that everyone is working as hard as they can; we want to try to help people work differently." —*Medical director*	• Help people work better by helping them work differently.
"Clear-cut protocols remove emotion [and let] us get to the facts, [let] us work on the real issues." —*Nurse director*	• Recognize the part of the work that is factual and objective.
"At this job, people take care of one another and the same spirit that takes care [of] them [serves] our clients. We don't, sort of, switch gears and not take care of one another. There's just a lot of care here. And it feels very much like a family. People are very interested. We celebrate everything." —*Staff member*	• Care for one another. • Demonstrate your interest in others. • Celebrate whatever you can.
"Being able to realize that you cannot provide care—you cannot care adequately for this person in front of you without the help of ten other people. And that is the realization that most physicians don't come with." —*Director*	• Recognize your interdependence.

(continued)

TABLE 3.2. TAKING ACTION IN CLINICAL MICROSYSTEMS: VIEWS ON LEADING QUOTED FROM OUR INTERVIEWS. (*Continued*)

Observations and Comments	Behaviors Illustrated
"I would never ask someone to do something I would not do myself." —*Nurse director*	• Lead by example.
"I wouldn't ask the staff to do something I could not do." —*Director*	• Ask others to do only what you would do yourself.
"[The director] never says this is how we are going to do it; instead it's, 'Here is what we have to do; how can we do it?'" —*Staff member*	• Be clear about *what* needs to be done, inviting people to contribute to *how* it might be done.
". . . taking a short-sleeve attitude." . . . —*Director, about his role*	• Recognize the need to be in the middle of the action.
". . . [realizing that] leadership was not usually one person." —*Director*	• Be aware of the others needed for leadership of the work.

It means making the values of the microsystem *come alive* in the daily work. It means liberating the potential in each member of the microsystem.

Reviewing and Reflecting: A View from the Balcony

When we pause to step out of the action and to get up on the balcony to look down on the action, what do we see? Analysis of the comments presented in Table 3.3 suggests that reviewing and reflecting in leading means creating a structure for reflection. This structure begins with having an image of what the clinical microsystem is trying to become. This vision provides insight into how the system's patterns, processes, and structure will enable the desired work to get done, what success will look like, and what will be next after that success is created. It means creating time—and geographical space—in which people can gather to have meaningful conversations about their work. Part of the structure of review and reflection is the leaders' awareness of the temporal limits on members' participation in the work of the microsystem, and their anticipation of the time when the current leaders' turns will be over (DeGeus, 1997).

Leading by reviewing and reflecting means having a process for honestly asking, "Is the work getting done?" and, "Is there a good match between the needs

TABLE 3.3. REVIEWING AND REFLECTING IN CLINICAL MICROSYSTEMS: VIEWS ON LEADING QUOTED FROM OUR INTERVIEWS.

Observations and Comments	Behaviors Illustrated
"They found that they needed to redefine success, particularly by extinguishing the prevalent desire to return to 'the good old days.' They continually exposed the staff to the real facts about the old system—marginal financial success, patient and staff dissatisfaction, and poor access—through data displays and frequent discussions." —*Staff member*	• Create definitions of *success* that serve the present and future best. • Ground interpretations of past and present in data and conversations grounded in the actual reality you face.
"He wants to put his microsystem into a position where they can't go back—by focusing on whole system redesign." —*Staff member*	• Foster an understanding of the imperative of leaving the past behind.
". . . [Dr.] _____ has developed . . . a monthly team meeting [. . . at which his department communicates with both the internal and external environment]. . . . This is a free-ranging half day when patients, representatives of other departments, even architects may be invited into the _____ Department microsystem to discuss and work on major new issues and to catch up on the latest news and data." —*Staff member*	• Create regular time for communication and conversation about the work. • Invite the *outside* connections of the microsystem to honor the time. • Let the reflective process serve the needs of the people involved.
"I think it goes back to that first meeting of how are we going to put the . . . center together when we drew the circle in the center: it was the patient, it wasn't the physician. And that has been a philosophy, that's been the vision, and that is how the leadership has taken us over time." —*Staff physician*	• Center the review on those served.
"We want to be the best neighborhood, where people want to come and visit, where people know when they come to this neighborhood, this microsystem, they are going to get a group of people who are highly qualified [and] have an interest in working together across disciplines to the benefit of a given patient's needs." —*Medical director*	• Recognize your microsystem as a *place* experienced by others. • Be mindful of the *signature* of your microsystem.
"Success is . . . seeing people happy and enjoying coming to work everyday." —*Director*	• Explore the relation between joy and success.
"I am here for a short time [life is short]." —*Medical director*	• Be explicit about the contributions that people can make to work that goes on beyond them.

(continued)

TABLE 3.3. REVIEWING AND REFLECTING IN CLINICAL MICROSYSTEMS: VIEWS ON LEADING QUOTED FROM OUR INTERVIEWS. (*Continued*)

Observations and Comments	Behaviors Illustrated
"I can continue to inspire and support and to lead, and lead not just from the top but lead from in the midst." —*Director*	• Review the positioning of leaders and followers.
"[It matters] that [the employees] know who they are and they know the mission that they're on and what they have to do. As well, I know who I am and what I have to do to help do my part. . . . And we all just come together . . . [and it] is beautiful." —*Director*	• Revisit the mission and the relation of the mission to what each person does. • Encourage reflection on the connection between individual's identity and the work itself. • Appreciate the aesthetics of interdependent work.
"They allow people to do things informally or formally to enhance professional development." —*Staff member*	• Focus on the enhancement of people as professionals—in both formal and informal ways.
"It's not about nursing care; it's not about medical care; it's really about patient care." —*Nurse director*	• Be mindful of the professional and disciplinary focus that can compete with attention to the patient.
"The group is very much on the edge of technology." —*Staff member*	• Explore the ways technology can help (and hinder) the work.
"[It is important to recognize] the changes in the environment that changed the leadership that was needed." —*Staff member*	• Regularly scan for the reality of the environment, and explore its implications for leading the work.
"[She helps us in] . . . remembering who we serve." —*Staff member*	• Help visualize, understand, and remember those served by the microsystem,—in the daily conversations about the work.
"[As a leader] . . . you have to visualize what happens after you succeed." —*Operations director*	• Be clear about what *next* will look like.
"We're changing ourselves; you know . . . it's a change from within." —*Staff member*	• Recognize change in your midst; certify it as the help it is.

TABLE 3.3. (Continued)

Observations and Comments	Behaviors Illustrated
"It's very important [for me] to hold the vision, be able to articulate it, to hold it, persevere and [have it] become part of how I worked as an individual. . . . The success is being able to hold that vision even when you are challenged." —Director	• Continually review the vision informing the direction of the work. • Explore the threats that erode a focus on the vision. • Have conversations about the competing commitments that *crowd* the vision.
"[We have to ask ourselves honestly] Is the work getting done?" —Staff member	• Create a safe, open place where truthful conversations about the facts of performance can occur.

of the patients (and other beneficiaries) and our work outputs?" It means that people are regularly invited to assess the degree to which their own professional growth and development is addressed. Exploring and noticing the predicted and unforeseen effects of change are additional parts of leaders' reflection on the work of the microsystem.

A final aspect of leading is reflecting on the patterns in practice and the assumptions driving them. This involves analyzing the ways in which the care and work processes connect to the structures of the microsystem. It calls for exploring the relationship of changes envisioned (or already made) in the microsystem's patterns, structures, and processes. It invites attention to the critical leadership task of framing and reframing the work (Bolman & Deal, 1991; Morgan, 1988).

Discussion

Approaches to the study of leaders have often focused on behaviors, traits, or styles (Blake & Mouton, 1985; Stogdill, 1948, 1974). Other approaches have explored situational and contingent leadership responses (which focus on linking the style and content of leadership to the situation facing the leader), *team* leadership, and a variety of other concepts (Fiedler, 1993; Graeff, 1997; Hackman, 2002, 1990; Northouse, 2001). Although helpful, these approaches have often made the daily actions of leading hard to recognize and even harder to improve. By focusing on the processes of leading, we believe we can complement these traditional approaches and offer a model that encourages change and improvement.

Leading and Being

It has been said that "leading is a state of being" (Helgeson, 1995). Our analysis underscores the wisdom of this point of view. In the high-performing microsystems we studied, the acts of leading were strongly associated with *being*, in the forms of building knowledge, taking action, and reviewing and reflecting. This linkage invites attending to the integrity and authenticity of the actions of the person who is the leader (Palmer, 2000). Leading and being was a consistent and continuous process among the set of leaders we studied, and was recognized by both the leaders and the led.

Leading Macrosystems to Foster Strong Microsystems

Outstanding leaders of the large systems in which clinical microsystems are embedded, those who pay attention to the *local* leadership within discrete microsystems, can enhance the functioning of these microsystems. The way they select the microsystem leaders and help them develop contributes enormously to the total organization's well-being. Leaders of this quality were not always present in the large organizations that hosted the microsystems that were the subject of this research. Some of the microsystems we observed perceived themselves as "islands" in the larger oceans of their macroorganizations. If it is true that the performance of the larger system can be no better than the performance of the smaller systems of which it is composed, then it is essential to have strong and effective leadership distributed throughout the entire macroorganization. In many health systems this fact is commonly known but not often acted upon.

It is noteworthy that in virtually all twenty of the microsystems studied, we found not a single leader but two or three coleaders who formed a powerful guiding force for their unit. This grouping often took the form of a physician leader and a nursing leader or an administrative leader, or both the nursing and the administrative leaders. These partnerships—often functioning like jazz ensembles—rounded out the work of leading these small clinical units.

Conclusion

Max De Pree has suggested that leadership is a matter of linking the leader's voice with the leader's touch (De Pree, 1992). Members of clinical microsystems have helped us understand what this means in their settings. In this chapter we have attempted to provide a framework for understanding the process of leading by emphasizing three fundamental processes of successful leadership—building knowledge, taking action, and reviewing and reflecting.

We have considered the leading of clinical microsystems primarily as a matter of process, but in doing so we do not wish to diminish the importance of leaders' personal attributes, such as energy, creativity, caring, and persistence (Deming, 1994; Greenleaf, 1977; Senge, 1990; Vaill, 1996). Nor do we intend to diminish the importance of leaders' personal and professional development as they strive to unify their heads, hands, and hearts in the daily work of attempting to care for patients and meet the needs of patients (Batalden & Leach, 2005). Nor do we mean to downplay in any way the obsession that superior leaders must have to identify and meet the current requirements of the current situation (Maslow, Stephens, & Heil, 1998). Rather, our focus on the processes of leading aims to enable more people to develop into leaders, more people to work on improving the processes of leading, and more people to share the roles of leading.

As you think about the process of leading in your own clinical microsystem, consider the knowledge you need to build, the actions you need to take, and the things you need to review and reflect on.

References

Ayto, J. (1991). *Dictionary of word origins* (1st U.S. ed.). New York: Arcade.

Barnhart, R. (2000). *Dictionary of etymology.* New York: Chambers.

Batalden, P., & Leach, D. C. (2005). The inner and outer life in medicine. In S. M. Intrator (Ed.), *Living the questions: Essays inspired by the work and life of Parker J. Palmer* (pp. 210–217). San Francisco: Jossey-Bass.

Batalden, P., & Splaine, M. (2002). What will it take to lead the continual improvement and innovation of health care in the 21st century? *Quality Management in Health Care, 11*(1), 45–54.

Blake, R. R., & Mouton, J. S. (1985). *The managerial grid III.* Houston, TX: Gulf.

Bolman, L. G., & Deal, T. E. (1991). *Reframing organizations: Artistry, choice, and leadership.* San Francisco: Jossey-Bass.

De Pree, M. (1992). *Leadership jazz.* New York: Doubleday, Currency.

DeGeus, A. (1997). *The living company.* Boston: Harvard Business School Press.

Deming, W. E. (1994). *The new economics for industry, government, education* (2nd ed.). Cambridge, MA: MIT Center for Advanced Engineering Study.

Denzin, N. K., & Lincoln, Y. S. (2000). *Handbook of qualitative research* (2nd ed.). Thousand Oaks, CA: Sage.

Fiedler, F. E. (1993). The leadership situation and the black box in contingency theories. In M. M. Chemers & R. Ayman (Eds.), *Leadership theory and research: Perspectives and directions* (pp. 1–28). New York: Academic Press.

Graeff, C. L. (1997). Evolution of situational leadership theory: A critical review. *Leadership Quarterly, 8,* 153–170.

Greenleaf, R. K. (1977). *Servant leadership: A journey into the nature of legitimate power and greatness.* New York: Paulist Press.

Hackman, J. R. (Ed.). (1990). *Groups that work (and those that don't): Creating conditions for effective teamwork.* San Francisco: Jossey-Bass.

Hackman, J. R. (2002). *Leading teams: Setting the stage for great performances.* Boston: Harvard Business School Press.

Heifetz, R. A. (1994). *Leadership without easy answers.* Cambridge, MA: Harvard University Press, Belknap Press.

Helgeson, S. (1995). *The female advantage: Women's ways of leadership.* New York: Doubleday, Currency.

Kelly, K. (1998). *New rules for the new economy: 10 radical strategies for a connected world.* New York: Viking.

Maslow, A. H., Stephens, D. C., & Heil, G. (1998). *Maslow on management.* Hoboken, NJ: Wiley.

Morgan, G. (1988). *Riding the waves of change: Developing managerial competencies for a turbulent world.* San Francisco: Jossey-Bass.

Northouse, P. (2001). *Leadership: Theory and practice* (2nd ed.). Thousand Oaks, CA: Sage.

Palmer, P. J. (2000). *Let your life speak: Listening for the voice of vocation.* San Francisco: Jossey-Bass.

Parks, D. S. (2005). *Leadership can be taught. A bold approach for a complex world.* Boston: Harvard Business School Press.

Patton, M. (1990). *Qualitative evaluation and research methods* (2nd ed.). Thousand Oaks, CA: Sage.

Revans, R. W. (1966). *Standards for morale: Cause and effect in hospitals.* London: Oxford University Press for the Nuffield Provincial Hospital Trust.

Schön, D. A. (1983). *The reflective practitioner: How professionals think in action.* New York: Basic Books.

Senge, P. M. (1990). *The fifth discipline: The art and practice of the learning organization.* New York: Doubleday.

Stogdill, R. M. (1948). Personal factors associated with leadership: A survey of the literature. *Journal of Psychology, 25*, 35–71.

Stogdill, R. M. (1974). *Handbook of leadership: A survey of theory and research.* New York: Free Press.

Vaill, P. B. (1996). *Learning as a way of being: Strategies for survival in a world of permanent white water.* San Francisco: Jossey-Bass.

Weick, K. E. (2002). The reduction of medical errors through mindful interdependence. In M. M. Rosenthal & K. M. Sutcliffe (Eds.), *Medical errors: What do we know? What do we do?* (pp. 177–199). San Francisco: Jossey-Bass.

CHAPTER FOUR

LEADING MACROSYSTEMS AND MESOSYSTEMS FOR MICROSYSTEM PEAK PERFORMANCE

Paul B. Batalden, Eugene C. Nelson, Paul B. Gardent, Marjorie M. Godfrey

Chapter Summary

Background. Building the capability to improve an entire health system requires intelligent leadership that is aligned with all levels of that system. This chapter provides ways to think about the system at different levels and describes the need for positive interrelationships that span these different levels, introduces alternative leadership frameworks, and offers suggestions on what senior leaders can do to create the conditions for peak performance throughout their entire organization.

Case study. A case study of a hospital CEO who is faced with a serious quality and revenue problem that threatens his hospital's survival is used to provide context for the leadership discussion that follows.

Review of leadership frameworks and complementary lenses. Seven different popular and powerful leadership frameworks are introduced to show that much is known about leadership and that a lot of helpful information is available to help leaders understand what their job is and what they might do to succeed as leaders. In addition, leaders can use many different lenses, or discipline-based perspectives, to increase their understanding of microsystems. Understanding that a specific thing can be viewed through multiple lenses and that each lens will reveal different characteristics of that specific thing helps leaders be more agile and better able to see the complexity of their own work in leading systems.

Suggestions for action. The last section of this chapter gives senior leaders some specific advice on what they can do to create the conditions that can catalyze high performance throughout their entire organization. These recommendations are based on observations of what works and what fails in the real world as well as on a synthesis of our understanding of the job of the senior leader in today's challenging and competitive health care environment.

Health care leaders must nurture their organization's capability to continuously improve the quality, reliability, and value of care. Leaders do so by engaging and energizing all the people striving toward the fundamental goal of providing high-quality services that meet patients' health needs. They need new ways of thinking, learning, and working to meet the three formidable challenges of today and tomorrow:

- Provide safe, timely, effective, equitable, efficient, and patient-centered care (Institute of Medicine, 2001).
- Attract and retain talented professionals and staff.
- Thrive in a new payment environment that rewards the higher-quality, lower-cost providers.

This chapter begins with a brief case study to frame the issues and a panoramic view of the challenges confronting today's health system leaders. We then review some relevant leadership frameworks and point out some unique features of the health care system structure that make it difficult for health care leaders to easily adopt these frameworks. Next we introduce some additional ways for health care leaders to learn and to gain a deep understanding of microsystems. We discuss what health care leaders can do to create the conditions for success, to execute strategic plans, and to create operational excellence at the front lines of care and throughout the organization. We conclude with a summary of take-home points and the real challenge for health care leaders—to adapt these ideas and approaches to the realities of their personal style and unique circumstances for the purpose of attaining peak reliable performance throughout the entire organization.

Case Study: A True Story, with Names Changed to Protect the Innocent

The following case is, in essence, true. It happened in the summer of 2004. The names and facts have been altered slightly to make it apply more closely to the conditions faced by many senior leaders of hospitals and health systems in the United States.

Jack Candoo, CEO of County Memorial Hospital and Health System (CMHHS), returned from his summer vacation and received some very bad news from his chief financial officer (CFO). While Candoo had been enjoying a much-needed beach holiday with his family, CMHHS had been informed by its largest purchaser that it was now classified as a Tier 2, rather than a Tier 1, health system and that reimbursement levels would be cut to reflect CMHHS's "suboptimal performance."

Initially, Candoo felt that the decision had come out of the blue and that the data were wrong. On further reflection, however, he roughly confirmed that the data were right. He started to think that this Tier 2 placement by one purchaser posed a much greater problem for the long-term future of CMHHS than it did for the next fiscal year. His reasoning behind this conclusion developed into the following internal monologue:

1. Looking at the data from the core measures from the Joint Commission on Accreditation of Healthcare Organizations (JCAHO)—and being honest about them—I realize that some of our numbers are excellent, some are average, and some are, frankly, shameful.
2. Patient satisfaction scores reflect a successful service excellence campaign—we now consistently rank above the 80th percentile, way up from the 45th percentile attained three years ago—but improving satisfaction has done nothing to improve clinical quality, costs per discharge, or costs per visit.
3. There is an aggravating and large gap—the Institute of Medicine (IOM) has even called it a *chasm*—between CMHHS's mission, vision, and rhetoric and its actual, honest-to-goodness, measured performance.
4. The performance gap is not just embarrassing and aggravating but has financial implications as well. The public can now view this gap because both the Joint Commission and the Centers for Medicare & Medicaid Services (CMS) publish our results, along with the results for every other health system in the United States, in the name of transparency. Our purchasers, who are getting serious about pay-for-performance and value-based purchasing programs, also use those results.
5. Today's gap could cause us huge problems tomorrow, given the ever-increasing number of gold-standard quality measures being published by the National Quality Forum (NQF)—hundreds of very specific quality measures are currently in development—and the reality that CMS leading the charge for all the pay-for-performance schemes. Unless things change for the better and for real at CMHHS, I could be out of a job, CMHHS's bond rating could plummet, and the survival of the whole organization that we have worked so hard to build up during the past decade could be mortally threatened.

Candoo thought that his reflections on current reality and future trends were fundamentally correct and deeply disturbing. He began to think that what he needed was a whole new way of thinking, acting, and leading. He knew from past experience that CMHHS could run a quality improvement project on this or that condition or item. Recently, it had been successful in improving Emergency Department (ED) and inpatient satisfaction, decreasing length of stay, and improving clinical quality for pneumonia and heart failure patients.

But his general observation was that CMHHS's work to improve quality and cut costs had been based on carrying out *projects*. These projects often succeeded in the short run but sometimes failed to hold the gains in the long run—and never did spread to other clinical processes or give rise to new, collateral improvements in other areas that also needed work. There just didn't seem to be fundamental improvement in the organization's capability to continually improve and adapt. He concluded that he needed a new and fresh way of leading his organization if it was to improve in all the ways that the future demanded. But he was wary of the management fads that he had seen come and go—continuous quality improvement, then total quality management, then reengineering, then Six Sigma, now lean thinking, and who knew what idea would be next.

Candoo felt that he needed not a new management craze but a durable and practical approach that (1) fit the special realities of health care, (2) was based on observations of what actually works, and (3) fit the health care system of the future. It was at this point in time that Candoo started to think more seriously about some conversations he had had with some friends at Dartmouth, a few articles he had read, and an intriguing book by a Dartmouth professor, James Brian Quinn, titled *Intelligent Enterprise* (Quinn, 1992). Candoo started to feel a bit less glum and began to think that maybe he could blaze a new path forward toward peak performance that would take his organization where it needed to go in executing strategic imperatives to meet staff needs and to exceed patient expectations.

Framing the Challenge

The situation facing Jack Candoo and CMHHS is not unique. In fact it is quite common today and will likely become the dominant reality tomorrow. The nation's health system is undergoing major changes. We seem to be entering an era that will be characterized by three new features:

- A new payment method: value-based, or pay-for-performance, purchasing
- A new paradigm: patient-centered care
- A new information environment: one that provides high-exposure, transparent outcomes data on quality and cost

FIGURE 4.1. A VIEW OF THE MULTILAYERED HEALTH SYSTEM.

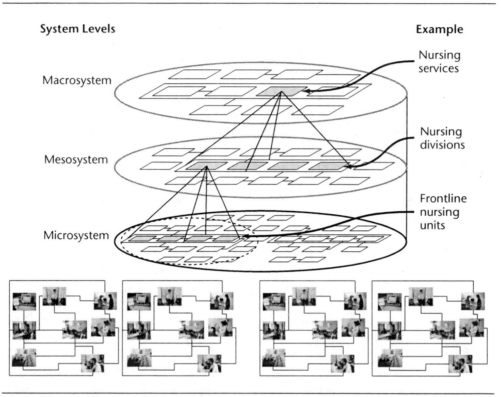

System Levels

Example

Nursing services

Macrosystem

Nursing divisions

Mesosystem

Frontline nursing units

Microsystem

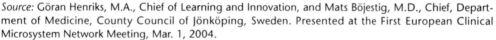

Source: Göran Henriks, M.A., Chief of Learning and Innovation, and Mats Böjestig, M.D., Chief, Department of Medicine, County Council of Jönköping, Sweden. Presented at the First European Clinical Microsystem Network Meeting, Mar. 1, 2004.

This new era will demand new, adaptive responses from health care; organizations will need to change and evolve, or they will fail. Peter Drucker, who was a leader in modern management thinking, once said about the need for change, "Every organization has to prepare for the abandonment of everything it does" (Gibson & Bennis, 1997).

Figure 4.1, which is based on work done in Jönköping, Sweden, and at Dartmouth-Hitchcock Medical Center in northern New England, provides a glimpse of the complicated, multilayered, and multifaceted job of senior, midlevel, and frontline leaders in health care. The figure represents the three levels in a typical integrated delivery system and gives an example of the linkages between levels.

1. The highest level, which can be referred to as the *macrosystem*, represents the whole of the organization and is led by senior leaders such as the CEO, chief

operations officer (COO), chief financial officer (CFO), chief medical officer (CMO), chief nursing officer (CNO), and chief information officer (CIO) and is guided by a board of trustees.

2. The second level, which may be termed the *mesosystem,* represents major divisions of the health organization, such as the department of medicine, the department of nursing, and information services as well as clinical service programs such as the oncology, cardiovascular, or women's health programs.

3. The third level, populated by what we call *clinical microsystems,* represents the frontline places where patients and families and careteams meet. They are the small functional units in which staff actually provide clinical care.

In this model the highest level of the delivery system, sometimes called the *blunt end,* contrasts with the lowest level, called the *sharp end* because it is the point where the patient directly contacts the system. The view shown in Figure 4.1 reflects a system of delivery that is exceedingly complex, which makes clear the need for a fresh approach that will reflect the intricacies of today's health care system while still focusing primary attention on the front lines of care where patients, families, and careteams meet.

Figure 4.2 provides another way to frame the challenge faced by health care leaders today. It retains the macro-, meso-, and microsystem format shown in Figure 4.1 but turns the image upside down. This diagram is based on the idea of the inverted pyramid and on Quinn's observations on the requirements needed to become a world-class leader in the service sector (Quinn, 1992). The inverted pyramid representation of a health care organization puts the patients and frontline staff at the top of the system and suggests that the rest of the organization really exists to support the myriad of important interactions that take place at the front line of care.

Clinical microsystems are the naturally occurring building blocks that form the front line of all health systems. These small systems form around the patient to provide care for shorter or longer periods of time, as health needs evolve. For example, if a person has an acute myocardial infarction (AMI) and survives, he or she will typically receive care in a series of clinical microsystems: paramedics stabilize, transport, and begin treatment; the ED diagnoses and treats; the catheterization lab assesses and treats as indicated; the cardiac care unit assesses and treats; the inpatient telemetry unit assesses, treats, and discharges; cardiac rehabilitation services assist with the full recovery; and the cardiology clinical practice, with or without the assistance of home health services in the community, follows the patient over time to minimize risk of a new cardiac event. All these microsystems act as the front line of care for that individual patient.

The quality and value of care for any single patient, or for a cohort of patients, such as people who have had an AMI, fully depends on the quality of

FIGURE 4.2. THE HEALTH CARE SYSTEM AS AN INVERTED PYRAMID.

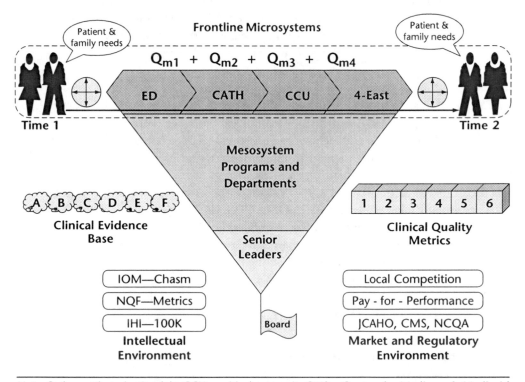

Note: Cath = catheterization lab; CCU = critical care unit; CMS = Centers for Medicare & Medicaid Services; ED = emergency department; IHI = Institute for Healthcare Improvement; IOM = Institute of Medicine; JCAHO = Joint Commission on Accreditation of Healthcare Organizations; NCQA = National Committee for Quality Assurance; NQF = National Quality Forum.

Source: Batalden, Nelson, Gardent, & Godfrey, 2005.

the health system. The quality of the health system (Q_{HS}) is a function of the quality of care provided within each contributing microsystem (Q_{m1}, Q_{m2}, Q_{m3}, and so forth) plus the quality of the handoffs and integration that occur in the organizational "white spaces" *between* microsystems (for example, handoffs of the patient, of information and data about the patient, and of services needed for the patient).

Clinical microsystems form the front line of the system—they represent the place where quality is made and costs are incurred. The special knowledge, skills, and resources of the clinical staff can be used in the clinical microsystem to meet the special needs of an individual patient. It is the place where innovation opportunities are most often uncovered. It is the place where, with discretion, things that should be flexible can be customized and where, with discipline, things that should be standardized can be made routine.

The inverted pyramid goes from the level of microsystem to the mesosystem and the macrosystem, respectively. The mesosystem includes the areas that contribute to the care of the patient, such as the following:

- Clinical departments (for example, medicine, nursing, surgery)
- Clinical support departments (for example, radiology, pathology, anesthesiology, pharmacy, medical information, care management)
- Critical midlevel structures (such as specific service line programs or centers for oncology, cardiovascular health, or women's health)

The macrosystem, at the bottom of the inverted pyramid, is populated by senior leaders (for example, the CEO, CFO, CMO, CNO, and CIO). In Figure 4.2 this section also contains a flag, representing a board of trustees that guides (and oversees) senior leaders in core areas such as vision, mission, values, guiding principles, strategy, and finance. Working down through the inverted pyramid can be compared with working through a root cause analysis that moves progressively away from the sharp end and toward the blunt end of the system as staff ask the *why* question repeatedly.

Implications for Health Care Leaders

The typical integrated delivery institution is thus a complex organization with three fundamentally important and different levels of systems: microsystem, mesosystem, and macrosystem. The inverted pyramid framework challenges leaders and leadership to act in a coordinated way at all levels to deliver high-quality and high-value care in order to succeed today and to find ways to innovate and improve in order to excel tomorrow. The inverted pyramid provides a panoramic viewpoint that frames the leadership challenge for macrosystem (or senior) leaders, mesosystem (or midlevel) leaders, and microsystem (or frontline) leaders.

The board of trustees and macrosystem senior leaders at the tip of the inverted pyramid must work together to establish the mission, vision, values, guiding principles, and strategy, all of which form the organizational context for the work of health care. They do this vital work looking inside the organization to assess both current and needed capabilities and by looking outside the organization to understand and to strategically react to major trends and issues in their organization's environment.

For example, the board and senior leaders may become aware that there is clinical evidence identifying the best practices for AMI care, practices that may or may not be designed into the patterns of care produced by the contributing clinical microsystems. At the same time, they may uncover gold-standard, evidence-based, clinical quality metrics that are generated by the patterns of AMI care and that emanate from the involved clinical microsystems. They may be cognizant of their local and regional competition, of the trend toward pay-for-performance reimbursement, and of the special requirements imposed by outside agencies such as the Joint Commission on Accreditation of Healthcare Organizations (JCAHO: http://www.jcaho.org), Centers for Medicare & Medicaid Services (CMS: http://www.cms.hhs.gov), and the National Committee for Quality Assurance (NCQA: http://www.ncqa.org). They may also be scanning the environment for powerful emerging forces that will shape the industry, such as the Institute of Medicine (IOM: http://www.iom.edu) and its special reports on quality and safety, the coming avalanche of gold-standard quality metrics promulgated by the National Quality Forum (NQF: http://www.qualityforum.org), and the work of high-profile health care organizations such as the Institute for Healthcare Improvement (IHI: http://www.ihi.org), which launched a campaign in December 2004 to save 100,000 lives and developed *whole system metrics,* a new way to measure the quality of an entire health system.

Leadership Frameworks: Some of the Best Approaches

Most successful macrosystem leaders know that the patient care their system provides is only as good as the clinical microsystems that make the care. Macrosystem leaders help create the environment inside the organization that enables, or diminishes, the work of the mesosystems and microsystems. Macrosystem leaders know that improvement means change.

What is the work of senior leaders and how might it be done? Many general leadership frameworks have been developed and popularized. Some of them explore challenges commonly found in health care and are described in the following sections. Although other frameworks are available, the ones discussed here illustrate some of the best approaches. Table 4.1 contains an overview of these frameworks and the relevant challenges.

Bossidy and Charan

According to Larry Bossidy and Ram Charan (2002, 2004), the job of macrosystem leaders is to establish a planning framework that confronts the reality of the situation they face and answers the following questions (Bossidy & Charan, 2002):

TABLE 4.1. LEADERSHIP FRAMEWORKS AND CHALLENGES.

Framework Author	Common Challenge
Bossidy and Charan	Making things happen amid current realities
Malcolm Baldrige National Quality Award	Assessing world-class levels of quality
Bolman and Deal	Framing leaders' work flexibly
Greenleaf	Being servant leaders
Kotter	Leading change
Weick	Improving reliability
Toyota	Linking work process, leadership development, and learning

- What's the nature of the game we're in?
- Where is it going?
- How do we make money in it?

Figure 4.3 represents Bossidy and Charan's model. Unless the *internal fundamentals* connect to the *external realities* facing the organization and unless appropriate connections are made to the organization's financial targets, it is doubtful that leaders will be able to create a sustainable, high-performing organization.

What might Figure 4.3 mean when applied to change and improvement at the level of the clinical microsystem? At a minimum it means that senior leaders have worked this framework out for the macrosystem and can share with leadership at other levels how the work of the microsystem connects with and contributes to the performance of the whole organization. Leaders must help the microsystem address the current reality, create a sustainable proposition for its work, and initiate the necessary changes and improvement. The Bossidy and Charan model can help connect the real work of the microsystem within the macrosystem environment. Absent this explicit awareness, leaders are likely to encounter difficulties in fully aligning their efforts for the microsystem and macrosystem.

Malcolm Baldrige National Quality Award

The framework of the Malcolm Baldrige National Quality Award and process (http://www.quality.nist.gov) reflects how leaders create conditions across the macrosystem for continuing improvement of daily work. The Baldrige model makes assumptions about what elements are needed to attain excellence and uses an assessment framework with seven criteria for the design, deployment, and continuous improvement of the results of each element. Figure 4.4 illustrates the general model.

FIGURE 4.3. BOSSIDY AND CHARAN'S FRAMEWORK FOR EXECUTION.

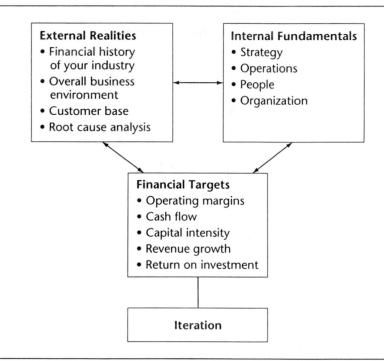

Source: Adapted from Bossidy & Charan, 2004.

A set of eleven values that macrosystem leadership must understand, embody, and establish throughout the organization supports performance excellence (Baldrige National Quality Program, 2006, p. 1):

- Visionary leadership
- Patient-focused excellence
- Organizational and personal learning
- Valuing staff and partners
- Agility
- Focus on the future
- Managing for innovation
- Management by fact
- Social responsibility and community health
- Focus on results and creating value
- Systems perspective

FIGURE 4.4. THE BALDRIGE PROCESS OF IMPROVEMENT.

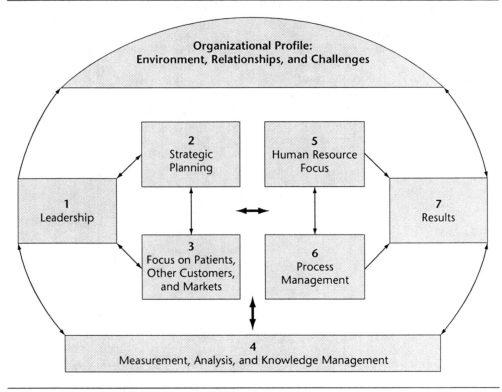

Source: Baldrige National Quality Program, 2006, p. 5.

These values and performance elements illustrate the organizational channels of interaction that senior leaders use to have good conversations and to promote continually improving results at the microsystem level.

Bolman and Deal

Lee Bolman and Terrence Deal (2003) assert that macrosystem leaders should begin their jobs by recognizing the uncertain and ambiguous nature of work today. Leaders must take a flexible approach to learning and taking action. They invite attention to the critical skill of framing and reframing work. Bolman and Deal use four frameworks—structure, human resource, political, and symbolic—to illustrate different ways of leading. Each framework has a unique set of assumptions, and each offers approaches for learning about performance and forming action strategies. Table 4.2 defines the four frameworks and outlines the differences in approach

TABLE 4.2. BOLMAN AND DEAL'S FOUR COMPLEMENTARY LEADERSHIP FRAMEWORKS, WITH BARRIERS AND STRATEGIES.

Frame	Effective Roles for Leaders	Effective Processes	Ineffective Roles for Leaders	Ineffective Processes	Barriers to Change	Essential Change Strategies
Structural	Analyst Architect	Analysis Design	Petty tyrant	Management by detail Arbitrary decrees	• Loss of clarity and stability • Confusion • Chaos	• Communicate • Realign • Renegotiate formal patterns and policies
Human Resource	Catalyst Servant	Support Empowerment	Weakling Pushover	Abdication	• Anxiety and uncertainty • People feel incompetent and needy	• Train to develop new skills • Encourage participation and involvement • Provide psychological support
Political	Advocate Negotiator	Advocacy Coalition building	Con artist Thug	Manipulation Fraud	• Disempowerment • Conflict between winners and losers	• Create arenas where issues can be renegotiated and new coalitions formed
Symbolic	Prophet Poet	Inspiration Framing experience	Fanatic Fool	Mirage	• Loss of meaning and purpose • Clinging to the past	• Create transition rituals • Mourn the past, celebrate the future

Source: Adapted from Bolman & Deal, 2003.

senior leaders will find as they use each framework to address organizational change and the making of *meaningful* work.

Greenleaf

In the middle of the twentieth century Robert Greenleaf began leadership training under the auspices of AT&T. Over time he worked with many different organizations. In 1969, he gave a series of lectures at Dartmouth College that were to form the basis of his later work on servant leadership and his view of a leader who encourages the whole person—head, hand, and heart—to show up for work. In those lectures he identified a number of personal attributes, strategies, themes, and approaches that leaders might take in their own organizations (Frick & Spears, 1996). Table 4.3 briefly recounts the themes from these lectures. These decades-old points still offer helpful counsel to leaders today.

Kotter

John Kotter developed a powerful method for leading change, basing it on his study of successful and unsuccessful efforts to transform organizations. His model offers a change process comprising sequential steps that often overlap, run in parallel, and interact with one another (Kotter, 1996). Exhibit 4.1 lists these steps. In 1999, Kotter assembled several of his previous writings and appended some reflective comments on the differences between managing and leading change. He stated that leaders (1) set a direction, (2) align people, and (3) motivate and inspire people. He noted that the powerful path of "see-feel-change" works more often than "analysis-think-change," and he went on to suggest ways leaders can vividly speak to the feelings of those they seek to lead (Kotter & Cohen, 2002). Many health care leaders have found these suggestions to be very helpful.

Weick

A renowned expert on the psychology of organizations, Karl Weick urges leaders to consider their assumptions when trying to foster change (Beer & Nohria, 2000; Weick & Sutcliffe, 2001). Weick believes that when leaders seek to make intentional change, they should assume that any model of change will do, as long as it accomplishes the following:

• Animates people and gets them moving and generating experiments that uncover opportunities
• Provides a direction

TABLE 4.3. HIGHLIGHTS OF ROBERT GREENLEAF'S DARTMOUTH COLLEGE LECTURES.

Theme	Description
Goal setting	Know what you are trying to do: the overarching purpose, the big dream, the visionary concept, the ultimate achievement that one approaches but never quite achieves. Goal setting's purpose is to excite the imagination. The right goal helps the rest of a leadership strategy to fall into place naturally.
Principle of systematic neglect	It is just as important to know what to neglect as to know what to do.
Listening	Listeners learn about people in ways that modify, first, the listener's attitude; then, his behavior toward others; and finally, the attitudes and behavior of others.
Language as a leadership strategy	A leader must articulate the goal. The effective use of language includes some estimate of what the listener's fund of experience is plus the art of tempting the listener into that leap of imagination that connects the verbal concept to the listener's own experience. One of the great communication arts is to say just enough to make that leap of the imagination feasible. In this process one must not be afraid of a little silence. In fact it is important to ask oneself, "In saying what I have in mind, will I really improve on the silence?" Recall that most of us don't like to be lectured to, but we all like to eavesdrop.
Values	We want a leader to be honest, loving, and responsible. Leaders are moved by the heart; compassion stands ahead of justice.
Personal growth	The leader must be a growing person.
Withdrawal	The best defense is to be able to withdraw, cast off the burden for a while, and relax. Optimum functioning includes carrying an unused reserve of energy in all periods of normal demand so that one has the resilience to cope with emergency.
Tolerance of imperfection	We must have a view, rooted deep in our interior, that people can be immature and ineffectual but that even imperfect people are capable of great dedication and heroism. A lot of people are in fact unqualified to lead because they cannot work through and with the people who are available to work with them.
Being your own person	Be the *natural* person you are, and realize that you own yourself.
Acceptance	When followers feel accepted, they tend to perform beyond their limits.
Foresight	What will happen in the future begins with a state of mind about *now.* The prudent person constantly thinks of now as . . . a moving concept—past, present moment, and future as one organic unity. This requires living by a sort of rhythm that encourages a high level of insight about the whole span of events, from the definite past through the present moment to the indefinite future. Leadership depends on intuiting the gap between the limit of the solid information and what is in fact needed for a dependable decision.

Source: Based on the material in Frick & Spears, 1996.

EXHIBIT 4.1. KOTTER'S EIGHT-STEP PROCESS FOR LEADING LARGE-SCALE CHANGE.

1. *Tension for change:* establishing a sense of urgency based on an understanding of realities of the market, crises, opportunities, and so forth
2. *Coalition:* creating a guiding coalition with enough power to lead the change
3. *Vision:* developing a vision and strategy that can direct the change effort, together with strategies for achieving that vision
4. *Communication:* communicating the change vision, using multiple modalities and vehicles for communication, and having the guiding coalition model the behaviors sought
5. *Empowerment:* empowering broad-based action while encouraging risk taking and removing barriers, obstacles, and undermining forces
6. *Early success:* generating short-term wins, and recognizing those wins and the people who contributed to making them
7. *Expanding change:* consolidating gains and producing more change to extend the vision for change beyond the initial targets and people
8. *Grounding:* anchoring the new approaches in the culture of the setting

Source: Adapted from Kotter, 1996.

- Encourages updating through improved situational awareness and closer attention to what's actually happening
- Facilitates respectful interaction in which trust, trustworthiness, and self-respect all develop equally and allow people to build a stable rendition of what they face

Weick observes that as leaders seek to change an organization, they can assume that their organization will observe the *either-or* states listed in Table 4.4. A model closer to the *either* side might drive a leader to carefully design and plan a change. If the reality facing the leader looks more like the *or* side, the leader must recognize that the primary job will be to certify the goodness of the changes actually made (Weick, 2000).

Further, both Weick (2001) and Scott (1987) note that settings in organizations vary in the degree to which they manifest tight or loose coupling, as shown in Table 4.5. The job of the leader seeking to foster change varies depending on the coupling phenomena present, as illustrated by the change strategies shown in Table 4.6. Weick (2001) notes that systems with loose coupling (high differentiation and low integration) may appear ineffective when assessed by criteria tied to efficiency but may be more effective when assessed against criteria that index flexibility, ability to improvise, and capability for self-design.

Improving these loosely coupled systems does not necessarily require making them into more tightly coupled systems. Indeed, as Weick (2001) suggests, "the loosely coupled system may be thought of as the social and cognitive solution to

TABLE 4.4. EITHER-OR STATES OF ORGANIZATIONAL CHANGE.

Either	Or
Move from one state to another in a forward direction through time.	Have repetitive periods of ebb and flow and of unraveling processes that then need to be reaccomplished.
Move from a less-developed state to a better-developed state.	Move in an orderly sequence through cycles whose disruption creates a crisis: try various strategies, remember, and repeat those that seem to work.
Move toward a specific end state, often articulated in a statement of vision.	Be preoccupied with journeys and directions rather than destinations and end states.
Move only when there is disruption and disequilibrium.	Consider change effective when change restores balance and adaptive sequences.
Move only in response to forces planned and managed by people apart from the system.	Accept the reality that nothing stays the same forever.

Source: Adapted from Weick, 2000.

TABLE 4.5. SYSTEM EXAMPLES ASSOCIATED WITH LOOSE AND TIGHT COUPLING.

System Characteristic	Loose Coupling	Tight Coupling
Interdependence of system elements	Parts are capable of semiautonomous action.	Parts are capable of contingent, dependent action.
Leadership	System has many *heads.*	System has one or few *heads.*
Stability of coalitions	Individuals and subgroups form and leave coalitions.	Individuals and subgroups form and maintain stable coalitions.
Role of coordination and control	Coordination and control are problematic.	Coordination and control are emblematic.
Boundaries	System boundaries are often amorphous.	System boundaries are pretty clear.
Operational alignments	Assignments of actors or actions to the organization or environment seem arbitrary.	Assignments of actors or actions to the organization or environment fit a rationale.
Role of structure and process	Shift in view from structure to process.	Focus on the structure, using the process to understand interdependencies.

TABLE 4.6. MATCHING CHANGE STRATEGIES
TO THE COUPLING SITUATION.

System Characteristic	Loose Coupling	Tight Coupling
Interdependence of system elements	Work on logic, purpose, socialization.	Change *parts*.
Leadership	Work via influence, charter, data.	Change leader's mind or change leader.
Stability of coalitions	Focus on orientation and roles of participants.	Pick participants well.
Role of coordination and control	Use data, shared reviews.	Establish clear accountability.
Boundaries	Work on purpose.	Change the *next* systems, or create a different context.
Operational alignments	Focus on *effects*.	Explore the role-rationale connection.
Role of structure and process	Focus on the paths of interaction with the STAR (*s*eparateness or differences, *t*alking and listening, *a*ction opportunities, *r*eason to work together) model.*	Work on structure and function.

* For the STAR model, see Zimmerman & Hayday, 1999.

Source: Adapted from Weick, 2001.

constant environmental change, to the impossibility of knowing another mind, and to limited information processing capacities" (p. 401).

When seeking high-reliability performance, as must be done in the organizations that Weick has studied in the nuclear power industry and on aircraft carriers, leaders have different concerns and often focus on what Weick and Sutcliffe call *mindfulness* (Weick & Sutcliffe, 2001). Leaders in high-reliability organizations share several characteristics:

- Preoccupation with failure
- Reluctance to simplify interpretations
- Sensitivity to operations
- Commitment to resilience
- Deference to expertise

Weick offers a vision of what the leader's work might be in complex organizations seeking highly reliable performance. Amalberti, Auroy, Berwick, and Barach (2005) note that in health care, some clinical microsystems, such as those engaged in blood banking or anesthesia for not-at-high-risk patients, operate in the zone of "highly safe, reliable" systems. However, most clinical medicine operates at much lower levels of reliability, with failure rates in parts per 10, 100, or 1,000. Weick offers leaders insight into the challenges of guiding high-reliability systems and into the process(es) of leading complex, adaptive systems.

Toyota Approach

Donald Berwick, president and CEO of IHI, has often said, "What we need in health care is a Toyota!" Because Toyota has had such profound worldwide influence on quality thinking and techniques, we will finish our brief review of leadership frameworks with this automaker's approach to a high-quality organization and will cover that approach in somewhat greater detail than we gave to those reviewed earlier. Three threads seem to contribute to the tapestry of Toyota's identity (Dixon, 1999; Fujimoto, 1999; Monden, 1993, 1998; Ohno, 1988; Toyoda, 1987; Womack & Jones, 1996):

- The way of work, or management philosophy, that the founders and their successors modeled
- The tools and methods of change, often described as the Toyota production system, or *lean manufacturing*
- The emergent learning process that—over time—has allowed deep organization learning to occur

Each is discussed in the following sections.

Way of Work. For more than twenty years Jeffrey Liker, a professor at the University of Michigan-Ann Arbor, has studied the Toyota way of work (Liker, 2004). He suggests that the Toyota way of work and the Toyota production system function as twin strands in the Toyota "DNA" (Monden, 1998; Ohno, 1988). Liker portrays his accumulated learning about the elements of Toyota's way of work and production systems with a pyramid (Figure 4.5) and with fourteen management principles (Exhibit 4.2), grouped according to the following four assumptions:

- The organization should be guided by a long-term philosophy.
- The right process will produce the right results.
- Add value to the organization by developing your people and partners.
- Continuously solving root problems drives organizational learning.

Liker (2004) also cautions that, "lean is not about imitating the tools used by Toyota in a particular manufacturing process. Lean is about developing principles

FIGURE 4.5. THE TOYOTA PYRAMID.

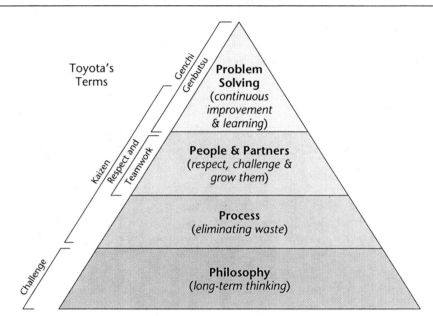

Source: Liker, 2004. Used with permission of the McGraw-Hill Companies.

that are right for your organization and diligently practicing them to achieve high performance that continues to add value to customers and society" (p. 41).

Tools and Methods of Change. The following list describes many of Toyota's numerous approaches to the reduction of waste in an organization, including methods such as smoothing the work flow, getting quality right, and standardizing work routinely employed in the Toyota production system (Fujimoto, 1999; Liker, 2004; Womack & Jones, 1996; Womack, Jones, & Roos, 1991). Many persons have worked hard to adapt these approaches to health care. Among the leading adopters of Toyota methods in health care are the Pittsburgh Regional Healthcare Initiative (http://www.prhi.org), Virginia Mason Medical Center (http://www.virginiamason.org), ThedaCare (http://www.thedacare.org), and IHI (http://www.ihi.org).

Toyota Production System Waste Reduction Methods

- Reduction of non-value–adding activities
- Foolproof prevention of defects
- Reduction of uneven pace of production
- Assembly line stop cord

EXHIBIT 4.2. TOYOTA'S FOURTEEN PRINCIPLES.

Philosophy
1. Base your management decisions on a long-term philosophy, even at the expense of short-term financial goals.

Process
2. Create continuous process flow to bring problems to the surface.
3. Use "pull" systems to avoid overproduction.
4. Level out the workload.
5. Build a culture of stopping to fix problems, to get quality right the first time.
6. Make standardized tasks the foundation for continuous improvement and employee empowerment.
7. Use visual control so no problems are hidden.
8. Use only reliable, thoroughly tested technology that serves your people and processes.

People and Partners
9. Grow leaders who thoroughly understand the work, live the philosophy, and teach it to others.
10. Develop exceptional people and teams who follow your company's philosophy.
11. Respect your extended network of partners and suppliers by challenging them and helping them improve.

Problem Solving
12. Go and see for yourself to thoroughly understand the situation.
13. Make decisions slowly by consensus, thoroughly considering all options, implement decisions rapidly.
14. Become a learning organization through relentless reflection and continuous improvement.

Source: Liker, 2004. Used with permission.

- Reduction of excessive workload
- Real-time feedback of production troubles
- Reduction of inventory by using the Kanban system (in which a replenishment signal transmits information, generally regarding the movement or production of products)
- On-the-spot inspection by direct workers
- Leveling of production volume and reduction of product mix
- Built-in quality
- Production plans based on order volume
- Cleanliness, order, and discipline on the shop floor
- Reduction of set-up change time and lot size
- Visual management
- Piece-by-piece transfer of parts between machines
- Frequent revision of standard operating procedures by supervisors
- Flexible task assignment for volume changes
- Quality circles

- Multitask job assignment along the process flow
- Standardized tools for quality improvement
- U-shaped machine layout that facilitates flexible and multiple task assignment
- Worker involvement in preventive maintenance
- Automatic detection of defects
- Low-cost automation or semiautomation with just enough functions
- Automatic shutdown of machines

Emergent Learning Process. Fujimoto (1999) notes that the Toyota manufacturing system today is not the result of a "grand design." Rather, he suggests that several manufacturing process elements have been adopted from other settings and combined with relentless reflection on the efforts needed to change, improve, and standardize work—yielding new insights into the process of system development.

This *emergent learning* fuses learning with continually improving operations and resembles Argyris's concept of *double loop learning:* that is, learning coupled with learning about learning (Argyris, 1991). Fujimoto suggests that the simple principle that permeates the complex structure of Toyota is the shared aim of "outperforming rivals in attracting and satisfying customers by all employees" (Fujimoto, 1999, p. 124). He claims that this is a key to maintaining the overall integrity of manufacturing routines. The comparable operating principle for health care might look something like the following:

BETTER PATIENT OUTCOME, BETTER SYSTEM
PERFORMANCE, BETTER PROFESSIONAL DEVELOPMENT
BY EVERYONE.

What might the tapestry of identity look like for health care leaders seeking organization-wide structures and processes with Toyota-like capability? Adopting Toyota ways is not the answer (Womack & Jones, 1996). Rather, weaving this tapestry may involve the following tasks:

- Identifying the roots and requirements of an *operating-learning* culture that makes local sense
- Demonstrating a theory of health care work that pursues never-ending improved patient outcomes by professionals working in reliable and efficient systems
- Securing a relentless commitment by all involved to reflect on the work and on the learning that arises from successful efforts to change and improve the work
- Using that learning and those reflective insights for the never-ending redesign of patient-centered care

Toyota has been an important contributor to some of the currently popular improvement methods such as lean design (Liker, 2004; Womack et al., 1991) and Six Sigma (Harry & Schroeder, 2000). It was and still remains true that the examples set by Toyota's founders guide the way work gets done. They modeled the improving and learning way of work at the local work site. Senior leaders in health care have an opportunity to model these practices and to create human resource systems that promote these actions throughout the organization. Macrosystem and mesosystem leaders (using Toyota as the exemplar) need to be able to teach these practices by sharing their own experiences with them and carrying them out in ways that are visible to all.

A Synopsis of Leadership Frameworks

The aforementioned experts who have written volumes on leadership and leading change offer a rich set of insights and possible paths of action. The following eight practices are particularly noteworthy for health care leaders:

1. Be clear about the current realities facing you now, including the assessments you make of your own organization's reliability.
2. Be prepared to use different and complementary frameworks for building knowledge, taking action, reviewing, and reflecting.
3. Link operations and learning at the site where the work is done.
4. Use balanced measures of outcome that reflect multiple, important dimensions of performance, and visually display the measures over time.
5. Infuse a coherent, understandable, dynamic, and uniting aim throughout the entire organization, forming a common interest around that aim.
6. Test change, learn from the effort(s), and engage in visibly leading the change.
7. Invite the whole person—cognitive ability, technical skill, values—to show up for work.
8. Practice vigilant, mindful operations.

Some Unique Features of the Health Care System

The leadership frameworks, which have much to offer health care leaders, have features in common as well as points of difference. For example, they are all based on observations of business and industry in general and are not grounded in the health care sector. So before we present our suggestions for health care macrosystem and mesosystem leaders, we look at what is different about health care. What are the factors that affect the challenges faced by its leaders? What might work perfectly for General Electric might fail miserably at County Memorial Hospital owing to fundamental differences in the two different sectors. This is not to say that health care leaders cannot learn from business leaders, but it is to emphasize that leadership approaches need to be thoughtfully adapted to the special circumstances of today's world of health care delivery.

A short list of some of these special features follows:

Role of health professionals in health care system. Change and improvement in health care services and health systems is inextricably connected with health care professionals. Changes must take into account the professional formation and professional identity of the persons whom patients depend on to provide needed care.

Patient-centered or provider-centered. In the past, care systems were often provider centered. In the future, the health system will become more visibly patient centered. The reality is that patients and careteams are part of the same system, as Lawrence Henderson observed in 1935. Health care is about relationships between patients and clinicians, between families and careteams, who share a common aim.

Endless need. Good health care is a societal goal and, many would say, a human right. Health care represents the conjunction of deep human needs, never-ending advancements in technology and science, and intelligent, creative people. This combination leads to the potential for unlimited costs, growth, and innovation.

Payment mechanisms. Attempts to contain health care growth and costs so far have concentrated on various reimbursement strategies to modify financial incentives—and more attempts will certainly be devised. The United States, which has gone from cost-plus reimbursement to price controls to managed care, now seems ready to move to pay for performance and value-based purchasing. We are entering a major change in the health care marketplace. Pay for performance represents a dramatic change in reimbursement, in which payment becomes contingent on quality and cost outcomes.

External agents. A diverse collection of accreditors, licensors, and regulators create an environment of rules, requirements, and measurements that exert a profound shaping effect on health care professionals and organizations.

Leading Large Health Systems to Peak Performance Using Microsystem Thinking

I prefer self-executing or self-implementing systems.

ROBERT GALVIN, FORMER CEO OF MOTOROLA,
PERSONAL COMMUNICATION TO PAUL BATALDEN, 1997.

In this section we provide our own leadership framework for leaders of macrosystems and mesosystems. This framework is based on our reflections on the general leadership frameworks and on our own experiences in working with hundreds of health care leaders who wish to have all parts of their systems provide care that is excellent in quality, safety, reliability, and cost. We first touch on the leadership process and then turn our attention to two specific facets of leadership—learning and doing.

Health care systems at all levels benefit from leadership because the work of health care at every system level is often ambiguous and uncertain (McCaskey, 1982; Weick & Sutcliffe, 2001). Steadfast aims and values that promote better quality, value, and flexibility to meet a particular patient's special needs, and also promote work settings in which professionals can experience growth and a sense of accomplishment, are necessary but not sufficient to achieve those outcomes. A leader is confronted with more invitations to act, more frustrations to address, more questions to answer, more information and measurement to interpret, and more problems to solve than he or she has time available to address. To simplify the challenge of leadership, recall that leading involves three fundamental processes: (1) building knowledge, or learning; (2) taking action, or doing; and (3) reviewing and reflecting (Batalden et al., 2003).

Learning: Understanding Microsystems by Using Multiple Frames

In performing these three fundamental processes leaders use *frames:* that is, a set of assumptions or mental models, that help them understand the work of the microsystem—the place where patients and careteams come together. All leaders know that they need to *learn*, to gain a deep understanding of that which they wish to change. Leaders can gain a deeper understanding of microsystems by using the eight frames discussed in the rest of this section.

The literature describes the many ways in which assumptions and paradigms shape what all of us think we know and what we do (Argyris & Schön, 1996; Bolman & Deal, 2003; Kahneman & Tversky, 1982; Kuhn, 1970; Lakoff, 2004; Lakoff & Johnson, 1999). Leaders with multiple ways of framing what they are trying to understand or improve have the benefit of increased versatility and have been empirically shown to be more effective in their work (Bensimon, 1989, 1990; Birnbaum, 1992; Bolman & Deal, 1991, 1992a, 1992b; Heimovics, Herman, & Jurkiewicz Coughlin, 1993, 1995; Wimpelberg, 1987). A leader might use the eight frames discussed here in exploring the work of a clinical microsystem, to inquire into what is happening, to construct options for action, and ultimately to make thoughtful, effective, and sustainable changes within an organization (Figure 4.6).

FIGURE 4.6. EIGHT FRAMES FOR EXPLORING MICROSYSTEMS.

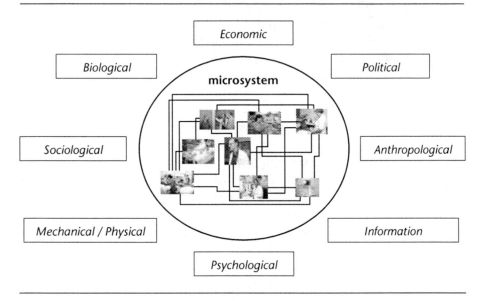

Biological system frame. This frame enables the leader to "see" evidence of vitality (Zimmerman, Lindberg, & Plsek, 1999). With this frame the clinical microsystem can be seen as a living, adaptive entity with the properties that complex adaptive systems have. It engages in generative work. It has emergent properties. It has structures, processes, and patterns, as do all other living systems.

Sociological system frame. Using this frame the leader might examine the relationships, the conversations, the interdependencies, the coupling, and the efforts to make sense and take meaning from the work of the clinical microsystem (Bolman & Deal, 2003; Scott, 1987; Weick, 1995).

Mechanical, or physical, system frame. With this frame the leader might look for the flow of the work, the temporal sequencing of the work, the spatial relationships involved among the people and equipment, and the integration of operations and logistics (Damelio, 1996; Hunt, 1996; Langley, Nolan, Norman, Provost, & Nolan, 1996; Oshry, 1996; Scholtes, 1988, 1998).

Psychological system frame. Adopting this frame the leader sees the clinical microsystem as a setting for behaviors, the interplay of the forces operating in a specific context the motivations behind the behaviors, and the personal and professional development of individuals (Barker & Schoggen, 1973; Batalden & Leach, 2005; Lewin, 1951; Lewin & Lewin, 1948).

Information system frame. Using this frame the leader can inquire into the flow of information and the obstructions to that flow, the cycle times of information and measurement, the ways measures reflect the work, the ways in which information is stored, the ways in which data are handled, and the ways in which information is displayed, analyzed, and used to inform the daily work (Centers for Medicare & Medicaid Services, 2006; Greif, 1991; Nelson, Splaine, Batalden, & Plume, 1998).

Anthropological system frame. This frame facilitates leaders' efforts to explore a microsystem's cultural milieu, the values, the symbols and artifacts, the rituals and ceremonies, the celebrations, and the way learning occurs (Bolman & Deal, 1984, 2003; Schein, 1999, 2003; Senge, Scharmer, Jaworski, & Flowers, 2004).

Political system frame. The leader can use this frame to inquire into the citizenship and equity, the coalitions, the power dynamics, the conflict and negotiating, the governance, and the way control operates in the daily work of the clinical microsystem (Bolman & Deal, 2003; Fisher, Kopelman, & Schneider, 1994).

Economic system frame. With this frame the leader assumes that what is *real* in the clinical microsystem is to be found in understanding the customers and suppliers, the inputs and outputs, and the costs, waste, and benefits of the work (James, 1993; James & Savitz, 2005; Liker, 2004; Monden, 1998; Ohno, 1988; Toyoda, 1987; Womack & Jones, 1996).

Examining a clinical microsystem with the aid of multiple frames allows the leader to understand it more deeply and to formulate more effective action strategies. Further, by making the assumptions and frames explicit the leader can invite others to a shared sense of the work and change. We are reminded of the truths in these observations made by Kofman and Senge (1993):

- Life (in this case, the clinical microsystem) cannot be condensed.
- We make models (that is, our understandings of the microsystem) of what is not condensable for our convenience and understanding.
- We attach measures to our models to assist us in conducting tests of change for improvement.
- In doing so we must avoid confusing our measures and models for the thing (the clinical microsystem) itself; to do that would be to confuse the map for the territory.

Doing: Leading Macrosystems by Deploying and Executing the Plan

So what might senior leaders *do* to lead macrosystems for microsystem peak performance? Leaders can use many useful frameworks, such as those listed earlier, to guide their mission critical work, that is, to take their system someplace else, to raise it to the next level of performance. The goal is to make lasting changes in the capability of the health care systems that they lead—to improve health outcomes by fostering safe, reliable, efficient, and flexible systems of care. Leaders could start in many ways, using a plethora of approaches, but we believe that it is wise to begin with the six action steps outlined in the rest of this section.

It would be smart and effective for Jack Candoo and his senior leadership team, described in the case study at the beginning of this chapter, to reflect on each of these six actions and to act on them in a way that fits the local culture. This would give them a sound path forward toward making the deep and lasting systemic changes that would profoundly improve the quality, reliability, and efficiency of their health system. Of course in making these changes they must also link the front office with the front line by working through the mesosystem, as discussed later, in the section titled "Connecting."

Action Step 1: Bring Meaning to the Work. Show frontline, midlevel, and senior leaders why the work they do makes a difference. Provide a worthy patient-centered aim that provides genuine meaning. Promote the worthy aim to animate and energize all the organization's staff to wish to excel because, in the end, their excellence benefits the people, the patients and families, that the organization exists to serve. Recognize that staff allegiance will naturally and more powerfully gravitate toward achieving a worthy patient-centered aim than toward fulfilling an organization's request for loyalty. Connect the organization's work to the aim by focusing on meeting the health needs of individual patients and families and the needs of communities. Create a simple, compelling story of a memorable (fictional) patient to describe what ideal patient-centered care looks like in a thoughtful, compassionate, and reliable environment. Tell this story at all levels of the organization to develop exemplary care, processes, and systems.

Connect the organization's work to core staff values, professional development, and the formation and personal growth of all staff. Challenge everyone to become personally engaged in safeguarding care and in improving care. Good people respond positively to worthwhile challenges. Recognize that challenges arising from the external environment (for example, public reporting of quality metrics, shifting to pay for performance, meeting new regulatory requirements) act as secondary motivators for most staff.

Action Step 2: Create the Context of the Whole. Establish a simple vision and strategy for the whole system, one that can be understood by all stakeholders and can be carried into every organizational unit. Consider using the image of the inverted pyramid (Figure 4.2), which puts the patients and those caring for patients at the top, highlights the handoffs between units and small systems, and recognizes the critical supporting roles played by the midlevel departments. Foster inquiry, learning, and change within, between, and across microsystems and mesosystems to achieve the worthy aims of the whole organization. Seek to engage every person—at the level and place of his or her own work—in the two fundamental tasks of (1) doing his or her work and (2) improving patient outcomes.

Action Step 3: Define Possibilities and Limitations. Share your views on the realities that the organization currently faces, and make the connection between those realities and the daily work of frontline microsystems. Make a distinction between what the system will do and what it will not do. Be clear about the contributions that the clinical microsystem can make to both advancing the worthy aim and enhancing the whole organization's well-being. Create an appreciation of the health care regulatory environment and the reimbursement mechanisms and the ways these external forces influence all levels of the health care system—micro, meso, and macro.

Action Step 4: Create Supportive Infrastructures for Health Information and Human Resources. Recognize that even though decisions about information technology and human resource policy are often made at the macrosystem level, they are acutely felt and have profound effects at the microsystem level. Take action to optimize the ability of these decisions to support frontline work.

Excellent health care requires excellent information. Information is at the heart of health care work. Making information readily accessible and ensuring that it contributes to the flow of good work in the clinical microsystem involves knowing the following:

- What the microsystem is trying to do
- How information helps and how it hinders doing what is needed at the point of care
- How information supports and how it limits efforts to improve care
- How information technology can reduce the workload in the clinical microsystem's daily functioning

Support doing the right thing at the right time by creating real-time, *feed forward* data flows—a method of collecting and using information as soon as it is needed and reusing it later in the process as needed. Create informative feedback data displays by developing a method of analyzing and displaying data to provide insights on past performance and on the relationship between processes and outcomes. Give people insight on performance and data they can use for maintaining quality or improving it through feedback that uses balanced metrics—a well-rounded set of measures that reflect important dimensions of quality and performance.

Excellent health care requires not only excellent information but also excellent staff. Creating a human resource value chain that will attract, select, orient, develop, and retain staff is essential to high performance. Align recognition, incentives, and rewards for individuals and groups to foster accountability for improving and maintaining quality, efficiency, and flexibility. Attaining the requisite alignment of incentives is complex and fraught with difficulties; therefore senior leaders will need to take the time to examine and understand how current incentives influence attitudes and behaviors and how revised incentives could be working, and then make adjustments appropriate for the culture of the organization.

Again, human resource policies set at the level of the macrosystem have great impact at the microsystem level. These policies may either contribute to or conflict with the creation of a work environment where every staff member can say he or she agrees with each of these challenges offered by Paul O'Neill (personal communication to M. Godfrey, 2003), past CEO of Alcoa:

- I'm treated with dignity and respect everyday by everyone I encounter . . . and it doesn't have anything to do with hierarchy.
- I'm given the opportunity and tools that I need to make a contribution and this gives meaning to my life.
- Someone noticed that I did it.

O'Neill also stated that a high level of worklife satisfaction is present when every employee can "strongly agree" with these three statements.

Action Step 5: Stay Connected. Stay connected to the clinical microsystem and create conditions to grow capability from the inside out. Show up at the site where the work is done and where learning and change must happen. Macrosystem leaders can offer their curiosity and their questions, encourage and develop staff, and recognize and celebrate gains. Foster and ensure good leadership in each and every microsystem. Create the conditions that bring action learning and reflection into the daily work environments of all staff. Promote the growth of the microsystems and the people who staff those systems.

Action Step 6: Drive Out the Fear of Change. Encourage staff to improve and innovate constantly. Challenge microsystem leaders and staff both to learn how to change and to actually make lasting change that optimizes performance. Promote frequent and rapid tests of change at all levels of the organization. Celebrate successful changes and also *learning from failures,* the unsuccessful changes that nevertheless provide valuable learning. Encourage inquiry and learning for improvement while diminishing the justifying and rationalizing behaviors that commonly limit learning and often lead to trapped thinking (Weick & Sutcliffe, 2003). Remind all staff at all levels that they have two jobs—to do their work and to improve the way they do their work—with a constant focus on best patient outcomes and greatest real value.

Connecting: Leading Mesosystems by Connecting the Front Office with the Front Line

In the image of the inverted pyramid, a large space separates senior leaders from the front line. This midlevel space is occupied by the intermediate levels of the organization, or the mesosystem. Health care macrosystems have many midlevel structures and leaders. As previously noted, examples include supporting functions (for example, human resources, information systems, medical records), clinical departments (for example, nursing, medicine, surgery, pharmacy, care management), and service line programs and centers (for example, oncology, women's health, primary care). Macrosystem leaders know that this level of their organization is critical for moving the organization's message between top and bottom and the mesosystem must be taken fully into account to create the conditions needed to generate high performance at the front line. The leaders of these vital midlevel systems face a wide variety of challenges and opportunities to improve the quality and value of patient care.

When a health care system seeks to execute its quality improvement strategy, it has to work through the midlevel systems to have the desired effect on the frontline microsystems. Although direct communication between the front office and the front line is desirable and often occurs, the mesosystem leaders need to buy into the strategic plan and carry the strategic message to the frontline leaders, as well as carry responses and concerns from frontline leaders back to senior leaders. To perform this important linking function well, mesosystem leaders need to attend to the fidelity of the message while also adapting the message to the recipients. Midlevel leaders require an understanding of and firm commitment to the strategic plan. They must also understand and support the microsystems to achieve success in the short run and sustain it in the long run.

The mesosystem leaders play a vital role in making the connection described by Bossidy and Charan (that is, the link between strategy, operations, and people) that is needed for successful execution. Midlevel leaders, in essence, mediate the cultural supports and the cultural changes a health care system requires if it is to move from providing care of erratic quality at the front lines to measurably improving the quality and value of that care. Midlevel leaders usually select the microsystem leaders, orient them, set their expectations, review their performance, and demand (or avoid) accountability for microsystem performance. The midlevel leader's personal style of work often speaks more convincingly about the desired way of work than any amount of words could.

All work in mesosystems must be undertaken with the clear understanding that the general aim is to improve patient care outcomes with more reliable and more efficient systems that are regularly reflected on and redesigned. Absent such a focus, understandings about work easily degrade into conversations about workload equity and problems of the past. Exhibit 4.3 displays commonly occurring needs, related skills, and helpful tips for mesosystem leaders.

Conclusion

Patients and payers demand better quality, better safety, and better value for their money. This pressure will likely intensify, which generates the widespread need to transform health systems, which in turn requires excellent leadership at all levels of the system—the macro-, meso-, and microlevels. System thinking at all levels can help leaders make this transformation. Using the image of the inverted pyramid, which places patients and frontline staff at the apex of the pyramid, leaders can communicate that systemic change runs top to bottom and side to side.

Changing large health care systems is a tall order. Fortunately, many thoughtful scholars and many renowned organizations provide useful frameworks that can be used to better understand the work of leading change in large, complex health care systems, and we reviewed a number of those frameworks at the beginning of this chapter. Because health care systems are unique, leaders can gain the most thorough understanding of clinical microsystems by using multiple complementary frames to analyze the current reality, and then they can take action to lead their macrosystems to microsystem peak performance.

The real challenge for leaders at all levels of the system is to make sense of the task by understanding the current reality, understanding the nature and magnitude of the changes that are taking place in the health care environment, creating frames for adapting ideas about effective leadership to their own settings, and getting on with the main work to ensure that every patient gets the best possible care for the

EXHIBIT 4.3. LEADING THE MESOSYSTEM.

Commonly Occurring Needs

- Develop vision for the desired microsystem and mesosystem future.
- Identify resource allocation strategies that address the functioning of the clinical microsystem and the optimal functioning of the whole mesosystem and macrosystem.
- Connect desired future to the current reality.
- Advocate for the microsystem within the macrosystem.
- Clarify implications of change(s).
- Develop measures of clinical microsystem performance.
- Generate ideas and options.
- Identify microsystem staffing and professional development needs.
- Design and conduct pilot tests of change.
- Integrate the professional education function with daily patient care realities.
- Balance local innovation, creativity, and the needs of the whole organization.
- Receive and process complaints.
- Standardize the work and work flow appropriately.
- Execute plans.
- Respond to signals that "all is not well."
- Convene microsystems and macrosystems.

Helpful Knowledge and Skills

- Develop knowledge of health care as a system and a process.
- Attract cooperation across health professional disciplinary traditions.
- Understand patient needs and illness burdens.
- Plan and work in a socially accountable way.
- Measure, display, and analyze variation in the daily processes of health care.
- Design and test change.
- Lead and follow.
- Link best-practice evidence to local processes and systems.

Helpful Tips

- Follow the patient's journey—especially between departments and into each different department.
- Establish ownership of the leverage processes in the space between microsystems.
- Look for ways interaction in the process could automatically generate data.
- Establish a process of review of shared care.
- Use data to understand unreliable, poor quality.
- Focus on flow of care, information, and patient need.
- Test changes in the process(es) of interaction.

Source: Adapted in part from Batalden et al., 1998.

best possible outcome in the most efficient way every time. This will occur only if senior leaders critically analyze and design the systems and processes that support and nurture the engagement of clinical microsystems within their organizations. To be successful, this commitment to microsystem excellence must be reflected in the active and ongoing involvement of individual senior leaders.

References

Amalberti, R., Auroy, Y., Berwick, D., & Barach, P. (2005). Five system barriers to achieving ultra-safe health care. *Annals of Internal Medicine, 142*(9), 756–764.

Argyris, C. (1991, May/June). Teaching smart people how to learn. *Harvard Business Review,* pp. 99–109.

Argyris, C., & Schön, D. A. (1996). *Organizational learning.* Reading, MA: Addison-Wesley.

Baldrige National Quality Program. (2006). *Health Care Criteria for Performance Excellence.* Retrieved September 1, 2006, from http://www.quality.nist.gov./PDF_files/ 2006_HealthCare_Criteria.pdf.

Barker, R. G., & Schoggen, P. (1973). *Qualities of community life.* San Francisco: Jossey-Bass.

Batalden P. B., Berwick, D., Bisognano, M., Splaine, M., Baker, G. R., & Headrick, L. (1998). *Knowledge domains for health professional students seeking competency in the continual improvement and innovation of health care.* Boston: Institute for Healthcare Improvement.

Batalden, P., & Leach, D. (2005). *The inner and outer life in medicine: Honoring values, relationships, and the human element in physicians' lives.* San Francisco: Jossey-Bass.

Batalden, P. B., Nelson, E. C., Gardent, P. B., & Godfrey, M. M. (2005). Leading the macrosystem and mesosystem for microsystem peak performance. In S. Berman (Ed.), *From front office to front line: Essential issues for health care leaders* (pp. 1–40). Oakbrook Terrace, IL: Joint Commission Resources.

Batalden, P. B., Nelson, E. C., Mohr, J. J., Godfrey, M. M., Huber, T. P., Kosnik, L., et al. (2003). Microsystems in health care: Part 5. How leaders are leading. *Joint Commission Journal on Quality and Safety, 29*(6), 297–308.

Beer, M., & Nohria, N. (Eds.). (2000). *Breaking the code of change.* Boston: Harvard Business School Press.

Bensimon, E. M. (1989). The meaning of "good presidential leadership": A frame analysis. *Review of Higher Education, 12*(2), 107–123.

Bensimon, E. M. (1990). Viewing the presidency: Perceptual congruence between presidents and leaders on their campuses. *Leadership Quarterly, 1,* 71–90.

Birnbaum, R. (1992). *How academic leadership works: Understanding success and failure in the college presidency.* San Francisco: Jossey-Bass.

Bolman, L. G., & Deal, T. E. (1984). *Modern approaches to understanding and managing organizations.* San Francisco: Jossey-Bass.

Bolman, L. G., & Deal, T. E. (1991). Leadership and management effectiveness: A multi-frame, multi-sector analysis. *Human Resource management, 30*(4), 509–534.

Bolman, L. G., & Deal, T. E. (1992a). Leading and managing: Effects of context, culture and gender. *Education Administration Quarterly, 28,* 314–329.

Bolman, L. G., & Deal, T. E. (1992b). *Reframing leadership: The effects of leaders' images of leadership.* Greensboro, NC: Center for Creative Leadership.

Bolman, L. G., & Deal, T. E. (2003). *Reframing organizations: Artistry, choice, and leadership* (3rd ed.). San Francisco: Jossey-Bass.

Bossidy, L., & Charan, R. (with Burck, C.). (2002). *Execution: The discipline of getting things done.* New York: Crown Business.

Bossidy, L., & Charan, R. (with Burck, C.). (2004). *Confronting reality: Doing what matters to get things right.* New York: Crown Business.

Centers for Medicare and Medicaid Services. Retrieved Oct. 19, 2006, from http://www.cms.hhs.gov/HospitalQualityInits/25_HospitalCompare.asp.

Damelio, R. (1996). *The basics of process mapping.* New York: Quality Resources.

Dixon, N. M. (1999). *The organizational learning cycle: How we can learn collectively* (2nd ed.). Brookfield, VT: Gower.

Fisher, R., Kopelman, E., & Schneider, A. K. (1994). *Beyond Machiavelli: Tools for coping with conflict.* Cambridge, MA: Harvard University Press.

Frick, D. M., & Spears, L. C. (Eds.). (1996). *On becoming a servant-leader: The private writings of Robert K. Greenleaf.* San Francisco: Jossey-Bass.

Fujimoto, T. (1999). *The evolution of a manufacturing system at Toyota.* New York: Oxford University Press.

Gibson, R., & Bennis, W. G. (1997). *Rethinking the future: Rethinking business, principles, competition, control & complexity, leadership, markets and the world.* Sonoma, CA: Nicholas Brealey.

Greif, M. (1991). *The visual factory: Building participation through shared information.* Cambridge, MA: Productivity Press.

Harry, M., & Schroeder, R. (2000). *Six sigma: The breakthrough management strategy revolutionizing the world's top corporations.* New York: Doubleday.

Heimovics, R. D., Herman, R. D., & Jurkiewicz Coughlin, C. L. (1993). Executive leadership and resource dependence in nonprofit organizations: A frame analysis. *Public Administration Review, 53*(5), 419–427.

Heimovics, R. D., Herman, R. D., & Jurkiewicz Coughlin, C. L. (1995). The political dimension of effective nonprofit executive leadership. *Nonprofit Management and Leadership, 5*(3), 233–248.

Henderson, L. (1935). Physician and patient as a social system. *New England Journal of Medicine, 212*(18), 819–823.

Hunt, V. D. (1996). *Process mapping: How to reengineer your business process.* Hoboken, NJ: Wiley.

Institute of Medicine (U.S.), Committee on Quality of Health Care in America. (2001). *Crossing the quality chasm: A new health system for the 21st century.* Washington, DC: National Academies Press.

James, B. C. (1993). Quality improvement in the hospital: Managing clinical processes. *The Internist, 34*(3), 11–13.

James, B. C., & Savitz, L. (2005). *Cost of poor quality and waste in delivery systems.* Paper presented at the *AHRQ Fourth Annual Meeting of the IDSRN,* Washington, DC.

Kahneman, D., & Tversky, A. (1982). The psychology of preferences. *Scientific American, 246*(1), 160–173.

Kofman, F., & Senge, P. M. (1993). Communities of commitment: The heart of learning organizations. *Organizational Dynamics, 22*(2), 5–21.

Kotter, J. P. (1996). *Leading change.* Boston: Harvard Business School Press.

Kotter, J. P. (1999). *John P. Kotter on what leaders really do.* Boston: Harvard Business School Press.

Kotter, J. P., & Cohen, D. S. (2002). *The heart of change: Real-life stories of how people change their organizations.* Boston: Harvard Business School Press.

Kuhn, T. S. (1970). *The structure of scientific revolutions* (2nd ed.). Chicago: University of Chicago Press.

Lakoff, G. (2004). *Don't think of an elephant! Know your values and frame the debate: The essential guide for progressives.* White River Junction, VT: Chelsea Green.

Lakoff, G., & Johnson, M. (1999). *Philosophy in the flesh: The embodied mind and its challenge to western thought.* New York: Basic Books.

Langley, G. J., Nolan, K. M., Norman, C. L., Provost, L. P., & Nolan, T. W. (1996). *The improvement guide: A practical approach to enhancing organizational performance.* San Francisco: Jossey-Bass.

Lewin, K. (1951). *Field theory in social science: Selected theoretical papers.* New York: HarperCollins.

Lewin, K., & Lewin, G. W. (1948). *Resolving social conflicts: Selected papers on group dynamics, 1935–1946.* New York: HarperCollins.

Liker, J. K. (2004). *The Toyota way: 14 management principles from the world's greatest manufacturer.* New York: McGraw-Hill.

McCaskey, M. B. (1982). *The executive challenge: Managing change and ambiguity.* Boston: Pitman.

Monden, Y. (1993). *The Toyota management system: Linking the seven key functional areas.* Cambridge, MA: Productivity Press.

Monden, Y. (1998). *Toyota production system: An integrated approach to just-in-time* (3rd ed.). Norcross, GA: Engineering & Management Press.

Nelson, E. C., Splaine, M. E., Batalden, P. B., & Plume, S. K. (1998). Building measurement and data collection into medical practice. *Annals of Internal Medicine, 128*(6), 460–466.

Ohno, T. (1988). *Toyota production system: Beyond large-scale production.* Cambridge, MA: Productivity Press.

Oshry, B. (1996). *Seeing systems: Unlocking the mysteries of organizational life.* San Francisco: Berrett-Koehler.

Quinn, J. B. (1992). *Intelligent enterprise: A knowledge and service based paradigm for industry.* New York: Free Press.

Schein, E. H. (1999). *The corporate culture survival guide: Sense and nonsense about culture change.* San Francisco, Jossey-Bass.

Schein, E. H. (2003). *DEC is dead, long live DEC: The lasting legacy of Digital Equipment Corporation.* San Francisco: Berrett-Koehler.

Scholtes, P. R. (1988). *The team handbook: How to use teams to improve quality.* Madison, WI: Joiner.

Scholtes, P. R. (1998). *The leader's handbook: Making things happen, getting things done.* New York: McGraw-Hill.

Scott, W. R. (1987). *Organizations: Rational, natural, and open systems* (2nd ed.). Upper Saddle River, NJ: Prentice Hall.

Senge, P. M., Scharmer, C. O., Jaworski, J., & Flowers, B. S. (2004). *Presence: Human purpose and the field of the future.* Cambridge, MA: SoL.

Toyoda, E. (1987). *Toyota: Fifty years in motion: An autobiography.* Tokyo and New York: Kodansha International.

Weick, K. E. (1995). *Sensemaking in organizations.* Thousand Oaks, CA: Sage.

Weick, K. E. (2000). Emergent change as a universal in organizations. In M. Beer & N. Nohria (Eds.), *Breaking the code of change* (pp. 223–241). Boston: Harvard Business School Press.

Weick, K. E. (2001). *Making sense of the organization.* Malden, MA: Blackwell.

Weick, K. E., & Sutcliffe, K. M. (2001). *Managing the unexpected: Assuring high performance in an age of complexity.* San Francisco: Jossey-Bass.

Weick, K. E., & Sutcliffe, K. M. (2003). Hospitals as cultures of entrapment: A reanalysis of the Bristol Royal Infirmary. *California Management Review, 45*(2), 73–84.

Wimpelberg, R. K. (1987). Managerial images and school effectiveness. *Administrator's Notebook, 32*(4), 1–4.

Womack, J. P., & Jones, D. T. (1996). *Lean thinking: Banish waste and create wealth in your corporation*. New York: Simon & Schuster.

Womack, J. P., Jones, D. T., & Roos, D. (1991). *The machine that changed the world: How Japan's secret weapon in the global auto wars will revolutionize western industry*. New York: HarperPerennial.

Zimmerman, B. J., & Hayday, B. (1999, July). A board's journey into complexity science: Lessons from (and for) staff and board members. *Group Decision and Negotiation, 8,* 281–303.

Zimmerman, B., Lindberg, C., & Plsek, P. (1999). *Edgeware: Insights from complexity science for health care leaders*. Irving, TX: VHA.

CHAPTER FIVE

DEVELOPING PROFESSIONALS
AND IMPROVING WORKLIFE

Thomas P. Huber, Marjorie M. Godfrey, Eugene C. Nelson,
Julie K. Johnson, Christine Campbell, Paul B. Batalden

Chapter Summary

Background. The chapters in this book focus on the success characteristics of high-performing clinical microsystems. Realization is growing about the importance of doing an excellent job of attracting, selecting, developing, and engaging professionals. By optimizing the work of all staff members and by promoting a culture where everyone matters, the microsystem can attain levels of performance not previously experienced.

Case study. At Massachusetts General Hospital Downtown Associates (Boston), a primary care practice, the human resource processes are specified and predictable, from a candidate's initial contact through each staff member's orientation, performance management, and professional development. Early on,

the new employee receives materials about the practice, including a practice overview and information about his or her typical responsibilities, the performance evaluation program, and the continuous quality improvement effort. Ongoing training and education are supported with skill labs, special education nights, and cross-training. The performance evaluation program, used to evaluate employees, is completed during the ninety-day orientation and training, then quarterly for one year, and then annually.

Conclusion. Some health care settings enjoy high morale, high quality, and high productivity, but all too many of them fail in this. The case study offers an example of a microsystem that has motivated its staff and created a positive and dynamic workplace.

There is a growing realization in health care systems about the fundamental importance of doing well at attracting, selecting, developing, and engaging staff in clinical settings. For instance, the Baldrige National Quality Program (2006) includes a *human resource focus*, which addresses "how your organization's *work systems* and your *staff learning* and motivation enable all *staff* to develop and utilize their full potential in *alignment* with your organization's overall objectives, strategy, and *action plans.* Also examined are your organization's efforts to build and maintain a work environment and *staff* support climate conducive to *performance excellence* and to personal and organizational growth." It has been observed that "workforce shortages, rising turnover, and sinking morale have a demonstrable negative effect on financial performance, quality of care, customer satisfaction, and market position" (Gelinas & Bohlen, 2002, p. 3) and that "many [nurses were] sacrificed before the now widespread realization that there is something wrong with the work environment" (Joint Commission on Accreditation of Healthcare Organizations, 2002, p. 10).

Without motivated and involved multidisciplinary staff, a microsystem cannot achieve the exceptional outcomes of which it is capable. By intentionally designing the workplace and paying attention to the workforce, leaders can "enable all staff to make the most out of their talent, training, and skills" (Godfrey, Nelson, Wasson, Mohr, & Batalden, 2003, p. 161) and optimize the clinical microsystem's outcomes.

The discussion in this chapter is based on the findings from our detailed qualitative study of twenty high-performing clinical microsystems and on listening to the people who staff these outstanding clinical units (Nelson et al., 2002). In this chapter we identify central success characteristics and focus on a case study to provide a real-world context for the guiding principles, useful insights, and practical methods that can help microsystem leaders improve their workforce and cultivate a positive working environment for their coworkers. We also provide staff comments that reveal the elements and the workings of the human resource value chain—that is, the comprehensive process to ensure the quality of the staff members—and of the success characteristics. By optimizing the work of each and every staff member and by promoting a culture where everyone matters, the microsystem can attain levels of performance not previously experienced.

Case Study: Staff Development at Massachusetts General Hospital Downtown Associates

This case study uses a fictional employee, medical assistant Anne Stirling, to examine the methods used by Massachusetts General Hospital Downtown Associates (MGH Downtown), a primary care practice in Boston, for developing its staff and improving staff members' work life.

The primary care clinic at MGH Downtown, located in the heart of the financial district of Boston, opened in April 1995. The clinic sees over 16,000 patients a year and has five physicians, one nurse, four medical assistants (MAs), and five patient services representatives (PSRs). MGH Downtown's efficient staff, technological resources, and innovative protocols and procedures allow it to operate at the cutting edge of modern medical care. A few of MGH Downtown's goals and aims follow:

- Treat each patient as a valued customer
- Provide the highest quality of health care support
- Improve constantly and forever the system of production and service to improve quality and productivity
- Provide the patients, physicians, and practice with a professionally trained support team that is empowered to exceed customer and patient service expectations

Anne Stirling, a recent graduate of a local, two-year college program for medical assistants, had applied for an MA position at MGH Downtown. She was prescreened by an outside agency to determine whether her personality, service background, and talents would be a good match for MGH Downtown. The agency discovered that Anne had worked for Ritz-Carlton, an organization known for its high-quality service delivery, before and during her educational program. On the basis of the prescreening, Anne was scheduled for an interview at MGH Downtown.

During the interview the MGH Downtown manager outlined the practice mission, philosophy, and culture and articulated its expectations—cross-functional activities, good teamwork, and patient-focused care. The manager reviewed the ninety-day orientation and training period and discussed the tasks and skills Anne would be required to perform. Once Anne's orientation was complete, the manager added, she would have the opportunity to attend additional skill laboratory and educational sessions to learn all aspects of overseeing a primary care practice. Anne was attracted to the MGH Downtown practice because a friend, also an MA, had worked there for five years and gained enough knowledge and experience to be hired as a practice manager in another health care organization.

Anne was hired, and both during and at the end of the orientation period, all staff participated in evaluating her on the basis of MGH Downtown's practice standards and expectations. Anne quickly experienced the importance of working in a team. The cross-training she received during her orientation allowed her to provide temporary assistance to a patient service representative (PSR) during a busy period of registration. Anne was able to use the electronic database and electronic medical record to assist a patient who was signing in and inquiring about a laboratory test result.

Communication within the practice was facilitated by e-mails and memos, which kept all staff and leaders informed on a timely basis regarding policies, procedures, ideas, and feedback. Anne attended the regular all-staff meetings to hear and discuss the latest updates and to review MGH Downtown's performance, including patient feedback and financial data. Anne believed that she was a valued member of the MGH Downtown team, and she was often encouraged to offer her ideas.

MGH Downtown encouraged Anne's continued development and growth through monthly dinner meetings, where a variety of topics was covered, and through the ongoing performance evaluation program (PEP). PEP reviews were conducted quarterly for the first twelve months of employment and then annually thereafter. The specified categories of performance were well defined, and Anne was able to set goals and target dates to advance her knowledge and skills.

After one year at MGH Downtown, Anne still found the work challenging and enjoyable; she was proud of the fact that she had contributed ideas (which were tested and used) to improve the flow of patients through the practice. Anne found that the variety of the roles she played and her opportunities to gain new knowledge and skills for managing a practice were challenging and enriching. She enjoyed caring for patients and experienced the benefit of working in an efficient, patient-centered, and team-oriented culture.

Comments

MGH Downtown's human resource processes are highly specified and predictable, from the initial contact with a candidate through each staff member's orientation, performance management, and professional development. Every employee knows what his or her role is, knows how to accomplish role-specific tasks, and is encouraged to develop in other professional areas. By specifying the desired behavior from day one and defining how everyone in the practice contributes to MGH Downtown's mission, the practice ensures that every staff associate knows what is expected and how to function in an environment that focuses on excellence in service and care.

The next section of this case describes the *links* in the human resource value chain—attraction, recruitment, and selection of staff; orientation; ongoing training and education; performance management; and information systems and electronic support to optimize staff roles—elements that can lead to an optimized, motivated, and satisfied workforce.

Recruitment, Attraction, and Selection of Staff

MGH Downtown uses an outside agency to prescreen support staff applicants on the basis of the practice's established service background and of personality profile attributes. Candidates are selected based on personality, talent, and skills. Intern and work-study programs have been established with local colleges and technical schools to produce potential candidates for employment. PSRs and medical services representatives are usually young and tend to work at MGH Downtown for two to four years. This relatively short time is not viewed as a negative. Rather, MGH Downtown leaders take pride in promising new staff the opportunity to be trained, on the basis of their individual interest and initiative, to run a "multimillion dollar" organization. MGH Downtown's reputation attracts young professionals because the organization makes it possible for all employees to obtain the skills and knowledge to achieve this goal.

Orientation of Staff

Preferred-vendor agreements have resulted in the use of standard equipment in several formal education programs, making them mirror the MGH Downtown setting; this results in more efficient training and orientation on equipment and software programs when MGH Downtown selects job applicants from these schools. Early on, a new employee receives materials about the practice, including a practice overview and information about the typical responsibilities of a PSR and MA, the customer service orientation, fiscal responsibility, the performance evaluation program, and continuous quality improvement. MGH Downtown attends to these key factors for a successful orientation:

- The orientation must be well defined; new employees must know what is expected of them in their role and within MGH Downtown's culture.
- New staff receive extensive training on the tasks and skills needed for their role.
- All staff evaluate the new employees, based on practice standards.
- All staff are encouraged to appreciate the individuality and interdependency of one another and to remain clear on the aim and objectives of the practice, as reflected in the expectation that staff will provide cross-coverage and contribute to each other's performance evaluations.

Ongoing Training and Education

Ongoing training and education are supported with skill labs, special education nights, and a rigorous performance evaluation program (PEP). During orientation everyone is cross-trained at each workstation in the practice (beyond the

TABLE 5.1. WORKSTATION ASSIGNMENTS AT MGH DOWNTOWN.

Patient Services	Clinical Services
In-processing	Phlebotomy
Referrals	Prescriptions
Future appointments	In-processing
Patient advocacy	Laboratory tests
Medical records	Diagnostic tests
Appointment confirmations	Inventory and supply ordering
	Examination room supply

individual person's specific role) so that staff members can assist or fill in for one another. After a year staff are given the opportunity to learn new administrative roles in addition to their daily workstation assignments (Table 5.1), which helps to fulfill MGH Downtown's promise that staff will be able to run a practice after five years of employment. One staff member commented: "We work as a team. We depend on each other. If the medical assistants are tied up, for instance, I can also take the patients back to the room, even though I technically work in patient services, and MAs can help if we're overloaded in the reception area."

Key elements that support cross-functioning include

- Standardized processes and protocols for each role that clearly define what is expected and how to accomplish various tasks for that role.
- Staff training at each workstation and continued on-the-job training.
- Skill labs in core subjects such as marketing, telecommunications, financial management, clinical procedures, customer management techniques, and information systems.
- Special education nights on topics such as variance reports and situations that fall outside normal protocol (for example, handling patient complaints).
- Regularly scheduled meetings to promote clear communication and to build esprit de corps. MAs meet once a month, PSRs meet twice a month, and an all-staff meeting is held once a month. Mutual respect between clinical and administrative staff is viewed as a critical success element for good staff inter-actions and relationships.
- Monthly dinner meetings to discuss any topics staff wish to discuss, such as hiring policies, salary administration, continuing education, and mentoring programs.
- The frequent use of memos by all staff members to communicate new ideas to make their work easier and smarter.

Performance Management

The PEP is an ongoing process used to evaluate the performance of all employees. The PEP is first completed during the ninety-day orientation and training period; it is then used quarterly for the first-year training period and after that is updated annually. A series of well-defined categories, such as practice knowledge, communication skills, and effective use of time, identify performance characteristics desired by MGH Downtown (Table 5.2).

The evaluator scores each staff member and provides specific observations and recommendations. When PEPs are started during the ninety-day orientation and training period, the clinical leader clearly states expectations and scores baseline performance. At the end of ninety days, MGH Downtown staff evaluate the new employee to see if the fit works from both new employee's and the organization's perspectives. PEPs are posted and list the evaluator and the person being evaluated; this offers all staff members an ongoing opportunity to offer advice and help one another grow in professional and personal skills, behaviors, and attitudes.

TABLE 5.2. EVALUATION SHEET FOR PERFORMANCE EVALUATION PROGRAM (PEP), SHOWING CATEGORIES AND DEFINITIONS.

Category	Definition	Value	Score	%
Attendance	• Punctuality • Paid-time-off requests provide coverage	25		
Attitude	• Self-motivation to accept and perform task • Willingness to help team members to learn new tasks and cross-train • Being a positive team player (willingness to assist team players wherever needed, with a positive attitude)	25		
Team effort	• Willingness to assist team members and physicians when needed • Consistently observe where help is needed by team members in both PSR and MSR workstations and assist where needed • Cross-train	25		
Patient care/ service	• Assisting patients in a professional manner • Observing any patient problems and offering assistance (requires special needs) • Assisting patients in several areas (referrals, acquiring phone numbers, explaining insurance benefits and coverage, providing directions to any site, and so on)	25		

(continued)

TABLE 5.2. (*Continued*)

Category	Definition	Value	Score	%
Effective use of time	• Perform all job responsibilities in a timely fashion • Observe where help is needed in all workstations • Assist team members where help is needed	20		
Practice knowledge	• Macrophilosophy • Utilization of systems • Cross-training • Provider protocols • Provider credentials • Which insurance plans are accepted at each site • Office knowledge (where supplies are kept, how to use all systems)	20		
Communication skills	• Proper phone etiquette (eight-ring policy, "May I place you on hold a moment?" "How may I assist you?") • Written memos • Proper chart documentation • Knowledge of physician protocols • Respond to voice mails in a timely fashion • Polite and courteous with patients • How constructive criticism is given and received	20		
Organizational skills	• Effective use of system organizers • Orderliness of office space • Ability to multitask	15		
Professional appearance	• Proper mannerisms, facial expressions, and communication skills with patients and doctors • Respect for patient confidentiality	15		
TOTAL		190		

Note: PSR = patient services representative; MSR = medical services representative.

Information Systems and Electronic Support to Optimize Staff Roles

Technology has been carefully designed into the practice and contributes to process flow and the success of the staff. All billing, scheduling, and medical record tasks are done electronically. The electronic medical record information system provides quick access to pertinent information, process guidelines, and clinical protocols. The information systems were designed to capture all aspects of a patient's contact with the practice, including voice mails, requests for prescription refills, orders for diagnostic tests, and requests for referrals and medical record information.

State-of-the-art software tracks patient messages and responses. A local software company customized an electronic system to support staff work and patient care, facilitating real-time documentation and tracking.

Tips from the Case Study

The MGH Downtown case study contains many useful tips and good practices that could be adapted to other practices. Here is a sampling of them:

Select for talent. For many positions it may be more important to hire people for their values, personality traits, and talents than for their skills and experience.

Consider that previous experience may not be needed. It may be beneficial to hire people without health care experience for support staff roles and to educate them using the practice values, goals, and expectations, in order to achieve high-quality, patient-centered care and services.

Cultivate your sources. Work *upstream* to identify potential sources of people to hire for your organization (for example, colleges and technical schools).

Offer comprehensive orientation and training. Develop an extensive orientation and training program to ensure that people understand essential knowledge, skills, work processes, and expectations. Horst Schulze (2003), founding president and COO of Ritz-Carlton, states that a new hire's first day of work is the most critical day; it should be used to set the expectations, values, and culture firmly in the new employee's mind.

Conduct 360-degree reviews. Involve all staff in the process of evaluating one another.

Hold town meetings. Hold monthly, all-staff meetings to foster good communications, relationships, esprit de corps, and continuous improvement.

The clinical microsystem staff we interviewed during our study of high-performing microsystems provided insight into the human resource value chain and clinical microsystem success characteristics. Table 5.3 shows both the human resource value chain elements and interviewees' statements that reflect on these elements. Table 5.4 lists microsystem success characteristic themes and quotes related comments from staff in the twenty microsystems. For example, one staff member commented: "This is the first place that I've ever worked where I could come to work and use my imagination in coming up with how to do something. Other places that I've worked, you have ideas, but . . . there's no point to bring it up because nobody is going to listen."

TABLE 5.3. STAFF COMMENTS THAT SUPPORT THE HUMAN RESOURCE VALUE CHAIN CONCEPT.

Value Chain Element	Comment
Attraction and recruitment	"We've managed to attract a group of individuals who are very excited and enthused about working here, and they've also kind of worked as group to make themselves better as individuals and as a group."
	"[In] job security and across the board our employees are on par with the external world in terms of reimbursement, but the quality of life and hours worked here [are] much better. For nurses we have a waiting list here; in the rest of the region there is a nursing shortage, but here we have a waiting line."
Selection	. . ."[We can] go with someone who does not have health care experience, someone that is open. It's better to work with them; we prefer to train them ourselves. We are looking for people that are interested, genuine, and enthusiastic; the rest we can train."
	. . . "I'd rather have the right fit, a person with the right values and philosophy. We can train them on all the skills later while they are here."
	"I think part of [selection] has to do with even the interviewing and recruitment staff, because some people just aren't the right ones to hire. And I think that you have to look at it and try to get a sense of what [people's] values are in the hiring and recruitment process. Because I don't think [individuals are] going to change just because they come to work at your place."
	"I look for an entrepreneur . . . someone who's a health care person, been doing this for a while, but has always wanted to own their own business or create that ideal workplace [where] everybody feels good when they come in."
Orientation of staff	"Once you educate staff as to requirements of their position, once you train them to the standards that you expect, once those standards are understood, you leave them alone. . . . By doing that, you show them that you have confidence in them, that you trust them to do the job. We focus a lot on training, so that the people in the practice–so that most of the people–are functioning at a higher level than they would otherwise."
	. . ."If the tech is busy . . . the charge nurse and the tech can kind of work together . . . one does one thing, the other does the other. . . . Everyone goes through the same orientation for both jobs and then they have a primary job code and a secondary job code to do those things."

(continued)

TABLE 5.3. STAFF COMMENTS THAT SUPPORT THE HUMAN RESOURCE VALUE CHAIN CONCEPT. (*Continued*)

Value Chain Element	Comment
Ongoing training and education	. . ."It's new and exciting here and it feels like you had an opportunity to grow. It feels like there's always something new coming up and, boy, if I want to, I can be part of it. I can help create it and craft it."
	"You can actually come here at entry level and, if you're very dedicated to your work and you like doing what you're doing, you can actually grow. And there are so many different departments here . . . that you would not run out of spaces [for] growing."
	. . . "They did the retraining and then most of our health assistants said, three weeks down the road, 'You know, my job is more interesting now. It's not as boring as it was before, because I can do more things.' . . . The job became more interesting–I really didn't work any harder but, boy, it was a lot more interesting. I got bored just doing two or three things all day long, with blood pressures and putting the chart here and moving it there. . . . We trained all our health assistants to draw blood."
Performance management	"Goals liberate the potential of people. There is so much potential out there that the quiet employee is as valuable as the extrovert. . . . You tap into people and find out what drives them and what moves them."
	"No one is here doing it for the money. No. None of us are. A paycheck is nice, but we're doing it for something bigger than that, and sometimes the public acknowledgment and support of that is very important."
	"We try to send people little things . . . like, if somebody's name gets mentioned in a satisfaction survey, we send them a gift certificate or something that says, you know, you're a star. You got recognized. . . . [We are] making people feel important."
Information systems and electronic support to optimize staff roles	"We're information oriented. We use computers and technology to help us in our work. We try to use it to our advantage and make things more effective."
	"I have so many things available; I am going to graduate school, working towards a PhD, doing research. I am in an environment where it is cool to do that and it is okay to do that."
	"This is the first time in many, many years that I've worked in an environment where you can see a potential for growth."

Principles

A deeper analysis of the MGH Downtown case study and findings from the nineteen other high-performing microsystems suggests four basic principles.

Mission, Vision, Principles (MVPs). Start by anchoring MVPs in your practice. Make the mission, vision, and guiding principles clear to each person; then specify

TABLE 5.4. STAFF COMMENTS THAT SUPPORT SUCCESS CHARACTERISTICS.

Success Characteristic Theme	Comment
Leadership	"The system has to offer the opportunity from all levels and you have to have the vision that you are building something that will enable those within the system to be successful in any way they want to be."
	"The managers seem to really take charge. . . . They are constantly trying to involve themselves with the staff and finding out what they need to better do their job on a daily basis."
	"The MD leader has always been supportive in anything I ever wanted to do. He has enabled me and empowered me to be able to do what I wanted to learn how to do and to do it well."
Staff	"I've always found that if people are part of the planning and having input into it and feel like they have ownership of it, they will try to make it succeed."
	. . . "[We] let people have input. . . . They all feel that their input counts and they can effect change within the organization that needs to occur. We don't want employees sitting around here just punching a time clock, putting in their eight hours and going home. We want employees to point out problems, point out inefficiencies, make suggestions. For the most part, people are pretty good at doing that."
	"It just seems like the staff here, from the doctors down to the custodians, everyone is very closely involved, and although this is a very large institution, I often feel like when I come upstairs here to this floor that this is our little sector, our own little part of the world–what I usually refer to as a finely tuned machine. It just seems like everything has its order and everything is very organized and the group as a whole is quite cohesive."
	. . . "[The] team support that we have within each other, that's real important. We are able to monitor each other and support each other as a unit; therefore we can go out and do what we need to do for these families."
	"People anticipate what each person is doing and respect each other. You know that people will be there for you when you need them."
	"What the other person sitting next to you does is so important to . . . how your day turns out."
	"Trust each other and be able to depend on each other when needed. Being a team, a true team, we collaborate and work together every day all the time."

(continued)

TABLE 5.4. STAFF COMMENTS THAT SUPPORT SUCCESS CHARACTERISTICS. (*Continued*)

Success Characteristic Theme	Comment
Patients	"[We have a] . . . connection to the community. . . . Outreach programs into the community are all over the place—and a philosophy to strengthen community, not just make the community dependent upon us."
Performance	"We are constantly trying to improve our performances and we are looking at any small changes in how we do things." "We have an atmosphere of constantly looking for ways to improve and make ourselves better. We do a lot of tests here where we trial something for a while. If it works we carry it out."
Information and information technology	"There is no way to interact without the computer for us. I can't make an appointment, I can't connect you, we are dependent on the computers, but the power and perks of having them is just tremendous."

the work role and show how the work of the individual contributes to the mission. Work to create a clear vision of excellence (doing the right things right) that staff members can use to navigate the correct path forward in their own work. Establish and anchor authentic guiding principles that reflect the core values and desired behaviors that are part of the bedrock for your local microsystem culture. Strive to connect the individual staff member with the mission and the vision and with core values to give him or her that deep sense of meaning that is capable of uniting the head, the hands, and the heart.

Climate. Create a positive, even joyful, working climate. Develop a social environment for working that exemplifies respect, interdependency, service, learning, growth, and joy in the work. Respect one another and what each one contributes individually to meet patients' needs. The working climate should generate patterns of respect—staff for other staff, staff for patients, staff for families—that enable all staff to handle turbulent times and situations effectively and empathically.

Value Chain. Refine your human resource value chain; it should be capable of attracting, selecting, orienting, and developing staff who see the vision and live the mission in their daily work. Align the work role with the individual's talents, education, and training. The aim is to enable everyone to play at the top of his or her game and to make the best use of his or her knowledge and skills. Learning is an essential part of the value chain and should be part of the work of the microsystem. External learning opportunities—for both personal and professional growth—can be used to foster lifelong learning that rebounds to improve people's work and their home microsystem. The goal is to enhance knowledge, skills, and attitudes that contribute to personal growth, professional development, career advancement, and an increasing capacity to provide needed services to patients.

Two Jobs. Make sure everyone knows that he or she has two jobs; staff members have to do their work and to improve their work (Tucker, Edmondson, & Spear, 2001). Providing high-quality care efficiently requires every person to do his or her work well all the time. Finishing today work that was started yesterday will not improve the system. Therefore it is important to create a community that has the ability to do today's work today and the ability to improve everyday work.

This list of principles could be expanded or contracted. It may be useful to consider to what extent individual clinical microsystems have patterns of practice, belief, sentiment, and performance that are in accord with these principles.

Helpful Resources and Methods

How does a clinical microsystem develop into a highly productive and satisfying work environment? How does one engage the head, the hands, and the heart of those involved in the delivery of exceptional health care? We recommend gaining knowledge of the clinical microsystem workplace and its individual staff and then planning action to improve the state of the workplace and its staff. Part Two of this book presents methods and tools for generating this knowledge.

Gaining Knowledge. It is important to understand the workplace's current state and staff capability before initiating efforts to improve them. Organizations frequently conduct staff satisfaction or morale surveys that can elucidate the current state of what it "feels like" to work in a particular clinical microsystem. For example, a revealing item in one tool, the Clinical Microsystem Short Staff Survey (Figure 5.1), asks staff, "How easy is it to ask anyone a question about the way we care for patients?" (Godfrey, Nelson, & Batalden, 2002). This question taps an important aspect of relationships in the microsystem; answers to it reveal whether the hierarchy within which physicians, associate providers, nurses, and secretaries interact inhibits or promotes inquiry among staff. Creating a joyful work environment starts with a basic understanding of staff perceptions of the organization. When clinical microsystems use a tool like this, every staff member should complete the survey, anonymously if desired, and a box should be provided where staff can

FIGURE 5.1. CLINICAL MICROSYSTEM SHORT STAFF SURVEY.

Clinical Microsystem Staff Survey   Choose only one response for items 1, 2, 3, and 4.

1. How stressful would you say it is to work in this practice?

☐ Very stressful   ☐ A little stressful

☐ Somewhat stressful   ☐ Not stressful

2. How would you rate other people's morale and their attitudes about working here?

☐ Excellent   ☐ Good   ☐ Poor

☐ Very good   ☐ Fair

3. I would recommend this practice as a great place to work.

☐ Strongly agree   ☐ Disagree

☐ Agree   ☐ Strongly disagree

4. How easy is it to ask anyone a question about the way we care for patients?

☐ Very easy   ☐ Difficult

☐ Easy   ☐ Very difficult

5. What would make this practice better for patients?

_____

_____

6. What would make this practice better for those who work here?

_____

_____

Source: Adapted from Godfrey et al., 2002.

drop off completed surveys. Many microsystems comfortable with electronics use Internet-based survey tools to conduct the same survey and eliminate the hard-copy process. For a longer version of this survey, see the Appendix, Figure A.7.

Another survey, the Personal Skills Assessment, can be used to help identify specific knowledge and skills an individual may need to perform better in a particular clinical microsystem (Godfrey et al., 2002). An example of this assessment is available in the Appendix, Figure A.8. Table 5.5 displays some examples of the personal skills a microsystem might assess. This survey also helps microsystems to

TABLE 5.5. EXAMPLES OF SKILLS ADDRESSED IN A PERSONAL SKILLS ASSESSMENT.

Personal Skills	Example
Technical skills	Capabilities with e-mail, dictation, handheld computer, fax, copier, phone system, and voice mail
Clinical information system skills	Capabilities with scheduling, test results, problem lists, direct entry, and template use
Meeting and interpersonal skills	Capabilities in meeting management: for example, using agendas with a clear aim and timed agenda items, understanding roles that lead to productive meetings, using brainstorming and multi-voting
Improvement skills and knowledge; process-mapping skills	Ability to use plan-do-study-act (PDSA) worksheets, fishbone (cause and effect) diagrams, and trend and control charts

Source: Adapted from Godfrey et al., 2002.

identify people who excel at certain skills and to whom others might turn for assistance. Managers can use survey results to facilitate discussion with individuals as they build their personal development plans.

Planning Action. Buckingham and Coffman (1999) have summarized extensive research on the things managers do to create outstanding workplaces, ones that achieve high levels of customer satisfaction, job satisfaction, productivity, and profitability. They contend that great managers create the conditions needed to generate superior performance. They suggest that managers need to focus on these basic tasks:

- Select for talent.
- Define the right outcomes.
- Focus on the strengths of individuals rather than the weaknesses.
- Find the right fit for individuals, based on their talent.

A staff member of a large, multispecialty health system recently said: "I used to love to come to work; I now come to pay my bills." This is a sad commentary: it suggests a rupture between one's personal values and one's work. There are many books and programs that can be used to involve staff and brighten the workplace (see, for example, Johnson, 2003; Johnson & Blanchard, 1998; Lundin, Paul, & Christenson, 2000; Roberts & Sergesketter, 1993).

Observations of high-performing clinical microsystems lead to these suggestions for local leaders:

- Know every individual in the clinical microsystem, and spend time to develop each person's potential.
- Set expectations and develop staff to encourage them to "be the best they can be" on the basis of education, training, talent, and licensure.
- Identify and design roles to meet patient and family needs (information to support this task comes from a study of the microsystem's 5 P's—*purpose, patients, professionals, processes,* and *patterns,* as described in Chapters Six and Thirteen) (Godfrey et al., 2003).
- Hold regular all-staff meetings, inviting everyone's participation. Use timed agendas with clear aims, and create a meeting environment that promotes learning and improving together.
- Actively develop supervisors and managers. Frequently the best and brightest physicians, nurses, and staff are promoted to leadership positions without leadership education. Consider studying "great" managers (Buckingham & Coffman, 1999).
- Try to develop coleaders in microsystems. Virtually all the best microsystems that we have studied enjoyed *shared leadership,* such as a physician leader who partnered with a nursing leader and or an administrative leader. These coleaders worked together to set expectations and hold staff accountable.

Conclusion

Some health care settings enjoy high morale, high quality, and high productivity, but all too often this is not the case. Many clinical microsystems suffer from high staff turnover, high absenteeism, and poor morale. The case study of developing staff and improving their work life at MGH Downtown offers good examples of ways to successfully activate staff and create a positive and dynamic workplace. Focusing on the elements of the human resource value chain can transform hiring practices into selection processes that match the organization's vision, goals, and values. Gaining insight into the current state of the staff and their work life is essential to developing a more engaging workplace that is characterized by high-performing, creative, and fully activated staff.

References

Baldrige National Quality Program. (2006). *Health Care Criteria for Performance Excellence.* Retrieved September 1, 2006, from http://www.quality.nist.gov./PDF_files/ 2006_HealthCare_Criteria.pdf.

Buckingham, M., & Coffman, C. (1999). *First, break all the rules: What the world's greatest managers do differently.* New York: Simon & Schuster.

Gelinas, L., & Bohlen, C. (2002). *Tomorrow's workforce: A strategic approach.* Irving, TX: VHA.

Godfrey, M. M., Nelson, E. C., & Batalden, P. B. (2002). *Assessing your practice workbook* (rev. ed.). Hanover, NH: Dartmouth College.

Godfrey, M. M., Nelson, E. C., Wasson, J. H., Mohr, J. J., & Batalden, P. B. (2003). Microsystems in health care: Part 3. Planning patient-centered services. *Joint Commission Journal on Quality and Safety, 29*(4), 159–170.

Johnson, S. (2003). *The present: The gift that makes you happy and successful at work and in life.* New York: Doubleday.

Johnson, S., & Blanchard, K. H. (1998). *Who moved my cheese? An amazing way to deal with change in your work and in your life.* New York: Putnam.

Joint Commission on Accreditation of Healthcare Organizations. (2002). *Healthcare at the crossroads: Strategies for addressing the evolving nursing crisis.* Retrieved August 31, 2006, from http://www.aacn.nche.edu/Media/pdf/JCAHO8-02.pdf.

Lundin, S. C., Paul, H., & Christenson, P. (2000). *Fish: A remarkable way to boost morale and improve results.* New York: Hyperion.

Nelson, E. C., Batalden, P. B., Huber, T. P., Mohr, J. J., Godfrey, M. M., Headrick, L. A., et al. (2002). Microsystems in health care: Part 1. Learning from high-performing front-line clinical units. *Joint Commission Journal on Quality Improvement, 28*(9), 472–493.

Roberts, H. V., & Sergesketter, B. F. (1993). *Quality is personal: A foundation for total quality management.* New York: Free Press.

Schulze, H. (2003, March 1). *Strategic leadership: Creating a passion for excellence.* Paper presented at the 2003 national conference of the American Medical Group Association, Hollywood, FL.

Tucker, A., Edmondson, A., & Spear, S. (2001, July 30). Why your organization isn't learning all it should. *HBS Working knowledge.* Retrieved November 8, 2005, from http://hbswk.hbs.edu/ archive/2397.html.

CHAPTER SIX

PLANNING PATIENT-CENTERED SERVICES

Marjorie M. Godfrey, Eugene C. Nelson, John H. Wasson, Julie K. Johnson, Paul B. Batalden

Chapter Summary

Background. Strategic focus on clinical microsystems—the small, functional, frontline units that provide most health care to most people—is essential to designing the most efficient, patient-centered services. The starting place for designing or redesigning clinical microsystems is to evaluate the 5 P's: the *purpose* of the microsystem, the *patient* subpopulations that are served by the microsystem, the *professionals* who work together in the microsystem, the *processes* the microsystem uses to provide services, and the *patterns* that characterize the microsystem's functioning.

Case study. The case study offered is an innovative primary care practice in Bangor, Maine, under the leadership of Charlie Burger, and exemplifies the process and outcome of providing patient-centered care based on detailed deep knowledge of its patient populations, optimization of professional roles, and processes through the use of information and information technology and study of patterns of outcomes, variation, and trends in services and care.

A developmental Journey. A clinical microsystem's developmental journey starts with assessment and diagnosis. Methods and tools have been developed for microsystem leaders and staff to use to assess the 5 P's in their microsystems and to design tests of change for improvement and innovation.

The next part of the journey is putting it all together. Once it has the results of the assessment, and diagnosis, a microsystem can help itself improve the things that need to be done better. The process of planning services is designed to improve the microsystem's ability to match the needs of distinct patient subpopulations with the services available to meet those needs, decrease unnecessary variation, facilitate informed decision making, promote efficiency by continuously removing waste and rework, create processes and systems that support staff, and design smooth, effective, and safe patient care services that lead to measurably improved patient outcomes.

Conclusion. The design of services leads to critical analysis of the resources needed for the right person to deliver the right care, in the right way, at the right time.

In this chapter we explore the challenge of gaining deeper knowledge of the 5 P's—the purpose, patients, professionals, processes, and patterns—of clinical microsystems. We identify the specific activities, information, and knowledge needed to design and plan patient-centered services and patient-centered care that meet or exceed patient expectations while also improving the work environment for staff.

The phrase *planning patient-centered services* refers to the analysis of the inner workings—the architecture and flow (or the *anatomy* and *physiology*)—of the microsystem for the purpose of making services available that best meet the needs of the distinct subpopulations served by that clinical unit. In contrast the phrase *planning patient-centered care* refers—in the context of a specific subpopulation—to the individualization of those services (whether offered by the microsystem itself or by other microsystems in the larger organization or the community) to best meet the changing needs of individual patients as their conditions, self-management skills, and desires change over time. By way of analogy we can say that to plan services is to plan the menu for prospective guests, whereas to plan care is to combine and deliver the menu offerings in a manner that meets the unique tastes and needs of each individual guest who requires service. The patient response that "they give me exactly what I want and need exactly when I want and need it" (Institute for Healthcare Improvement, 2000) will not be heard in any real-world clinical setting unless its services have to a large extent been designed to be there for the patient on demand. This chapter focuses on planning patient-centered services.

Planning Patient-Centered Services and the 5 P's

The planning of patient-centered services requires knowledge of (1) the needs of the major patient subpopulations served by the clinical microsystem, (2) the ways the people in the microsystem interact with one another, and (3) the ways the people in the microsystem interact with the processes that unfold to produce critical outcomes. This knowledge comes from both formal analysis and tacit understanding of the clinical unit's structure, its patients, its processes, and its daily patterns of work and interaction.

When planning services for their patients, members of the microsystem benefit by mastering the 5P's:

- *Know your purpose.* Answer these questions: What is our aim? What do we actually intend to *make*? As we think of the people we care for and what we are trying to create, what is our intention? Our system exists to _____. Remember that this purpose exists within the context of the population the microsystem seeks to serve.
- *Know your patients.* Answer these questions: Whom are we caring for? Are there subpopulations we could plan services for differently? What are the most common patient diagnoses and conditions in our practice? What other microsystems support what we do to meet patients' needs? How satisfied are patients with our microsystem?
- *Know your professionals.* Answer these questions: Who provides patient care, and who are the people supporting the clinical careteam? What skills and talents do staff members need to provide the right service and care at the right time? What is the morale of our team? What is the role of information technology as a team member?
- *Know your processes.* Answer these questions: How do we deliver care and services to meet our patients' needs? Who does what in our microsystem? Do our hours of operation match the needs of our patients? What are our core and supporting processes? How does technology support our processes? How do we learn from failures or near misses?
- *Know your patterns.* Answer these questions: What are the health outcomes of our patients? What are the costs of care? How do we interact within our microsystem? What are the regularly recurring associated or sequential work activities? What does it feel like to work here? What are the costs in our microsystem? Do information systems provide data and information in a timely way to inform us about the impact of our services? How do we stay mindful of the possibility of our efforts failing?

When members of a clinical microsystem work together to gain information about their purpose, patients, professionals, processes, and patterns, they acquire knowledge that can be used to make long-lasting improvements in the clinical microsystem.

Case Study: Planning Services for Subpopulations of Patients to Best Provide Care for Individual Patients

One clinical microsystem, Evergreen Woods, a primary care practice that is part of Norumbega Medical in Bangor, Maine, has been evolving for more than a decade to plan for the future by designing services that are there on demand to provide outstanding care for individual patients when they need it.

A Typical Visit

When a patient calls the office with a medical problem, a patient representative triages him or her using the Triage Coupler. This software program is driven by protocols that can handle a broad spectrum of problems, from the common cold to complex chest pain, and services, such as standardized protocols to help people prepare for overseas travel and providing prescription refills. If the patient needs to be seen, prompts suggest questions to ask and diagnostic tests that might be required before the patient comes to the office. Sometimes the patient can be provided with a standard treatment and does not need to make an office visit. This information system supports highly trained individuals, who do not have medical degrees, in safely and competently making direct decisions about clinical care at the point of contact with the patient. If a patient questions the advice being given, then an appointment can be booked.

A patient with an appointment is asked to arrive at the office thirty minutes before the appointment time to complete a survey of his or her physical and mental health status, medical history, presenting problems, and current functioning. Medical assistants escort the patient to the exam room, where they use Problem-Knowledge Couplers (PKCs) to verify patient history, to enter current assessment data in the medical record, and to enter any available test results.

The Problem-Knowledge Coupler is software that provides guidance from an extensive medical database that is customized to individual patients based on their unique patient information. The patient information is matched to the latest medical information to result in patient-specific advice, including potential causes, treatments, and management strategies (see www.pkc.org).

This information allows the physician or nurse practitioner to spend more time with the patient on unique issues, shared medical decision making, and patient education. The provider reviews the findings for possible diagnoses and potential care options. To finish the appointment the patient is given printed information about his or her condition, as well as a copy of the visit note that is stored in the patient's electronic medical record.

Evergreen Woods collects extensive data on patient demand for office visits. These data, which include trend charts by session, day of week, and month of year, allow the staff to deploy the practice's resources to match demand. Evergreen Woods uses continuous feed-forward information and planned feedback systems (Nelson et al., 2003), as well as extensive databases, to aid planning and improvement. The practice staff use a *data wall,* posted information that reports performance measures, to monitor progress for the clinical team and to identify improvement ideas and actions (Nelson, Splaine, Batalden, & Plume, 1998).

Evergreen Woods's pattern of staff interaction includes weekly team meetings, frequent e-mail communications, and many off-hour get-togethers. Continuous training is conducted to train every member on effective interpersonal communication skills. Additional facts that are key elements in the success of Evergreen Woods, along with their relationship to the 5 P's, are shown in Table 6.1.

Comments

Evergreen Woods is an exemplary model of office efficiency and advanced design. Although the practice has invested heavily in technology, most clinical settings— be they rural, urban, academic, inpatient, or outpatient—can learn and adapt the following tips:

Integrate data into the flow of work to support the work. Data collection is integrated into the design of patient care and operations. There are methods and ways to achieve similar results and tracking without advanced information technology. Decision making without data is not acceptable in this clinical environment.

Enable all staff to make the most of their talent, training, and skills. Optimization of staff roles, through detailed training and education of each individual, leads to increased staff abilities to cross-cover for one another, engage in improvement work, and feel a sense of accomplishment and self-worth on a daily basis.

Provide strong leadership. The leader's example and vision guide the common goals and values of the group.

The next section builds on this case study and explores methods and tools that can be used to promote *guided discovery* for staff to gain knowledge about the population they serve, the processes for providing services, and the different patterns that (1) spin off good or bad outcomes for patients and (2) engender a generative or a toxic work environment for staff.

TABLE 6.1. EVERGREEN WOODS'S ADDITIONAL SUCCESS ELEMENTS AND THEIR LINKS TO THE 5 P'S.

Key Elements of Success	Know Your Purpose	Know Your Patients	Know Your Professionals	Know Your Process	Know Your Patterns
Computer terminals are placed in every room to support scheduling, record keeping, telephone triage, shared decision making, and patient education.		X		X	X
Staff use e-mail to communicate among themselves. There is open discussion about their shared work life, including improvement opportunities, difficult communications, conflicts, and celebrations of group successes.	X		X		X
Patients and providers use e-mail to communicate about medical problems, medication refills, referrals, test results, and other matters.		X	X	X	X
Patients complete a health status survey.		X			X
Specially trained patient service representatives triage patients using the Triage Coupler to support decision making.			X	X	
Staff training is ongoing and rigorously based on performance and competency. Computer tools coupled with this training allow all staff to function at an advanced level with high morale and low turnover.			X	X	
After six to twelve months with the practice, employees enroll in a total quality management course at the local community college.			X	X	X
All staff are encouraged to use a standardized form to suggest practice improvements. This form, based on the plan-do-study-act (PDSA) format, is				X	X

(continued)

TABLE 6.1. EVERGREEN WOODS'S ADDITIONAL SUCCESS ELEMENTS AND THEIR LINKS TO THE 5 P'S. (*Continued*)

Key Elements of Success	Know Your Purpose	Know Your Patients	Know Your Professionals	Know Your Process	Know Your Patterns
designed to help the creation of a disciplined community of scientists. The form is circulated to all staff for input prior to the weekly staff meeting, where final revisions and decisions are made.					
The staff meet weekly to evaluate practice performance. They also attend a yearly off-site meeting for the purpose of team building.			X	X	X
Staff hold daily *huddles* to evaluate the prior day, the current day, and the future.				X	X
Problem-Knowledge Couplers (PKCs) *couple* patient-specific data with current biomedical knowledge to support evidence-based practice in routine care. The *couplers* are updated at 6-month intervals.			X	X	
The practice has an extensive *data wall* that is used daily to track numerous indicators such as Health Plan Employer Data and Information Set (HEDIS) technical quality metrics (Nelson, Splaine, Batalden, & Plume, 1998).		X		X	X
The data wall also displays statistical process control charts and measures of process and clinical outcomes as essential measures to manage and improve the practice (Langley, Nolan, Norman, Provost, & Nolan, 1996).				X	X
The electronic medical record alerts staff to unique needs of patient sub-populations, such as the diabetic population, and tracks essential interventions that benefit those populations.		X	X	X	X

A Developmental Journey: Beginning to Assess, Understand, and Improve a Clinical Microsystem

Build knowledge of the core processes and outcomes of your microsystem to foster the continual improvement and innovation necessary to meet and exceed patient needs (Nelson, Batalden, Mohr, & Plume, 1998).

Getting Started: Diagnosing and Treating a Clinical Microsystem

Methods and tools have been developed for microsystem leaders and staff to use (or to adapt to local circumstances) to assess their microsystems and design tests of change for improvement and innovation. The aim is to increase each microsystem's capacity to better realize its potential and to better relate to other microsystems that come together with it to form the service continuum.

Every person and microsystem is unique. The tools and questions found in the second part of this book and the Appendix (and at http://www.clinicalmicrosystem.org) are intended to provide guidance and provoke thinking about essential information that can improve a microsystem. The "Primary Care Workbook" in the Appendix at the end of this book provides a framework for diagnosing the 5 P's of a microsystem—the purpose, patients, professionals, processes, and patterns—which are described in the following sections. Workbooks for other types of microsystems are available at http://www.clinicalmicrosystem.org.

Know Your Purpose. Being clear about your aim guides the relationship between the microsystem's work processes and the population's need. The purpose describes the microsystem's orientation—its *true north*—for improvement and development of the work processes and systems.

Know Your Patients. Be relentless in the pursuit of patient knowledge—what patients need, what they get, and how they fare. For almost one hundred years, from Ernest A. Codman (1914/1996) to John E. Wennberg (Wennberg, Freeman, Shelton, & Bubolz, 1989), it has been understood that most practitioners have lacked data on the vital details of the patient populations they cared for. Further, they knew even less about distinct subpopulations of patients, whose care can now be planned proactively. Key to planning services is knowledge of the subpopulations served. Table 6.2 offers examples of some of the data that clinical microsystems should know about the patients they serve.

Gaining this information has helped practice members explore new ways to improve their delivery system. Thedacare, based in Kimberly, Wisconsin, learned that approximately 3 percent of the patients in its health plan were diabetic. In

TABLE 6.2. KNOW THE P'S FOR CLINICAL MICROSYSTEMS ACROSS THE HEALTH CONTINUUM.

Primary Care

Patients
- Age distribution and % of females?
- Patient population with seasonal fluctuations?
- Most frequent diagnoses?
- Frequent users of services?
- How satisfied are our patients with our services?

Professionals
- Who are the people in our clinical microsystem?
- What roles and functions do we currently have, and how do they relate to our main aim or purpose?
- What information technology do we depend on to support care?
- Where do our staff spend their time (for example: teaching or outreach)?
- What resources do we have available daily to provide patient care?
- What is the morale of our staff?
- Are health profession students part of our team?

Processes
- Who are our supporting departments?
- What are our key supporting processes?
- What is our interdependence (linkages) with other microsystems?
- What is our dependence on our macrosystem?
- What is our cycle time?
- Are staff knowledgeable about our key processes?
- What is our demand?
- What are our indirect patient pulls?

Patterns
- What are our disease-specific health outcomes?
- What is the number of out-of-practice visits?
- What is our margin after costs?
- What is the number of encounters per year?

Inpatient Care

Patients
- Age distribution and % of females?
- Patient population with seasonal fluctuations?
- Most frequent diagnoses?
- Frequent users of services?
- How satisfied are our patients with our services?

Professionals
- Who are the people in our clinical microsystem?
- What roles and functions do we currently have, and how do they relate to our main aim or purpose?
- What information technology do we depend on to support care?
- Where do our staff spend their time?
- What resources do we have available daily to provide patient care?
- What is the morale of our staff?
- Are health profession students part of our team?

Processes
- Who are our supporting departments?
- What are our key supporting processes?
- What is our interdependence (linkages) with other microsystems?
- What is our dependence on our macrosystem?

Patterns
- What are our census numbers by hour, day, and week, and what is the variation?
- What is the number of discharges per day, per week, per month, and what is the variation?
- What is the average length of stay?

Home Health Care

Patients
- Age distribution and % of females?
- Patient population with seasonal fluctuations?
- Most frequent diagnoses?
- Frequent users of services?
- How satisfied are our patients with our services?

Professionals
- Who are the people in our clinical microsystem?
- Where do our staff spend their time (for example: homes, driving, public transportation)?
- What is the morale of our staff?
- Are health profession students part of our team?

Processes
- Who are our supporting departments?
- What are our key supporting processes?
- What is our interdependence (linkages) with other microsystems?
- What is our dependence on our macrosystem?

Patterns
- What are our census numbers by hour, day, and week, and what is the variation?
- What is the number of discharges per day, per week, per month, and what is the variation?
- What is the average length of stay?

Nursing Home Care

Patients
- Age distribution and % of females?
- Patient population with seasonal fluctuations?
- Most frequent diagnoses?
- Frequent users of services?
- How satisfied are our patients with our services?

Professionals
- Who are the people in our clinical microsystem?
- What roles and functions do we currently have, and how do they relate to our main aim or purpose?
- What information technology do we depend on to support care?
- Where do our staff spend their time?
- What resources do we have available daily to provide patient care?
- What is the morale of our staff?
- Are health profession students part of our team?

Processes
- Who are our supporting departments?
- What are our key supporting processes?
- What is our interdependence (linkages) with other microsystems?
- What is our dependence on our macrosystem?

Patterns
- What are our census numbers by hour, day, and week, and what is the variation?
- What is the number of discharges per day, per week, per month, and what is the variation?
- What is the average length of stay?

Specialty Care

Patients
- What are our most frequently referred patient types?
- What % of patients referred require the special skills and knowledge of our specialty?
- Number of patients returned to referring providers per week?

Professionals
- Who are the people in our clinical microsystem?
- What roles and functions do we currently have, and how do they relate to our main aim or purpose?
- What information technology do we depend on to support care?
- Where do our staff spend their time?
- What resources do we have available daily to provide patient care?
- What is the morale of our staff?
- Are health profession students part of our team?

Processes
- What is the cycle time for usual episode of care?
- Who are our supporting departments?
- What are our key supporting processes?
- What is our interdependence (linkages) with other microsystems?
- What is our dependence on our macrosystem?

Patterns
- Who are the most frequent referring providers?
- What is the satisfaction rating of our referring providers?
- What are the services of satisfaction and of dissatisfaction for our referring providers?

partnership with the health plan, Thedacare created a registry to track evidence-based interventions. Group visits evolved through a primary care practice exploring innovative care models. The outcomes for patients in the group visits improved significantly. For example, glycosylated hemoglobin (HbA1c) levels <8 improved by 4 percent, low-density lipoprotein (LDL) levels <130 mg/dl improved 32 percent, and the overall quality of care being rated by patients as "excellent" improved 14 percent (Thedacare Diabetes Cooperative, 2000). The reason for these improvements is that the clinical microsystem made an innovation in service delivery; it moved from sole reliance on one type of service (one-on-one visits with a physician) to offering a second type of service (group visits with standardized tracking and interventions customized to the individual patient's needs and wishes) that complemented the traditional one-on-one visit.

Clinical microsystems need to be acutely aware of how patients perceive the care they receive. When patient satisfaction surveys are conducted, the results are often sent back to microsystems many months after the surveyed set of patients was seen; this makes it difficult to take timely action to improve services. A brief, point-of-service patient satisfaction survey, such as that found in Figure A.3 (in the Appendix of this book) and in Godfrey, Nelson, and Batalden (2005), can be used to provide timely, patient-based feedback.

Know Your Professionals. Many members of clinical microsystems do not see their own work and the roles and functions of others as interdependent, as the collaborative work of a group of professionals with a shared aim and a system for providing care to distinct subpopulations of patients. What are the morale and the level of stress in your clinical setting? What is the turnover rate? Is the right person doing the right thing at the right time for patient care? Is there an appropriate match between function and roles, based on talent, education, training, and licensure? What are the roles in care and services occurring apart from the visit? The staff in the clinical microsystem make or break the processes of service delivery. Without them, good system functionality cannot exist. Managing staff as vital resources, basing decisions on detailed data on patients' needs and demand for services, is essential.

Know Your Processes. Many health professionals are *process illiterate* (Batalden & Stoltz, 1994). The best way to eliminate process illiteracy is to use flowcharting or process mapping. How much time does it take for patients to receive services? How much undesirable variation in processes exists? How much waste and rework occurs, making the day more frustrating? How do core and supporting processes get accomplished? Are they done in the same way by every member of the team? Are patients assessed in a standard way? Do clinical support staff perform activities that anticipate the arrival of patients? How does technology support work flow and care delivery (also see Table 6.2)?

Variation in clinical services is often related to a physician's preference about the way things are done rather than to a decision about the best process for the patient. Table 6.3 provides an assessment tool to help clinical microsystems evaluate the services they provide. All staff members (1) complete the assessment tool, (2) determine which process to improve (the highest-ranked problem process), and (3) begin to test changes by modifying the flowchart of the current process using the scientific improvement method to reach hoped-for improvement (also see the following box).

Analysis and Improvement of Processes

A general internal medicine practice analyzed current processes and identified improvements that could lead to better efficiencies and reductions in waste. Every member of the practice—including physicians, nurse practitioners, nurses, and secretaries—completed the Practice Core and Supporting Processes Assessment (Table 6.3). This revealed that the diagnostic test reporting process needed to be improved by shortening the time taken to report results to providers and patients. After flowcharting the process—which revealed rework, waste, delay, and long cycle times—the group brainstormed and then rank-ordered improvement ideas. It decided to test the idea of holding a *huddle* at the beginning of each day to review diagnostic test results and to specify actions to take. The aim was to eliminate extra phone calls from the patients and delays in taking action due to waiting for the provider to respond. All the group members would know the action plan after huddling with the provider.

Using the plan-do-study-act (PDSA) method the team conducted its small test of change. Within two weeks patient phone calls for laboratory results had decreased, reflecting the fact that staff were now calling patients in a timely manner about their results. (For more information about analysis and improvement see Nelson, Splaine, et al., 1998; Langley, Nolan, Norman, Provost, & Nolan, 1996.)

Know Your Patterns. Each microsystem's particular combination of patients, professionals, and processes creates patterns that reflect routine ways of thinking, feeling, and behaving on the part of both patients and staff in that system. The patterns are also related to the typical results and outcomes—and variations thereof—associated with the microsystem's mission. Some patterns will be well known and talked about (for example, hours of service, busy times of the day or week, common hassles, and bottlenecks). Some patterns may be well known and never discussed (sacred cows). And some may be unrecognized by staff and patients but nevertheless have powerful effects (for example, mistrust stemming

TABLE 6.3. PRACTICE CORE AND SUPPORTING PROCESSES ASSESSMENT.

Process	Works Well	Small Problem	Real Problem	Totally Broken	Cannot Rate	We're Working on It	Source of Patient Complaint
Appointment system							
Answering phones							
Messaging							
Scheduling procedures							
Reporting diagnostic test results							
Prescription renewals							
Making referrals							
Preauthorization for services							
Billing and coding							
Phone advice							
Assignment of patients to our practice							
Orientation of patients to our practice							
New patient workups							
Education for patients and families							
Prevention assessment and activities							
Chronic disease management							

Note: Each of the processes is rated by each staff member using the categories shown. If the process is a source of patient complaint, that is also noted.

from a local culture dominated by historical divides that separate staff with different educational backgrounds, such as nurses, receptionists, physicians, and technicians). Answering the following questions will reveal important underlying patterns in the microsystem:

- Who is the leader?
- What is the leadership style?
- How do we *act out* the mission of our clinical microsystem every day?
- What are the cultural patterns (the norms, sentiments, and beliefs) in our practice setting?
- What barriers tend to separate health professionals and administrative support staff?
- How easy is it to ask a question about patient care?
- How often does the entire staff meet for the purpose of planning services that are patient centered?
- How satisfied are patients with their access to services?
- How do patients feel about the goodness of their outcomes and the costs of receiving care?
- How do we respond to disruptions of our routines?
- How do we *notice* the failure of our systems that we depend on to prevent accidents and harm to our patients?

Putting It All Together: Planning Services

Based on its assessment, or diagnosis, a microsystem can now help itself improve the things that need to be done better. Once we have knowledge of the purpose, patients, professionals, processes, and patterns, what can we proactively plan for in our daily work to enhance the functioning of our microsystem? Planning services is designed to do the following:

- Decrease unnecessary variation.
- Build feed-forward and feedback mechanisms for informed decision making.
- Promote efficiency by continuously removing waste and rework.
- Create processes and systems that support staff to be the best they can be.
- Design smooth, effective, and safe patient care services that lead to measurably improved patient outcomes.
- Flowchart or specify core processes, supporting processes, and playbooks.

Figure 6.1 offers a panoramic view of a primary care clinical microsystem. It suggests the interplay of patients with practice staff and with processes, which in

FIGURE 6.1. HIGH-LEVEL VIEW OF A PRIMARY CARE CLINICAL MICROSYSTEM.

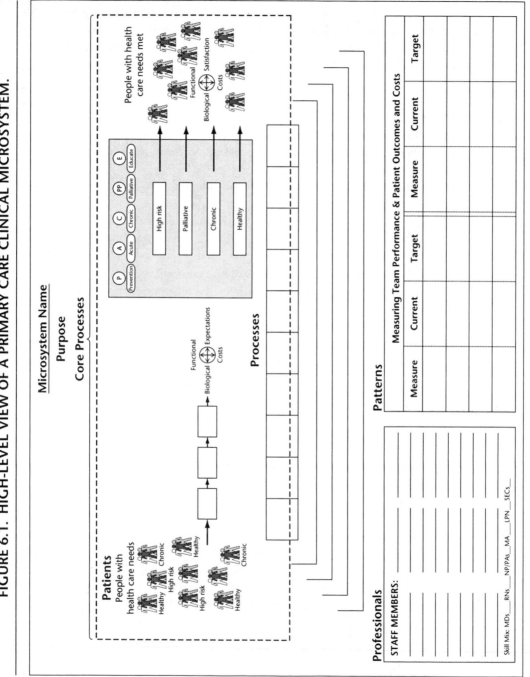

turn produces patterns that characterize the microsystem's performance. Managing these patterns can result in the best health care for patients and for microsystem staff. Typical supporting processes in a primary care practice include such activities as renewing prescriptions, reporting diagnostic test results to patients, and making referrals.

Flowcharts can be used to diagram and diagnose each process to learn how to redesign it to maximize efficiency. This tool is particularly valuable with core or supporting processes whose patterns are characterized by hassles, bottlenecks, and mistakes. Many clinical microsystems have used the methods in Part Two of this book for guided discovery and for taking actions to redesign their services; some examples of their work are provided in Table 6.4.

A review of some of the microsystem improvement efforts to which we have contributed has uncovered many common sources of waste. Table 6.5 summarizes some of these sources and recommends ways to reduce waste and improve efficiency.

A clinical microsystem might ultimately build its own *playbook*—an organized collection of flowcharted processes that can be used for training, performance management, and improvement. The playbook can be used for educating new staff, cross-training staff, managing performance, and troubleshooting because it describes how processes should work.

Discussion

To be able to intentionally plan services and care for populations of patients and individual patients, high-performing clinical microsystems meet regularly to review current process and outcomes to match with patient needs.

Intentional Planning of Services and the Value of Meeting for Service Planning. Our study of microsystems in health care revealed that high-performing units intentionally designed patient-centered services to support patients and families and the staff providing care. As shown in the Evergreen Woods case study, planning services can be intentional and well orchestrated. Moreover, it should be supported by a continuous flow of data (for example, data can be produced throughout the day to identify unfilled appointment slots) to inform every member of the microsystem, to drive corrective actions (any staff person can schedule patients into unfilled slots anytime during the day), and to spawn improvements (at monthly all-staff meetings and annual retreats).

The service sector has many examples of people coming together to plan the services they deliver. In good restaurants, waiters, cooks, and hostesses preview the menus for the day and cover strategies to ensure that the meal service is

TABLE 6.4. ASSESSING YOUR PRACTICE DISCOVERIES AND ACTIONS: THE P'S.

Know Your Patients	Discoveries	Actions Taken
1. Age distribution	30% of our patients are > 66 years old	Designed special group visits to review specific needs of this age group, including physical limitations, dietary considerations.
2. Disease identification	We do not know what percentage of our patients have diabetes.	Team reviewed coding and billing data to determine approximate numbers of patients with diabetes.
3. Health outcomes	Do not know what the range of HbA1c is for our patients with diabetes, or if they are receiving appropriate ADA-recommended care in a timely fashion.	Team conducted a chart audit with 50 charts during a lunch hour. Using a tool designed to track outcomes, each member of the team reviewed 5 charts and noted the findings on the audit tool.
4. Most frequent diagnosis	We learned we had a large number of patients with stable hypertension and diabetes seeing the physician frequently. We also learned that during certain seasons we had huge volumes of pharyngitis and poison ivy.	Designed and tested a new model of care delivery for stable hypertension and diabetes, optimizing the RN role in the practice using agreed-upon guidelines, protocols, and tools.
5. Patient satisfaction	We don't know what patients think unless they complain to us.	Implemented the point of service patient survey, patients completed and left in a box before leaving the practice.

Know Your Professionals	Discoveries	Actions Taken
1. Provider FTE	We were making assumptions about provider time in the clinic without really understanding how much time providers are out of the clinic with hospital rounds, nursing home rounds, and so on.	Changed our scheduling process; utilized RNs to provide care for certain subpopulations.
2. Schedules	Several providers are gone at the same time every week, so one provider is often left and the entire staff work overtime that day.	Evaluated the scheduling template to even out each provider's time to provide consistent coverage of the clinic.
3. Regular meetings	The doctors meet together every other week. The secretaries meet once a month.	Began holding an entire practice meeting every other week on Wednesdays to help the practice become a team.
4. Hours of operation	The beginning and the end of the day are always chaotic. We realized we are on the route for patients between home and work and they want to be seen when we are not open.	Opened one hour earlier and stayed open one hour later each day. The heavy demand was managed better and overtime dropped.
5. Activity surveys	All roles are not being used to their maximum. RNs only room patients and take vital signs, medical assistants doing a great deal of secretarial paperwork, and some secretaries are giving out medical advice.	Roles have been redesigned and matched to individual education, training, and licensure.

Know Your Processes	Discoveries	Actions Taken
1. Cycle time	Patient lengths of visits vary a great deal. There are many delays.	The team identified actions to eliminate and steps to combine and learned to prepare the charts for the patient visit before the patient arrives. The team also holds daily *huddles* to inform everyone on the plan of the day and any issues to consider throughout the day.
2. Key supporting processes	None of us could agree on how things get done in our practice.	Detailed flowcharting of our practice to determine how to streamline and do in a consistent manner.
3. Indirect patient pulls	The providers are interrupted in their patient care process frequently. The number one reason is to retrieve missing equipment and supplies from the exam room.	The team agreed on standardization of exam rooms and minimum inventory lists that were posted on the inside cabinet doors. A process was also determined for *who* would stock exam rooms regularly and *how* the rooms would be stocked, and through the use of an assignment sheet, people for this task were identified and held accountable.

Know your Patterns	Discoveries	Actions Taken
1. Demand on the practice	There are peaks and lows for the practice, depending on day of the week, session of the day, or season of the year.	The team identified actions to eliminate and steps to combine, and learned to prepare the charts for the patient visit before the patient arrives. The team also holds daily huddles to inform everyone on the plan of the day and any issues to consider throughout the day.
2. Communication	We do not communicate in a timely way, nor do we have a standard forum in which to communicate.	Every other week practice meetings are held to help communication and e-mail use by all staff and to promote timely communication.
3. Cultural	The doctors don't really spend time with nondoctors.	The team meetings and heightened awareness of behaviors have helped improve this.
4. Outcomes	We really have not paid attention to our practice outcomes.	Began tracking and awareness and posting results on a data wall to keep us alert to outcomes.
5. Finances	Only the doctors and the practice manager know about the practice money.	Finances are discussed at the team meetings and everyone is learning how all of us make a difference in practice financial performance.

Note: HbA1c = glycosylated hemoglobin; ADA = American Diabetes Association; URI = upper respiratory infection.

TABLE 6.5. ASSESSING YOUR PRACTICE DISCOVERIES AND ACTIONS: COMMON OVERSIGHTS AND WASTES.

Common High-Yield Wastes	Recommended Methods to Reduce Waste	Traps to Avoid
1. Exam rooms not stocked or standardized: missing equipment or supplies.	• Create standard inventory of supplies for all exam rooms. • Design process for regular stocking of exam rooms, with accountable person. • Standardize and utilize all exam rooms.	• Don't assume rooms are being stocked regularly—track and measure. • Providers will use only "their own" rooms. • Providers cannot agree upon standard supplies—suggest "testing."
2. Too many appointment types, which creates chaos in scheduling.	• Reduce appointment types to 2 to 4. • Use standard building blocks to create flexibility in schedule.	
3. Poor communication among the providers and support staff about clinical sessions and patient needs.	• Conduct daily morning *huddles* to provide a forum to review the schedule, anticipate the needs of patients, and plan supplies and information needed for a highly productive interaction between patient and provider.	• People are not showing up for the scheduled huddle—gain the support of providers who are interested; test the idea and measure the results. • Huddle lasts longer than 15 minutes—use a worksheet to guide the huddle.
4. Missing information or chart for patient visits.	• Review patient charts *before* the patient arrives—it is recommended this be done the day before to ensure information and test results are available to support the patient visit.	• Avoid doing chart review when patient is present. • If you have computerized access to test results, don't print the results.
5. Confusing messaging system.	• Standardize messaging process for all providers. • Educate and train on messaging content. • Use a process with a prioritization method, such as a *bin* system in each provider office	• Providers may want their own way—this adds confusion for supply staff and decreases cross-coverage capacity. • Content of message can't be agreed upon—test something!
6. High number of prescription renewal requests via phones.	• Anticipate needs of the patients. • Create *reminder* systems in the office, such as posters, screen savers. • Standardize the information support staff obtain from patients before the provider visit—include prescription information and needs.	• It doesn't need to be the RN who takes the call—medical assistants can obtain this information.

7. Staff frustrated in roles and unable to see new ways to function.	• Review current roles and functions, using activity survey sheets. • Match education, training, licensure to function. • Optimize every role. • Eliminate functions.	• Be sure to focus on talent, training, and scope of practice, not on individual people.
8. Appointment schedules have limited same-day appointment slots.	• Evaluate follow-up appointment and return visit necessity. • Extend the intervals of standard follow-up visits. • Consider RN visits. • Evaluate the use of protocols and guidelines to provide advice for home care—www.icsi.org	• Do not set a certain number of same-day appointments without allowing for variations throughout the year.
9. Missed disease-specific or preventive interventions and tracking.	• Use flowcharts to track preventive activities and disease-specific interventions. • Use "stickers" on charts to alert staff to preventive or disease-specific needs. • Review charts before patient visit.	• Be alert to creating a system for multiple diseases, and do not use many stickers and many registries.
10. Poor communication and interactions between members.	• Hold weekly team meetings to review practice outcomes, staff concerns, improvement opportunities.	• Hold weekly meetings on a regular day and at a regular time and place. • Do not cancel—make the meeting a new habit.
11. High no-show rate among patients.	• Consider improving same-day access.	• Automated reminder telephone calls are not always well received by patients.
12. Patient expectations for visit not met, resulting in phone calls and repeat visits.	• Use CARE vital sign sheet. • Evaluate patient at time of visit to determine whether their needs were met.	• Use reminders to question patients about needs being met. • New habits not easily made.

flawless. Plans are made to cover breaks, and what-if scenarios are rehearsed. Flight crews routinely preview the flight plan, use checklists to prepare for take-off, and review flights after their completion, because they know all of this contributes to a culture of trust, reliability, and safety.

Similarly, high-performing clinical microsystems have learned to reap the benefits of daily meetings, or huddles, to plan the day and weekly or monthly meetings to strategize and manage improvement, as described by the plastic surgery team in the boxed example that follows. Holding regular sessions to advance patient-centered care and services has several benefits. It can

- Promote collegiality and create an environment of equality.
- Improve communications.
- Make visible the team of interdisciplinary professionals engaged in planning and providing care for patients and families.
- Keep staff members *patient focused.*

A Huddle in Plastic Surgery

During the IHI IDCOP collaborative, many primary care practices adapted the military crew resource management concept of "huddles" to their own practice to take advantage of the benefits of huddles, such as preplanning for the day and review of roles, processes, and updates, to name a few benefits.

The design of the huddle was adapted from the IDCOP (idealized design of clinical office practices) literature on primary care huddles and the benefits of huddles to the practice and patients. Drawing from that experience the lead team in the Plastic Surgery Section designed a huddle process to pilot with Dr. Ryan, the lead physician.

Dr. Ryan instituted two huddles for her practice. One was a fifteen- to twenty-minute weekly huddle with a nurse, a clinic appointment scheduler, and a surgical scheduler. The substance of their meeting was to review the upcoming appointments and surgeries projected for the next two weeks in order to identify potential errors in scheduling (such as overbooking or underbooking) and to determine the specific information that needed to be gathered on patients prior to their visit. These huddles enabled timely action and learning—allowing everyone on the team to do his or her job better because they increased everyone's understanding of the challenges of the roles played by others.

The second huddle was held daily, taking five to ten minutes and involving Dr. Ryan and her nurse and the LNA (licensed nurse assistant) team assigned to her that day. The aim of this huddle was to preview the coming day's activities and anticipate needs for that single day.

Success of the Pilot Huddles

The huddles resulted in improved communication, decreased work stress, and increased opportunities for teaching, planning the day's work, adjusting the schedules, and thinking ahead to meet patients' needs while improving efficiency.

Given this success, the huddles were replicated with all the providers and their clinical teams in the section.

Benefits

All the clinicians in the Plastic Surgery Section now conduct interdisciplinary huddles. Here are some of the observed benefits:

- Efficiency is built into the system; work is now done mindfully, in advance, rather than under pressure on the day of a patient's visit.
- Teaching of future physicians is done by modeling the need and benefits of interdisciplinary teamwork.
- Better knowledge and improved communication are achieved because staff understand the work of other team members and they see how their actions affect the whole patient experience.
- Stronger relationships are built among team members, which contributes to greater worklife satisfaction.
- Scheduling errors are reduced and information gathering is improved, resulting in a decline of required tasks per huddle, from five or six down to one or two.

Key Learnings Noticed

- Huddles educate the staff—both newcomers needing orientation and long-time members needing continued learning.
- Huddles offer an easy way to make a significant difference in the staff's daily work and to craft a team approach to patient care.
- Huddles strengthen team health—team members have better communications, an understanding of one another's roles, more respect for and appreciation of what each contributes to the care of the patients.
- Huddles promote interdisciplinary communication on a regular, structured basis.
- Huddles generate flow—the sense of smooth and coordinated service delivery.

Inside-Out Planning. A microsystem's attention is often focused on market-driven service lines or traditional departments—which reflect the strategic plan and the organization chart—rather than on meeting patients' needs through an array of superlative services. Yet focusing attention first and foremost on the patient and family and how they present their health needs to the system, makes it relatively easy to identify the microsystems that provide services and to determine how the best services can be designed within each microsystem and how these services can be best linked together.

The staff in many microsystems work in a complex environment characterized by competing interests, inefficiencies, hassles, and frustrations due to poorly operating processes. They may feel helpless or that they cannot make the system work correctly because the system is run by outsiders. This feeling can be counteracted by working from the inside out, meaning that staff learn about their own patients and their microsystem—and then make improvements—as they go about their work, rather than being told what to do by those outside the microsystem.

Interdependency and Involvement. It is rare for staff to realize that they are part of a microsystem that renders identifiable care to subpopulations of patients and that they are fully interdependent with one another and the patients. The whole of the practice can be only as good as its individual components. Staff are often so busy trying to do "the job" that they have no time to reflect on the work they do, how they do it, and what the outcomes of their efforts are. Involvement of all members of the microsystem is essential to render the best patient services.

Conclusion

Knowledge of the purpose, patients, professionals, processes, and patterns of a clinical microsystem drives the design, redesign, and creation of patient-centered services. The design of services leads to critical analysis of the resources needed for the right person to deliver the right care, in the right way, at the right time. Tools and methods to support the transformation of clinical microsystems so they yield better results for patients and staff have been described here and offered for widespread use and adaptation.

The next chapter will show how a microsystem can blend the services it offers together in order to plan care to best meet the needs of each individual patient.

References

Batalden, P., & Stoltz, P. (1994). Fostering the leadership of a continually improving healthcare organization. *Quality Letter for Healthcare Leaders, 6*(6), 9–15.

Codman, E. A. (1996). *A study in hospital efficiency: As demonstrated by the case report of the first five years of a private hospital.* Oakbrook Terrace, IL: Joint Commission on Accreditation of Healthcare Organizations. (Originally published in 1914)

Godfrey, M., Nelson, E., & Batalden, P. (2005). *Clinical microsystems: A path to healthcare excellence: Improving care within your inpatient units and emergency department.* Workbook. Hanover, NH: Dartmouth College.

Institute for Healthcare Improvement. (2000). *Idealized design of clinical office practices.* Boston: Author.

Langley, G. J., Nolan, K. M., Norman, C. L., Provost, L. P., & Nolan, T. W. (1996). *The improvement guide: A practical approach to enhancing organizational performance.* San Francisco: Jossey-Bass.

Nelson, E. C., Batalden, P. B., Homa, K., Godfrey, M. M., Campbell, C., Headrick, L. A., et al. (2003). Microsystems in health care: Part 2. Creating a rich information environment. *Joint Commission Journal on Quality and Safety, 29*(1), 5–15.

Nelson, E. C., Batalden, P. B., Mohr, J. J., & Plume, S. K. (1998). Building a quality future. *Frontiers of Health Service Management, 15*(1), 3–32.

Nelson, E. C., Splaine, M. E., Batalden, P. B., & Plume, S. K. (1998). Building measurement and data collection into medical practice. *Annals of Internal Medicine, 128*(6), 460–466.

Thedacare Diabetes Cooperative. (2000). *Thedacare diabetes cooperative care storyboard.* Storyboard presented at the Idealized Design of Clinical Office Practices: Prototype Session 5, of the Institute for Healthcare Improvement, Tampa, FL.

Wennberg, J., Freeman, J., Shelton, R., & Bubolz, T. (1989). Hospital use and mortality among Medicare beneficiaries in Boston and New Haven. *New England Journal of Medicine, 320,* 1183–1211.

CHAPTER SEVEN

PLANNING PATIENT-CENTERED CARE

John H. Wasson, Marjorie M. Godfrey, Eugene C. Nelson,
Julie K. Johnson, Paul B. Batalden

Chapter Summary

Background. Clinical microsystems are the essential building blocks of all health systems. At the heart of an effective microsystem is a productive interaction between an informed, activated patient and a prepared, proactive practice staff. Support, which increases the patient's ability for self-management, is an essential result of a productive interaction. This chapter describes how high-performing microsystems design and plan patient-centered care.

Planning patient-centered care. Well-planned, patient-centered care results in improved practice efficiency and better patient outcomes. However, planning this care is not an easy task. Excellent planned care requires that the microsystem have services that match what really matters to a patient and family and protected time for staff to reflect and plan. Patient self-management support, clinical decision support, delivery system design, and clinical information systems must be planned to be effective, timely, and efficient for each individual patient and for all patients.

Conclusion. Our study of twenty high-performing clinical microsystems demonstrated that excellent planned services and planned care are attainable today in microsystems that understand what really matters to a patient and family and have the capacity to provide services to meet each and every patient's needs.

Effective microsystems are designed with the patient, or recipient, in mind (Nelson et al., 2002). Today many of the most progressive microsystems design care or improve their existing design of care not only with the patient in mind, but also with patients and families serving as full members of the team. These exemplary microsystems know how to make their services best meet the needs of the distinct subpopulations they serve. In this chapter we focus on the way effective microsystems *individualize* their services (and sometimes the services offered by other microsystems in the macrosystem or the community as well) to best meet a patient's needs.

In Chapter Six we described how microsystem awareness of the 5 P's—purpose, patients, professionals, processes, and patterns—can result in greater efficiency. Planned services result in less unwanted variation and waste, smoother process flow, more effective use of information, and better matching between staff roles and work.

This chapter describes how a self-aware microsystem can ground efficient services in the patient-centered planned care model. Planned care results in productive patient-provider communication and improved patient self-management. The natural synergy between planned services and planned care results in doing it right the first time for every single patient.

Decades of clinical research confirm the power of productive interactions between informed, activated patients and clinical staff. This research is summarized in a planned (or chronic) care model (Bodenheimer, Wagner, & Grumbach, 2002a, 2002b). The planned care model has several critical components that support a productive interaction (Figure 7.1), and there is considerable overlap between the planned care model and the microsystem framework. In an effective microsystem, self-management support, decision support, delivery system design, and clinical information systems are planned to be effective, timely, and efficient for each individual patient and for all patients. In an effective microsystem, planned services evolve to fit the care needs of an individual patient like a glove fits a hand.

Planning Care Well: Exemplary Clinical Microsystems

In this section we provide a brief description of several microsystems that excel at planning care. In planning care the Dartmouth-Hitchcock Spine Center, in Lebanon, New Hampshire, uses a computer with a touch-screen monitor to collect information on each patient's general and disease-specific health status; this information then provides a sound basis on which the patient and the clinicians can engage in shared decision making to best match the patient's changing needs with

FIGURE 7.1. SCHEMATIC OF THE PLANNED (CHRONIC) CARE MODEL.

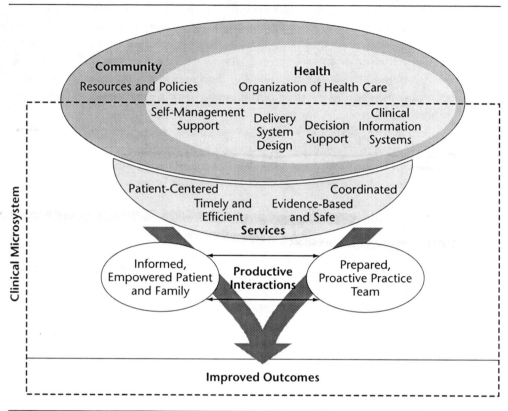

Source: Wagner, 1998.

the preferred treatment plan. At the Intermountain Health Care Shock Trauma Intensive Care Unit (IHC STRICU), in Salt Lake City (Nelson et al., 2003), predetermined protocols, data collection, and feedback among all care staff help staff tailor the planned services into unique, patient-centered planned care. (These two organizations are also discussed in Chapter Nine.)

A patient who visits the Dartmouth-Hitchcock Spine Center uses a touch-screen computer that inquires about his or her symptoms, functional status, expectations for care results, and results of past treatment. Clinical staff use a summary of this information to guide the patient's evaluation and treatment. When possible, clinical staff employ additional technology to guide the evaluation and management of the patient's concerns. Most of the care is preplanned for the most common types of spine patient problems. For example, if the patient has low back pain, the clinician will ask the patient to view shared decision-making video programs that customize clinical management of the patient's condition to the individual patient's needs (Barry, 2003). Effective and safe care is designed so that little of the evaluation and management work is left to chance. A patient receives phone follow-up to ensure that the information and management plan are understood and are in place. At subsequent office visits the patient's symptoms, function, and response to treatment are reassessed, again using the touch-screen computer.

Any patient sent to the twelve-bed IHC STRICU is critically ill; about 15 percent of the time, she or he may not survive. Many standard protocols are used. Computers are at the bedside of every patient, and the staff have developed several long (two-hour) and short (ten-minute) reporting formats to augment the information contained in the bedside electronic medical record. Data elements tracked over time for improvement purposes include the usual physiological measures (for example, vital signs, blood gases, intake-output), thirty types of errors, eleven distinct bacterial infections, and administrative information (diagnoses, treatments, costs, staffing). The information flow ensures that everyone knows which particular management plan has been chosen for each patient and what each staff member must do to deliver the planned care. Staff also have the ability to complete shift reports on unstable patients within minutes. Despite all the activity and technology, the STRICU preserves a very close and caring interaction with family members, who can visit the patient at any time.

A patient calling the Norumbega Evergreen Woods primary care office, in Bangor, Maine, is interviewed by a patient representative who uses a software program called the Problem-Knowledge Coupler (PKC; http://www.pkc.com) to guide the interview. This program uses protocols that address everything from a simple cough to complex chest pains and prompt staff to order needed diagnostic tests before the patient comes to the office. The program also helps staff schedule patients in time slots according to the severity of their conditions. Patients complete standard, program-based questions that inquire about the mental and physical components of their problem. The software also displays an evidence-guided list of possible diagnoses for the problem, organized for easy review, and suggests possible courses of action.

Each examination room contains a computer that is used for patient records, scheduling patient visits, telephone triage, and decision support and also for displaying patient education programs. Staff use the patient education software to manage patient concerns and generate information for the patient about his or her problems. Statistical process control charts of clinic performance are posted, and measures of preventive interventions are available automatically from the PKC. (This microsystem is also discussed in Chapter Six.)

On Lok SeniorHealth, which is located in San Francisco, provides a program of all-inclusive care for the elderly that is intended to optimize each patient's quality of life, sense of independence, and physical and cognitive function and to maintain the patients in their communities and homes. (*On lok* means "place of peace and happiness" in Cantonese.) A standard assessment of physical and mental health and social functioning is completed on enrollment to determine the services best suited to meet patient and family needs. All patient information is entered into a computer system, where it can be accessed by interdisciplinary staff. The information system is used to document care, transmit medication orders to local pharmacies, and ensure feedback of performance measures to staff members.

These four exemplary microsystems know their 5 P's. They have the information and knowledge needed to plan efficient services for the benefit of both patients and staff. They have rejected many of the common myths that underlie much of current clinical practice (Table 7.1).

Exemplary microsystems reject the notion that they must have an advanced information system before they can provide great care and service. In fact, an inappropriate information system can make inefficient processes more difficult to change. It is best to learn how to optimally match work to patient needs before committing to an information system. The information systems of the exemplary microsystems described here resulted from months and years of doing tests, so that each microsystem was sure it understood its 5 P's.

As described in detail in Chapter Six, exploring the 5 P's deepens a clinical microsystem's knowledge of the patients who are the beneficiaries of care, the professionals providing care, the processes used to provide services, and the patterns of social interactions, health outcomes, and process measures. This knowledge positions the microsystem to engage in meaningful improvements. The microsystem becomes informed, aware of its identity as a system, and curious to try out improvements based on this new information.

Exemplary microsystems reject the notion that factors such as educational level will automatically affect a patient's ability to absorb information or to act on information. They know that patient self-management is critical to effective planned care (Bodenheimer, Lorig, Holman, & Grumbach, 2002). The belief that particular types of patients (or their families) are "too limited" to self-manage their problems is a myth.

Exemplary microsystems reject the notion that new approaches will not work for a particular setting or for certain types of patients. Self-management support and monitoring of progress is increasingly facilitated by the telephone, patient registries, e-mail, and Web-based technologies. Technology facilitates the extension of care beyond the office. Innovative microsystems learn that electronics are right

TABLE 7.1. COMMON MYTHS REJECTED BY EFFECTIVE CLINICAL MICROSYSTEMS.

Negative Attitude or Myth	More Useful Reality
Advanced information systems are needed before services and care can be improved.	Better to understand purpose, patients, professionals, processes, and patterns; test changes; retest changes; then build information systems to make the best processes more efficient.
Patient self-management skills are dependent on education, income, language, and so on.	Better to realize that patient self-management skills can be learned and that the microsystem has a central role in supporting these skills.
"Electronics are not right for my patients." Many practices assume that they have to spend money for hardware and software and the space and personnel to maintain this technology.	Better to realize that a rapidly increasing number of patients will welcome patient-centered electronic methods for getting information and engaging in self-management. Because the patients can do a lot of the data entry, the practice flow immediately benefits.
Ambulatory care is visit based. Fee-for-service practices most often build patient flow around visits because that is how they are paid.	Better to think about what each patient needs to attain high levels of self-management, so inefficient rework is minimized. Many revisits "clog" the system with low reimbursement care.
All paths lead to a doctor. When patients need help, they need a doctor.	Better to think about what has to be done to serve patient needs and deliver efficient effective care. Once the *what* is answered, the *who* often turns out not to be the doctor.
Demand is patient driven. When patients need help, they go and get it.	Better to realize that many demands are caused by professional habits and rework. Once rework is reduced and demand is managed, the microsystem will have enough time to plan how to do the right thing at the right time.
Resources are needed to help patients develop their self-management skills.	Better to have planned services; the efficiencies will result in more resources and capacity to plan care.
A designated person to plan care (for example, the care manager) will correct a practice's deficiencies.	Better to make planned care part of planned service (for example, involves all roles and all "work").
All resources and capacity to support patient care exists within the four walls of the practice.	Better to explore resources within the practice and outside the four walls, in the community.

for many of their patients; that patient-centered technology can build patient self-management support into everyday practice. And for those patients who may not be able to use electronics, family members and community organizations can be encouraged to offer assistance.

Exemplary microsystems reject the notion that all care must be visit based. They know there are many ways to provide planned care; it is seldom confined to an office visit, nor is it confined to the care provided by a physician. Physician-centered care often results in bottlenecks, but these can be minimized by the use of other professionals, peers, and community services. Providing only physician-dominant, visit-based care is often more costly and less complete for patients, and it may, paradoxically, reduce net practice revenue.

Exemplary microsystems also reject the notion that aiming to care for patients when patients want to receive care will overwhelm an ambulatory care practice. They know that current patient demand largely results from the way the microsystem has operated in the recent past; demand will change to match the way services and care are planned in the future (Schwartz, Woloshin, Wasson, Renfrew, & Welch, 1999; Wasson et al., 1992).

Finally, exemplary microsystems use the efficiencies of their planned services to improve their capacity to provide care. This capacity is spread across microsystem staff as they develop the new roles and tasks needed to help patients become better self-managers.

Planning Care in Any Microsystem

Effective microsystems are designed with the patient, or recipient, in mind (Nelson et al., 2002). Today many of the most progressive microsystems design care or improve their existing design of care not only with the patient in mind but also with patients and families serving as full members of the team. The worksheets in the Appendix "Primary Care Practice Patient Viewpoint Survey" (Figure A.4) and "Through the Eyes of Your Patients" (Figure A.5) are helpful tools to gain deeper insight into the patient and family experience to enable "just right" improvements based on direct patient feedback.

Microsystem staff must make sure that as they develop more efficient services, they focus on the provision of planned care. Attributes of planned care and planned services designed to meet individual patient needs are summarized in Figure 7.2 and Table 7.2. By incorporating components of the planned care model into its practice, a clinical microsystem promotes productive interactions between patients and clinical staff. (Additional information about the planned [chronic] care model and practice assessment forms can be found at http://www.improvingchroniccare.org.)

FIGURE 7.2. PLANNING CARE AND PATIENT SELF-MANAGEMENT: SERVICE AND INFORMATION FLOW IN A MICROSYSTEM.

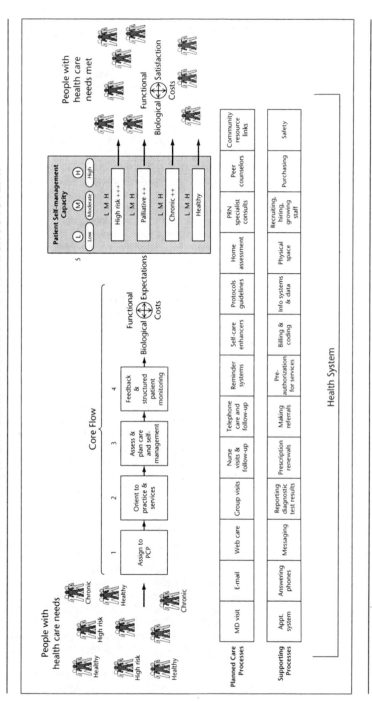

Note: PCP = primary care physician; PRN = as needed.

TABLE 7.2. ATTRIBUTES OF PLANNED CARE.

Element of the Planned Care Model	Attributes
Health Care Organization	• The business plan includes measurable goals for system improvement. • Senior leaders visibly support system improvement. • Effective improvement strategies aim for comprehensive system change. • Open and systematic handling of errors is encouraged, with a view to improving quality of care. • Provider incentives and avoidance of disincentives encourage better care. • Developing staff and integrating them into the culture is an organizational priority. • Leadership develops relationships that facilitate care coordination.
Community Resources and Policies	• Effective programs are identified and patients are encouraged to participate. • Partnerships are formed with community organizations to support or develop interventions that meet patient needs.
Self-management Support	• Each patient's central role in managing his or her illness is emphasized. • Patient self-management knowledge, behaviors, confidence, and barriers are assessed. • Effective behavioral change interventions and ongoing support with peers or professionals are provided. • Culturally competent and linguistically appropriate approaches are used in patient interactions. • The organization ensures collaborative care planning and problem solving by the team.
Delivery System Design	• Team roles are defined, and tasks are delegated among team members. • Staff are employed to the extent of their scope of practice. • Demand is measured, and master schedules are developed that match capacity and demand. • Patients have access to care when they want it. • Complex patients receive clinical case management services; this includes communicating with other settings where these patients are receiving care. • Planned visits are used to support evidence-based care. • Patients are assured of regular follow-up by the primary care team. • Interpretive services are provided for non-English speakers and low-literacy patients.

(continued)

TABLE 7.2. (*Continued*)

Element of the Planned Care Model	Attributes
Decision Support	• Evidence-based guidelines are embedded in daily clinical practice. • Linkages are established between primary care and specialty providers in order to facilitate care coordination. • Specialist expertise is incorporated into primary care. • Proven provider education modalities are used to support behavioral change. • Patients are informed about guidelines pertinent to their care. • Staff use standing or standard orders.
Clinical Information System (IS)	• IS includes a registry function that summarizes clinically useful and timely information on all patients with particular characteristics. • IS provides timely reminders and feedback for providers and patients and provides protection against errors. • Registry can identify relevant patient subgroups for proactive care. • Registry facilitates individual patient care planning. • IS facilitates timely sharing of information between care settings.

Many clinical groups currently do not get the right information to the right place, do not match staff roles to the work, and do not build efficiency and effectiveness into practice flow. Furthermore, for a significant number of issues, clinicians do not know what matters to their patients (Braddock, Edwards, Hasenberg, Laidley, & Levinson, 1999; Magari, Hamel, & Wasson, 1998; Nelson et al., 1983). In the absence of a deep understanding of what matters to a patient, interactions are unlikely to be productive.

It is imperative that clinical microsystems plan services that match the needs of their patients. Because a patient with a chronic condition must manage it for many years, the microsystems must provide sufficient patient self-management support (as exemplified in Table 7.2). The microsystem must provide care for the illness and guidance so that the patient can live as normal a life as possible and mitigate the psychosocial impact of the condition.

The "Assessment of Care for Chronic Conditions" (Figure A.7) is a helpful tool in the appendix to begin to learn the patient perspective about chronic disease care to support improvement and redesign the roles and process to better meet patient needs.

As a general rule, the less ready the patient is for self-management, the more resources the microsystem needs to devote to this process. Resources are most effective when they seamlessly support self-management during assessment, management, and follow-up. As previously noted, the microsystem's staff resources go well beyond the number of available physicians.

In many clinical settings patient and information flows follow the pattern illustrated in Figure 7.2; for almost every clinical need of a patient, a microsystem must ask itself who and what will meet that need and when, where, and how will that need be met.

For example, when an inquisitive microsystem is concerned about the best way to manage a patient who has pain, it confronts a series of questions about assessment and the planning of care. For example:

1. Who will identify the patient with pain? Will this be done by interview or by a self-assessment tool?
2. With what measure will the pain problem be identified? Will the measure be paper based or electronic? Will it assess other problems that matter to the patient at the same time?
3. When will the pain be identified? Will it be identified during or before an office visit?

After the microsystem has developed answers to these questions, it can conduct a few tests with a few patients to see which answers will lead to the most efficient and effective processes. The same question and test process is used to discover the best approaches for the management of patient needs. Finally, the microsystem has to consider follow-up and monitoring: who, what, when, where, and how? Again, the preliminary answers to these questions need to be tested with a few patients.

A Low-Tech Example for Ambulatory Services: CARE Vital Signs

The technology-rich microsystem examples of the Spine Center, STRICU, Norumbega, and On Lok might support the myth that advanced information systems are a prerequisite for excellent patient-centered care. We now describe a process called CARE Vital Signs to illustrate how microsystem services and staff resources can improve their matching with ambulatory patient needs *without* employing expensive technology. CARE is an acronym for Check, Activate,

Reinforced, Engineering. Each column signals activity that can occur for different roles in the microsystem. *Check* is intended for a medical assistant to begin the vital sign review and also make assessments of other important patient measures. *Activate* indicates teaching and follow-up that can be initiated to "activate" the patient and family. *Reinforced* refers to the health care provider follow-up and reinforcement with the patient. *Engineering* refers to redesign and system improvements to ensure the process of care is embedded in the microsystem and new innovative processes of care help to support the patient and follow up.

In almost every ambulatory care practice, someone obtains vital signs and moves patients to rooms. These people are usually certified medical assistants (CMAs) or licensed practical nurses (LPNs). When you compare what CMAs, LPNs, and even registered nurses (RNs) do in practice to what they have the education and training to do, you find that they are usually greatly underutilizing their skills and training.

In *usual care,* after the nurse or medical assistant obtains vital signs, most paths lead to the physician. This approach is usually inefficient, incomplete, and often leads to bottlenecks. Opportunities to promote patient self-management are often limited to what happens in the "black box" of the physician's private examining room. The assessment, monitoring, and education needed by patients who have important preventive care needs and chronic diseases often get short shrift.

In contrast to usual care, the CARE Vital Signs process offers an explicit plan for checking, activating, reinforcing, and engineering.

Checking

As patients come to the practice, they are routinely screened to see if they have issues that might benefit from a standardized self-management program. The LPN or CMA checks for important preventive and patient-relevant issues while obtaining the patient's weight, blood pressure, and pulse. For patients nineteen to sixty-nine years old, staff usually inquire about the presence of three to five common chronic conditions, pain, health habits, feelings, medication problems, the patient's confidence about his or her self-management skills, and age- and gender-specific completion of necessary preventive tests.

Activating

When an issue is identified during this CARE Vital Signs process, the LPN or CMA informs the patient about valuable resources for self-management and brings the issue to the attention of the clinician.

Reinforcing

When the clinician is alerted about an important issue, she or he is in a powerful position to activate the patient toward self-management and to reinforce the importance of planned care. Goals and priorities are identified at this point.

Engineering

Engineering refers to systematically incorporating components of planned care into the roles of practice members, into the planned services, and into the flow of practice processes. Patients with significant needs are usually asked to register for brief programs in which the LPN or CMA phones to check the patients' understanding of self-management and their completion of self-management goals.

An example of the CARE Vital Signs form is shown in Figure 7.3. A patient may have a few needs for self-management, some needs, or many needs. When no or few needs are identified and the patient is confident about his or her self-management skills, the visit proceeds in the usual way except that the relatively healthy patient is given the completed CARE Vital Signs form and is urged to use free, Web-based materials for an additional assessment and individualized information. The hypothetical patient described in Figure 7.3 has been found to have problems with emotions, pain, and confidence in managing her health problems. Given these findings the practice is prepared to offer her special follow-up care to improve self-management of these conditions. The circled areas on the figure indicate follow-up areas and patient instructions. Engineering options include phone follow-ups, nurse visits, e-mail, and group visits.

For a patient who has some needs for self-management, brief, prescheduled telephone follow-up is used to reinforce goals over time and to adjust the goals to changing circumstances. For the patient with many needs or limited self-management skills, intensive monitoring and assistance are scheduled. A mnemonic is helpful to describe the focus of good self-management support, which can be thought of in terms of the 5 As—*assess, advise, agree, assist,* and *arrange* (Glasgow et al., 2002).

A low-tech microsystem can refer patients to http://www.howsyourhealth.org for an extensive assessment of their health status and education tailored to their health needs. When the CARE Vital Signs process is used, about half of a typical ambulatory care population of patients aged nineteen to sixty-nine will be found to have important needs: about 40 percent of these patients will be quite confident and 10 percent will have little confidence that they can self-manage their problems. The generic question for members of the microsystem is, How can

FIGURE 7.3. EXAMPLE OF USING A CARE VITAL SIGNS FORM.

CARE Vital Signs Form (front)

CARE VITAL SIGNS (FOR ADULTS AGED 19+)
PROVIDER COPY: Complete on new patients or if not completed in past year

Patient Name: _____Cindy Jones_____ Date: __1/1/02__ ID #: 0097007

What does patient want to discuss or expect to be done at this visit:
Wants to deal (finally) with the feelings that have been upsetting her for a long time

MEASURE OR QUESTION CHECK	CLINICAL FLAG ACTIVATION (Circle when noted)	PLANNED CARE STANDING ORDERS	
		REINFORCED WEB-BASED*	ENGINEERING PRACTICE-BASED**
Height __5-5__ BMI __22__ Weight __130__	BMI 25–30 → BMI 30+ →.	HYH: Exercise/Eating add Diet Evaluation	
BP __130/70__	>140/80 → <100/60 →	HYH: Common Medical	
Pulse __70__ RR __14__	<50; >100; irregular short of breath		
Any of the following: ❑ Hypertension ❑ Cardiac/Vascular Disease ❑ Diabetes ❑ Lung Problems/Asthma ❑ Other	Any concerns: ———————— ———————— ———————— Or no previous use HYH Condition Form	For condition management use www.howsyourhealth.com HYH: Common Medical	
Feeling Score 5 (see reverse)	4 or 5 →	HYH: Feelings/Emotion Evaluation	Phone follow-up for patients with Feelings/Emotion
Pain Score 4 (see reverse)	4 or 5 →	HYH: Pain Evaluation	Phone follow-up for patients with Pain
Are your Pills making you ill? (Yes, no, maybe, not taking)	Yes or Maybe	HYH: Common Medical	
Not Good Health Habits 2 (see reverse)	4 or 5 →	HYH: Health Habits	
How confident are you that you can control and manage most of your health problems? (Very, Somewhat, Not at All)	Somewhat or Not →	HYH: Self-Management Module	

Prevention: Circle if not completed. _____ _____

	19–49	50–69	70+
Female Only**		Mammogram q1 yr Pap q 3 yr	
Male Only**			
Both**		Hemoccult q 1 yr	

Patient Instructions: Based on Discussion with your Provider. Any checks or circles above? Go to the web site before our next visit or phone contact.

After today's visit, we will call you twice to check on your progress; please use the problem solving form on the web when you talk to us.

*When instructed for the reasons listed above, OR for a general health "check-up," OR the HYH Chapters, OR other special forms recommended by the office, go to **www.howsyourhealth.com** and type in _____ when you are asked for your pass code.
**Criteria to be completed by the office. Some Engineering options include phone follow up, nurse visits, e-mail and group visits.

(continued)

FIGURE 7.3. EXAMPLE OF USING A CARE VITAL SIGNS FORM. (*Continued*)

Height in Shoes	Weight Range "Normal"*	BMI 30+ Seriously Overweight
4'10"	91–119	145
4'11"	94–124	150
5'	97–128	156
5'1"	101–132	162
5'2"	104–137	187
5'3"	107–141	173
5'4"	111–146	179
5'5"	114–150	184
5'6"	118–155	190
5'7"	121–160	195
5'8"	125–164	200
5'9"	129–169	206
5'10"	132–174	212
5'11"	136–179	217
6'	140–184	223
6'1"	144–189	229
6'2"	148–195	234
6'3"	152–200	240
6'4"	156–205	245
6'5"	160–211	250
6'6"	164–216	255

*(BMI 25–29 "overweight" is between upper range of normal and BMI 30+ "seriously overweight")

PAIN

During the past 4 weeks…
How much bodily pain have you generally had?

No pain		1
Very mild pain		2
Mild pain		3
Moderate pain		4
Severe pain		5

FEELINGS

During the past 4 weeks…
How much have you been bothered by emotional problems such as feeling anxious, depressed, irritable, or downhearted and blue?

Not at all		1
Slightly		2
Moderately		3
Quite a bit		4
Extremely		5

HEALTH HABITS

During the past month, how often did you practice good health habits such as using a seat belt, getting exercise, eating right, getting enough sleep, or wearing safety helmets?

All of the time		1
Most of the time		2
Some of the time		3
A little of the time		4
None of the time		5

Source: www.clinicalmicrosystem.org (under Tools).

we provide services and plan care over the next year or two to increase self-management competencies among patients with needs?

A microsystem will usually phase in the use of CARE Vital Signs. For example, by introducing CARE Vital Signs just for patients aged fifty to fifty-five, practice staff test their capacity to provide planned care. After successfully identifying and managing the needs of this group of patients, practice staff can then use CARE Vital Signs with another age group, repeating this cycle every three to four months until all age groups are using CARE Vital signs and are experiencing better assessment, better advice, agreement on goals, assistance with self-management, and effectively arranged follow-up to support self-management.

CARE Vital Signs is an example of how a generic approach can address many patients' needs and incorporate necessary screening and management functions into the everyday work of a busy microsystem. The CARE Vital Signs approach is an efficient, standardized gateway to effective patient self-management. However, it is also evident that the use of a CARE Vital Signs form will not make planned care happen. Planned care requires that interdisciplinary staff plan regular time to meet, design planned care services, and make the attributes of the planned care model vital components of everything they do.

Conclusion

In this chapter, as in Chapter Six, we described some ways that exemplary clinical microsystems have found to escape the *glue* that many clinical units are stuck in: traditional roles, undesigned processes, frequent hassles, and myriad workarounds. Working inefficiently, they struggle just to get through the day. They believe that they are unable to change because they do not understand how to overcome the mismatch between what they provide and what their patients really need. Exemplary clinical microsystems simply design their planned services to be there to meet individual patients' needs like a glove fits a hand.

References

Barry, M. (2003). Health decision aids to facilitate shared decision making in office practice. *Annals of Internal Medicine, 136*(2), 127–135.

Bodenheimer, T., Lorig, K., Holman, H., & Grumbach, K. (2002). Patient self-management of chronic disease in primary care. *Journal of the American Medical Association, 288*(19), 2469–2475.

Bodenheimer, T., Wagner, E., & Grumbach, K. (2002a). Improving primary care for patients with chronic illness. *Journal of the American Medical Association, 288*(14), 1775–1779.

Bodenheimer, T., Wagner, E., & Grumbach, K. (2002b). Improving primary care for patients with chronic illness: The chronic care model, Part 2. *Journal of the American Medical Association, 288*(15), 1909–1914.

Braddock, C. R., 3rd, Edwards, K. A., Hasenberg, N. M., Laidley, T. L., & Levinson, W. (1999). Informed decision making in outpatient practice: Time to get back to basics. *Journal of the American Medical Association, 282*(24), 2313–2320.

Glasgow, R. E., Funnell, M. M., Bonomi, A. E., Davis, C., Beckham, V., & Wagner, E. H. (2002). Self-management aspects of the improving chronic illness care breakthrough series: Implementation with diabetes and heart failure teams. *Annals of Behavioral Medicine, 24*(2), 80–87.

Magari, E. S., Hamel, M. B., & Wasson, J. H. (1998). An easy way to measure quality of physician-patient interactions. *Journal of Ambulatory Care Management, 21*(3), 27–33.

Nelson, E. C., Batalden, P. B., Homa, K., Godfrey, M. M., Campbell, C., Headrick, L. A., et al. (2003). Microsystems in health care: Part 2. Creating a rich information environment. *Joint Commission Journal on Quality and Safety, 29*(1), 5–15.

Nelson, E. C., Batalden, P. B., Huber, T. P., Mohr, J. J., Godfrey, M. M., Headrick, L. A., et al. (2002). Microsystems in health care: Part 1. Learning from high-performing front-line clinical units. *Joint Commission Journal on Quality Improvement, 28*(9), 472–493.

Nelson, E., Conger, B., Douglass, R., Gephart, D., Kirk, J., Page, R., et al. (1983). Functional health status levels of primary care patients. *Journal of the American Medical Association, 249*(24), 3331–3338.

Schwartz, L. M., Woloshin, S., Wasson, J. H., Renfrew, R. A., & Welch, H. G. (1999). Setting the revisit interval in primary care. *Journal of General Internal Medicine, 14*(4), 230–236.

Wagner, E. H. (1998, August). Chronic disease management: What will it take to improve care for chronic illness? *Effective Clinical Practice, 1*(1), 22–24.

Wasson, J., Gaudette, C., Whaley, F., Sauvisgne, A., Baribeau, P., & Welch, H. G. (1992). Telephone care as a substitute for routine clinic follow-up. *Journal of the American Medical Association, 267*(13), 1788–1793.

CHAPTER EIGHT

IMPROVING PATIENT SAFETY

Julie K. Johnson, Paul Barach, Joseph P. Cravero,
George T. Blike, Marjorie M. Godfrey, Paul B. Batalden,
Eugene C. Nelson

Chapter Summary

Background. This chapter explores patient safety from a microsystem perspective and from an injury epidemiology perspective and shows how to embed safety into a microsystem's operations.

Microsystem patient safety scenario. Allison, a five-year-old preschooler with a history of "wheezy colds," and her mother interacted with several microsystems as they navigated the health care system. At various points the system failed to address Allison's needs. We apply the Haddon matrix, a useful framework for analyzing medical failures in patient safety, to this scenario, showing how this process sets the stage for developing countermeasures.

Case study. The case of JH, a child with congenital abnormalities, shows the types of failures that can occur in complex medical care settings such as those associated with pediatric procedural sedation. Six patient safety principles, such as "design systems to identify, prevent, absorb, and mitigate errors," can be applied in a clinical setting. In response to this particular case, the subsequent analysis of the case, and the application of microsystems thinking, the Anesthesiology Department of the Children's Hospital at Dartmouth (part of the Dartmouth-Hitchcock Medical Center) developed the PainFree Program to provide optimal safety for sedated patients.

Conclusion. Safety is a property of a microsystem, and it can be achieved only through thoughtful and systematic application of a broad array of process, equipment, organizational, supervision, training, simulation, and teamwork changes.

This chapter explores safety in the context of clinical microsystems. In 1999, the Institute of Medicine (IOM) report *To Err Is Human* estimated that 44,000 to 98,000 people die each year from medical errors (Kohn, Corrigan, & Donaldson, 1999). Although the topics of safety, medical errors, and patient harm have been on some agendas for decades (Bates et al., 1997; Brennan et al., 1991; Cook, Woods, & Miller, 1998; Leape, 1994; Leape et al., 1991; Perrow, 1999), the release of the IOM report brought national attention to the subject (Berwick & Leape, 1999; Helmrich, 2000; Mohr & Batalden, 2002; Reason, 2000; Reason, Carthey, & de Leval, 2001).

Clinical microsystems provide a conceptual and practical framework for thinking about the organization and delivery of care. The purpose of this chapter is to explore patient safety from a microsystem perspective as well as from an injury epidemiology perspective and to address the tensions that exist between the conceptual theory and the daily practical applications, tensions that raise such questions as how are we to embed safety into a microsystem's developmental journey and how are we to promote system resilience, given the many transitions of care (gaps and handoffs) among various microsystems.

The chapter begins by presenting a hypothetical scenario (Figure 8.1) that we have used to teach health professionals how to apply some of what is known about systems safety to the microsystem concept. We examine these ideas further with a case study of the PainFree Program at the Dartmouth-Hitchcock Medical Center in Lebanon, New Hampshire. Several safety principles can be elicited from the scenario and the case study, and we list and describe these principles.

Finally, we link important characteristics of high-performing microsystems to specific design concepts and actions that can enhance patient safety in microsystems.

Microsystem Patient Safety Scenario

Figure 8.1 illustrates a hypothetical scenario that volume authors Julie K. Johnson and Paul Barach have used to connect patient safety principles with clinical microsystems thinking. In this scenario the patient is Allison, a five-year-old preschooler with a history of "wheezy colds." As we follow the scenario, it is clear that Allison and her mother interact with several microsystems as they navigate the health care system in an attempt to address Allison's illness—the hypothetical community-based pediatric clinic (which we call Mercy Acute Care Clinic) and several overlapping microsystems within the university hospital.

While working through this scenario, the reader will see many obvious points where the system *failed*, where it did not address Allison's needs. What are the ways to think about these system failures? Many valuable tools are available for

FIGURE 8.1. MICROSYSTEM PATIENT SAFETY SCENARIO.

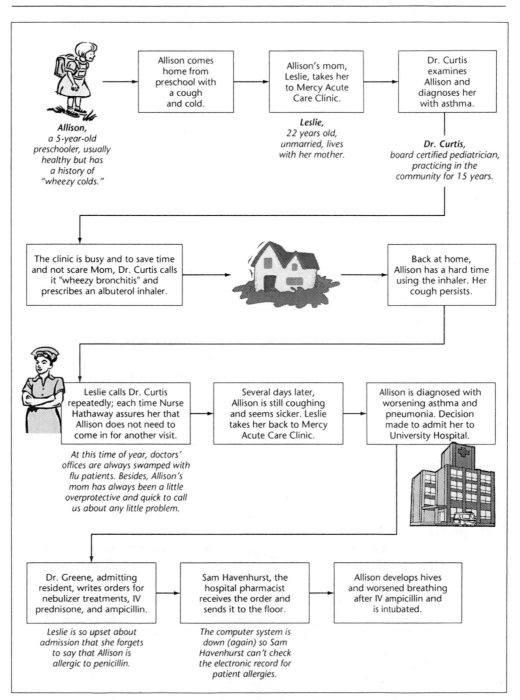

Allison, a 5-year-old preschooler, usually healthy but has a history of "wheezy colds."

Allison comes home from preschool with a cough and cold.

Allison's mom, Leslie, takes her to Mercy Acute Care Clinic.

Leslie, 22 years old, unmarried, lives with her mother.

Dr. Curtis examines Allison and diagnoses her with asthma.

Dr. Curtis, board certified pediatrician, practicing in the community for 15 years.

The clinic is busy and to save time and not scare Mom, Dr. Curtis calls it "wheezy bronchitis" and prescribes an albuterol inhaler.

Back at home, Allison has a hard time using the inhaler. Her cough persists.

Leslie calls Dr. Curtis repeatedly; each time Nurse Hathaway assures her that Allison does not need to come in for another visit.

At this time of year, doctors' offices are always swamped with flu patients. Besides, Allison's mom has always been a little overprotective and quick to call us about any little problem.

Several days later, Allison is still coughing and seems sicker. Leslie takes her back to Mercy Acute Care Clinic.

Allison is diagnosed with worsening asthma and pneumonia. Decision made to admit her to University Hospital.

Dr. Greene, admitting resident, writes orders for nebulizer treatments, IV prednisone, and ampicillin.

Leslie is so upset about admission that she forgets to say that Allison is allergic to penicillin.

Sam Havenhurst, the hospital pharmacist receives the order and sends it to the floor.

The computer system is down (again) so Sam Havenhurst can't check the electronic record for patient allergies.

Allison develops hives and worsened breathing after IV ampicillin and is intubated.

analyzing medical errors, such as morbidity and mortality conferences, root cause analysis, and failure mode and effects analysis. Although it is tempting to rely on one or two tools in an attempt to simplify the complexity involved in understanding errors and patient harm, the challenge for most health care professionals is to preface the search for root causes with a broader look that will help them place the error in context. One method that we have found to be useful for taking this broader look builds on William Haddon's overarching framework for injury epidemiology (Haddon, 1972).

As the first director of the National Highway Safety Bureau (1966 to 1969), Haddon was interested in the broad issues of injury that results from the transfer of energy in such a way that inanimate or animate objects are damaged. Haddon (1973) identified ten strategies for reducing losses:

1. Prevent the marshaling of the energy.
2. Reduce the amount of energy marshaled.
3. Prevent the release of the energy.
4. Modify the rate or spatial distribution of release of the energy.
5. Separate in time and space the energy being released and the susceptible structure.
6. Use a physical barrier to separate the energy and the susceptible structure.
7. Modify the contact surface or structure with which people can come in contact.
8. Strengthen the structure that might be damaged by the energy transfer.
9. When injury does occur, rapidly detect it and counter its continuation and extension.
10. When injury does occur, take all necessary reparative and rehabilitative steps.

These strategies have a logical sequence that can be described in terms of pre-injury, injury, and post-injury.

The Haddon framework is a 3 × 3 matrix in which the factors involved in an automobile injury (*human, vehicle,* and *environment*) head the columns, and the phases of the event (*pre-injury, injury,* and *post-injury*) head the rows. Figure 8.2 shows a completed Haddon matrix. It focuses the analysis on the relationships among the three factors and the three phases. A mix of countermeasures derived from Haddon's strategies is necessary to minimize loss. Furthermore countermeasures can be designed for each phase—pre-event, event, and post-event. This approach confirms what is known about adverse events in complex environments: it takes a variety of strategies to prevent or mitigate harm. Understanding injury in its larger context helps leaders and staff recognize the basic fragility of systems and the importance of mitigating inherent hazards by increasing the resilience of the system (Dekker, 2002).

FIGURE 8.2. HADDON MATRIX ANALYZING AN AUTO ACCIDENT.

	Factors		
	Human	**Vehicle**	**Environment**
Pre-injury	Alcohol intoxication	Braking capacity of motor vehicles	Visibility of hazards
Injury	Resistance to energy insults	Sharp or pointed edges and surfaces	Flammable building materials
Post-injury	Hemorrhage	Rapidity of energy reduction	Emergency medical response

Source: Haddon, 1972.

FIGURE 8.3. COMPLETED SAFETY MATRIX FOR ALLISON'S SCENARIO.

	Factors		
	Provider	**Patient and Family**	**System and Environment**
Pre-event	Physician decision about diagnosis	Child with history of wheezy colds	Busy primary care clinic University hospital
Event	IV ampicillin	Allergy to penicillin	Computer systems down
Post-event	Intubation	Hives, difficulty breathing	Hospital—team response to allergic reaction

Building on injury epidemiology, we can also use the Haddon matrix to think about analyzing medical injuries (Layde et al., 2002). To translate this tool from injury epidemiology to patient safety, we have revised the phase descriptions from *pre-injury, injury,* and *post-injury* to *pre-event, event, and post-event.* We have revised the factor descriptions from *human, vehicle,* and *environment* to *provider, patient and family, and system and environment.* In this latter factor, *system* refers to the processes and systems that are in place for the microsystem. *Environment* refers to the context within which the microsystem exists. We added *system* in order to recognize the significant contribution that systems make toward harm and error in a microsystem. Figure 8.3 shows a completed matrix derived from Allison's scenario and illustrating how the Haddon matrix may be adapted for analysis of medical injuries.

The next step in learning from errors and adverse events is to develop countermeasures to address the issues in each cell of the matrix. To examine this step and further describe safety issues in microsystems, we will move from the hypothetical scenario to the following case study.

Case Study: Dartmouth-Hitchcock PainFree Program

JH is a four-year-old white girl with a history of multiple congenital abnormalities. Most notably, she has had developmental delays, unusual facial appearance, and absence of the corpus callosum. She does not have an identifiable syndrome. At home on the day before admission, her mother noticed the onset of three generalized seizures, each seizure lasting ten minutes and terminating on its own. JH was admitted for further evaluation and a magnetic resonance imaging (MRI) scan. Because the MRI scanner had a full schedule for the day and the technicians did not want to inconvenience the elective patients, JH was scheduled to be scanned at 7:00 P.M. on the evening of admission. Sedation was to be delivered by the pediatric house officer because the anesthesia team that worked on the elective cases during the day was not available at night.

The primary sedation provider was a first-year resident. He had been advised by his senior resident to give a combination of midazolam hydrochloride and fentanyl for the sedation and to titrate to effect. The patient actually proved to be quite irritable, and she was difficult to sedate. She seemed to have a paradoxical reaction to the 2 mg of midazolam, which was titrated in more than thirty minutes; she became irritable and was crying and inconsolable. Fentanyl titration was then started. During the course of the next 30 minutes, the child received 4 mcg/kg of fentanyl. She became sleepy and was placed in the MRI scanner. Four minutes after the scan was started, O_2 saturation levels were noted to be 75 percent, and the child was pulled out of the scanner when it was noted that she was apneic. A code blue was called, and the pediatric code team responded. A significant (four-minute) delay occurred while a discussion ensued over whether the patient should be taken out of the scanner area during this code because of equipment considerations or should be taken care of in the scanner area. Eventually, JH was moved out of the scanner area and fully resuscitated, and reversal medications were administered. She recovered without difficulty and was scanned two days later, without incident, with an anesthesia team (physician anesthesiologist and resident) administering the sedation.

Discussion

The case study illustrates the type of failures that can occur in complex medical care settings such as those associated with pediatric procedural sedation. A gap was evident between the state-of-the-art resources available for the work and the systems to ensure that the best people, tools, and environmental conditions were used.

To respond to the gap between the current state and the future desired state, two of the chapter authors [G.T.B. and J.P.C.], who are members of the Anesthesiology Department, launched a project to redesign the pediatric sedation process. This work ultimately resulted in the design of a completely new clinical microsystem that intentionally promoted safety and reliability.

The first goal for these two leaders of redesign in understanding this event (and preparing to commence the redesign work) was to characterize the *problem space* sedation providers contend with. They used a human factors approach, videotaping and evaluating sedations as they were performed by a variety of providers (nurses and physicians) in a variety of settings (radiology, pediatric cardiology, pediatric oncology, and pediatric anesthesiology) (Blike, Cravero, & Nelson, 2001; Coté, Karl, Notterman, Weinberg, & McCloskey, 2000; Wickens, Gordon, & Liu, 1998).

In response to this particular case, its subsequent analysis, and the application of microsystems thinking, the Anesthesiology Department of the Children's Hospital at Dartmouth developed the PainFree Program. The PainFree Program became operational in October 2001, funded with a combination of charitable funds and clinical revenue, and it currently services approximately 1,800 patients annually. Staff now include a registered nurse (RN), a patient care technician, a dedicated anesthesiologist, and a secretary. Resident and certified RN anesthetist (CRNA) staffing is variable and on an as-available basis.

This newly designed microsystem—works in this way. All children requiring sedation for diagnostic or therapeutic procedures are designated to come through the PainFree Program. Preprocedural education, admission, sedation, and recovery services are the responsibility of PainFree Program staff and are designed specifically to meet the needs of sedation patients. All sedation is provided by pediatric anesthesiologists in conjunction with nurse anesthetists and residents. Pediatric residents participate in this service with a monthlong sedation and pain management rotation during their first year. Child life specialists—health care professionals with training and certification in reducing child and family stress associated with health care experiences—are consulted on all patients, and primary pediatric providers are solicited for input on the management of patients. When appropriate, children receive their tests and procedures with distraction techniques as the only intervention. When required, general anesthesia with endotracheal intubation is provided. All intermediate levels of sedation are also provided, depending on the requirements of the procedure to be done. A shared decision-making model has been adopted, so that parents and the patients themselves are informed of the nature of the intervention to be undertaken and the options for management.

The PainFree Program is intended to provide optimal safety for sedated patients. It reflects the recognition that errors in medication delivery and sedation will occur, but there is a focus on the ability of the team to recover from these events. The advantages of the PainFree Program over the previous system lie in the fact that the providers who are most able to resuscitate patients after errors in sedation delivery (pediatric anesthesiologists who possess the most expertise and experience in delivering medications for sedation) are now present at the point of sedation delivery. Also, the nursing staff and technicians are fully trained on sedation recovery criteria and management, and this is the only care they provide.

Although the orientation and training provided by the PainFree Program led to a deeper understanding of sedation practices among its staff, it was widely recognized that one cannot assume safety simply because there is an absence of critical events. Said another way, there is a risk of *operational complacency* when an organization is successful (Weick & Sutcliffe, 2001).

The lessons learned from the comprehensive reorganization involved in the design of the PainFree Program are reflected in the following actions. They show that the patient in the case study would be treated quite differently today.

- Staff have adopted the motto "Do today's work today." This means that they work emergency cases into each day's schedule through a flexible staffing system with the Anesthesiology Department.
- An anesthesiologist, with expertise in pediatric care, uses the newest and shortest-acting sedative agents available to allow rapid emergence from sedation.
- Pediatric sedation is now a centralized process that uses anesthesia providers and postanesthesia nursing staff. The PainFree Program is an intentionally designed and innovative clinical microsystem built to do the work of pediatric sedation for procedures and examinations. Rather than fit this work into the Anesthesiology Department's structure, the program has made the pediatric population that is in need of care the driver of the design of the work.
- In the case of a sedation complication the anesthesiologist is present to manage the airway, using proven equipment and techniques that he or she practices every day.

Principles for Safety in Clinical Microsystems

Drawing on our experience with multiple microsystems across diverse settings and our understanding of the patient safety literature, we offer the following six safety principles, which may be used as a framework for adapting patient safety concepts into clinical microsystems.

Principle 1: Errors Are Human Nature and Will Happen Because Humans Are Not Infallible. Errors are not synonymous with negligence. Medicine's ethos of infallibility leads, wrongly, to a culture that sees mistakes as individual problems or weaknesses and remedies them with blame and punishment. Instead people should be looking for the multiple contributing factors, which can be resolved only by improving systems.

Principle 2: The Microsystem Is the Key Unit of Analysis and Training. Organizations can train microsystem staff to include safety principles in their daily work through rehearsing scenarios, conducting simulations, and role playing. The goal is for the microsystem to behave as a robust, high-reliability organization—an organization that is preoccupied with the possibility of failure or with chronic unease about safety breaches (Wickens et al., 1998).

Principle 3: Design Systems to Identify, Prevent, Absorb, and Mitigate Errors. Identify errors by establishing effective, sustainable reporting systems that encourage and support transparency and freedom from punitive actions and empower workers to feel comfortable with speaking up, even if that means they will challenge the authority gradient. Design work, technology, and work practices to uncover, mitigate, or attenuate the consequence of error. There are many approaches that reduce the impact of errors by simplifying and standardizing the systems and processes people use. For example, tools such as checklists, flowcharts, and ticklers compensate for deficiencies in vigilance and memory. Improve access to information and information technology. Systems should be designed to absorb a certain amount of error without harm to patients. Key buffers might include, for example, time lapses (built-in delays to verify information before proceeding), redundancy, and forcing functions.

Principle 4: Create a Culture of Safety. A safety culture is one that recognizes that the most important part of making health care safer is a transparent climate that supports reporting errors, near misses, and adverse events and treats these events as opportunities for learning and improving (Reason, 1997; Westrum, 1992). Embrace and celebrate storytelling by patients and clinicians that clarifies where safety is made and where it is breached and that provides opportunities for learning.

Principle 5: Talk to and Listen to Patients. Patients have much to say about safety. When a patient is harmed by health care, all details of the event pertaining to the patient should be disclosed to the patient and his or her family. This disclosure should include

- A prompt and compassionate explanation of what is understood about what happened and the probable effects
- An assurance that a full analysis will take place to reduce the likelihood of a similar event happening to another patient
- An assurance that there will be a follow-up based on the analysis
- An apology

Principle 6: Integrate Practices from Human Factors Engineering into Microsystem Functioning. Design patient-centered health care environments that are based on human factors principles. Design for human cognitive failings and the impact of performance-shaping factors such as fatigue, poor lighting, and noisy settings.

A discussion of patient safety in clinical microsystems cannot be complete without acknowledging how characteristics of high-performing microsystems can be used in shaping any microsystem's response to the challenge of embedding safety into the daily work of caring for patients. Table 8.1 lists primary and additional success characteristics of high-performing microsystems (identified in Chapter One) and provides specific actions that can be further explored in your own clinical microsystems. This list of actions is not intended to be exhaustive but rather to represent a place to start when applying patient safety concepts to microsystems.

Conclusion

As the patient safety scenario, the clinical case study, and the design of an innovative microsystem—the PainFree Program—illustrate, safety is a dynamic property of each clinical microsystem.

An understanding of local conditions that jeopardize safety and reliability can be acquired by using a variety of powerful tools and techniques, such as the Haddon matrix, root cause analysis, and failure mode and effects analysis. However, improvements in safety will not happen absent active and intelligent systemic changes. These can best be achieved through thoughtful and systematic application of a broad array of process, equipment, organizational, supervision, training, simulation, and teamwork changes at the level of the frontline clinical microsystems that constitute the sharp end of the delivery system, where quality, safety, and reliability flourish or fail.

TABLE 8.1. LINKAGE BETWEEN MICROSYSTEM CHARACTERISTICS AND PATIENT SAFETY.

Microsystem Characteristic	Specific Actions for Patient Safety
Leadership	• Define the safety vision of the organization. • Identify existing constraints in the organization. • Allocate resources for safety plan development, implementation, and ongoing monitoring and evaluation. • Build in microsystem participation and input to plan development. • Align organizational quality and safety goals. • Provide updates to the board of trustees.
Organizational support	• Work with clinical microsystems to identify patient safety issues and make relevant local changes. • Put the necessary resources and tools into the hands of individuals; this action needs to be real, not superficial.
Staff focus	• Assess current safety culture. • Identify the gap between the current culture and the safety vision. • Plan cultural interventions. • Conduct periodic assessments of culture.
Education and training	• Develop a patient safety curriculum. • Provide training and education of key clinical and management leadership. • Develop a core of people with patient safety skills who can work across microsystems as a resource.
Interdependence of the Care Team	• Build the plan-do-study-act (PDSA) or standardize-do-study-act (SDSA) approaches into debriefings. • Use daily huddles for after-action reviews, and celebrate identifying errors.
Patient focus	• Establish patient and family partnerships for safety. • Support disclosure and truth around medical error.
Community and market focus	• Analyze safety issues in the community, and partner with external groups to reduce risk to populations.
Performance results	• Develop key safety measures. • Create the *business case* for safety.
Process improvement	• Identify patient safety priorities based on assessment of key safety measures. • Address the safety work that will be required at the microsystem level. • Establish patient safety *demonstration sites.* • Transfer the learning across microsystems.
Information and information technology	• Enhance error-reporting systems. • Build safety concepts into information flow (for example, checklists, reminder systems, and the like)

References

Bates, D., Spell, N., Cullen, D. J., Burdick, E., Laird, N., Petersen, L. A., et al. (1997). The costs of adverse drug events in hospitalized patients. *Journal of the American Medical Association, 277*(4), 307–311.

Berwick, D., & Leape, L. (1999). Reducing errors in medicine. *British Medical Journal, 319,* 136–137.

Blike, G., Cravero, J., & Nelson, E. (2001). Same patients, same critical events—different systems of care, different outcomes: Description of a human factors approach aimed at improving the efficacy and safety of sedation/analgesia care. *Quality Management in Health Care, 10*(1), 17–36.

Brennan, T., Leape, L. L., Laird, N. M., Hebert, L., Localio, A. R., Lawthers, A. G., et al. (1991). Incidence of adverse events and negligence in hospitalized patients: Results of the Harvard Medical Practice Study I. *New England Journal of Medicine, 324*(6), 370–376.

Cook, R., Woods, D., & Miller, C. (1998). *A tale of two stories: Contrasting views of patient safety.* Retrieved June 20, 2003, from http://www.npsf.org/exec/front.html.

Coté, C., Karl, H. W., Notterman, D. A., Weinberg, J. A., & McCloskey, C. (2000). Adverse sedation events in pediatrics: Analysis of medications used for sedation. *Pediatrics, 106*(4), 633–644.

Dekker, S. (2002). *The field guide to human error investigations.* Burlington, VT: Ashgate.

Haddon, W. (1972). A logical framework for categorizing highway safety phenomena and activity. *Journal of Trauma, 12*(3), 193–207.

Haddon, W. (1973). Energy damage and the ten countermeasure strategies. *Human Factors, 15*(4), 355–366.

Helmrich, R. (2000). On error management: Lessons learned from aviation. *British Medical Journal, 320*(7237), 781–785.

Kohn, L. T., Corrigan, J. M., & Donaldson, M. S. (Eds.). (1999). *To err is human: Building a safer health system.* Washington, DC: National Academies Press.

Layde, P., Cortes, L. M., Teret, S. P., Brasel, K. J., Kuhn, E. M., Mercy, J. A., et al. (2002). Patient safety efforts should focus on medical injuries. *Journal of the American Medical Association, 287*(15), 1993–1997.

Leape, L. L. (1994). Error in medicine. *Journal of the American Medical Association, 272*(23), 1851–1857.

Leape, L. L., Brennan, T. A., Laird, N., Lawthers, A. G., Localio, A. R., Barnes, B. A., et al. (1991). The nature of adverse events in hospitalized patients: Results of the Harvard Medical Practice Study II. *New England Journal of Medicine, 324*(6), 377–384.

Mohr, J. J., & Batalden, P. B. (2002). Improving safety on the front lines: The role of clinical microsystems. *Quality & Safety in Health Care, 11*(1), 45–50.

Perrow, C. (1999). *Normal accidents: Living with high-risk technologies.* Princeton, NJ: Princeton University Press.

Reason, J. (1997). *Managing the risks of organizational accidents.* Burlington, VT: Ashgate.

Reason, J. (2000). Human error: Models and management. *British Medical Journal, 320,* 768–770.

Reason, J., Carthey, J., & de Leval, M. (2001). Diagnosing "vulnerable system syndrome": An essential prerequisite to effective risk management. *Quality in Health Care, 10*(Suppl. 2), ii21–ii25.

Weick, K. E., & Sutcliffe, K. M. (2001). *Managing the unexpected: Assuring high performance in an age of complexity.* San Francisco: Jossey-Bass.

Westrum, R. (1992). Cultures with requisite imagination. In J. Wise, D. Hopkin, & P. Stager (Eds.), *Verification and validation of complex systems: Human factors issues* (pp. 401–416). New York: Springer-Verlag.

Wickens, C., Gordon, S., & Liu, Y. (1998). *An introduction to human factors engineering.* Reading, MA: Addison-Wesley.

CHAPTER NINE

CREATING A RICH INFORMATION ENVIRONMENT

Eugene C. Nelson, Paul B. Batalden, Karen Homa,
Marjorie M. Godfrey, Christine Campbell, Linda
A. Headrick, Thomas P. Huber, Julie K. Johnson,
John H. Wasson

Chapter Summary

Background. A rich information environment supports the functioning of the small, functional, frontline units—the microsystems—that provide most health care to most people. Three settings offer case examples of how clinical microsystems use data in everyday practice to provide high-quality and cost-effective care.

Case studies. At the Dartmouth-Hitchcock Spine Center, Lebanon, New Hampshire, a patient value compass, a one-page health status report, is used to determine whether the care and services are meeting the patient's needs. In Summit, New Jersey, Overlook Hospital's Emergency Department (ED) uses real-time process monitoring of patient care cycle times and tracks quality, productivity, and patient and customer satisfaction. These data streams create an information pool that is actively used in this ED microsystem—minute by minute, hourly, daily, weekly, and annually—to analyze performance patterns and spot flaws that require action. The Shock Trauma Intensive Care Unit (STRICU) at Intermountain Health Care, Salt Lake City, uses a data system to monitor the "wired" patient remotely and share information at any time in real time. Staff can complete shift reports in ten minutes.

Discussion. Information exchange is the interface that connects staff to patients and staff to staff within the microsystem; microsystem to microsystem; and microsystem to macrosystem.

In the first chapter of Part One the research findings on twenty high-performing microsystems from the care continuum were outlined (Nelson et al., 2002). The strategic and practical importance of focusing on the small, functional, frontline units that provide most health care to most people was stressed. This, the last chapter in Part One, further advances microsystem knowledge by demonstrating the importance of creating a rich information environment that supports microsystem functioning.

Some medical practices, clinical programs, and clinical units consistently generate superb health care, based on science, on compassion, and on specific and unique knowledge of what "this patient" wants and needs right now. These same microsystems consistently use data to review their performance—to monitor, manage, and improve quality, safety, and efficiency. This is exceptional. As an Institute of Medicine (IOM) report shows, it is not the way things work in most clinical units (Institute of Medicine [U.S.], Committee on Quality of Health Care in America, 2001). Most microsystems use data today the same way they did decades ago, with little thought given to planning the flow of information to support clinical decision making and to optimize total practice performance.

Three case examples of clinical microsystems that are using data in everyday practice to provide high-quality, cost-effective care are presented in this chapter. Afterward, the principles for using data in microsystems and a discussion of some useful concepts and frameworks are offered.

Case Study 1: Specialty Care: Dartmouth-Hitchcock Spine Center

We needed a language to work with our patients. The value compass provides the language that helps our multidisciplinary team work with our patients to get them back to work, back to play, one back at a time.

JAMES WEINSTEIN, SPINE CENTER FOUNDER

A Typical Illness Episode: Health Outcomes Tracking and More

A patient comes for his first visit to the Dartmouth-Hitchcock Spine Center in Lebanon, New Hampshire. He is greeted by the receptionist, given a touch-screen computer, and asked to use the computer to answer a set of important questions about his health before seeing the physician. He takes less than twenty minutes to answer questions about his back problem, functional status, expectations for treatment, and working status. When the patient finishes, he hands the computer back to the receptionist. The receptionist transfers the survey data to the reception desk computer, which has a custom-designed database application for processing and printing a *patient value compass* (PVC) in the form of a one-page summary report (Figure 9.1). The PVC provides a balanced view of clinical and functional status, patient expectations for and satisfactions with her or his clinical care management, and other data on work status and costs of care. The PVC is used to enhance communication between the provider and patient to better meet the patient's needs. It is placed on the front of the medical record, and when the patient sees the physician for an initial assessment, they review the PVC, which describes the patient's health status specific to the spine and also related areas, such as bodily pain, physical health, mental health, and role performance compared to an average person of her or his age and sex.

The sample PVC in Figure 9.1 shows not only that the patient is suffering from acute back pain but also that he has an extreme sleeping problem, is possibly suffering from depression, has been unable to work at his job for three weeks because of his back problem, and has had chronic back pain for more than three years. The patient and physician discuss these results, and after gathering additional data through history taking and physical examination, they develop a care plan that is based on the patient's preferences and health needs and that blends behavioral medicine, physical therapy, and occupational therapy.

On each subsequent visit to the Spine Center during the next two months, the patient uses the touch-screen computer to record his current health status; this updates the changes in such health outcomes as back pain, physical functioning, and mental health that he has achieved. After six months the patient is back on the job, is free from depression, and has pain that is only slightly worse than that of the average adult (Weinstein, Brown, Hanscom, Walsh, & Nelson, 2000).

Other Facts About the Spine Center

- The Spine Center uses a *data wall* to display important indicators of clinical outcomes, patient satisfaction, and business performance. (A data wall displays key measures for use by the clinical team; these measures show current performance and trends over time.) The various data displays create a *story* about practice performance, which can be viewed by the entire practice staff.
- The Spine Center views statistical process control charts and measures of processes and outcomes as essential keys to practice management and improvement.

FIGURE 9.1. PATIENT VALUE COMPASS FOR A TYPICAL SPINE PATIENT.

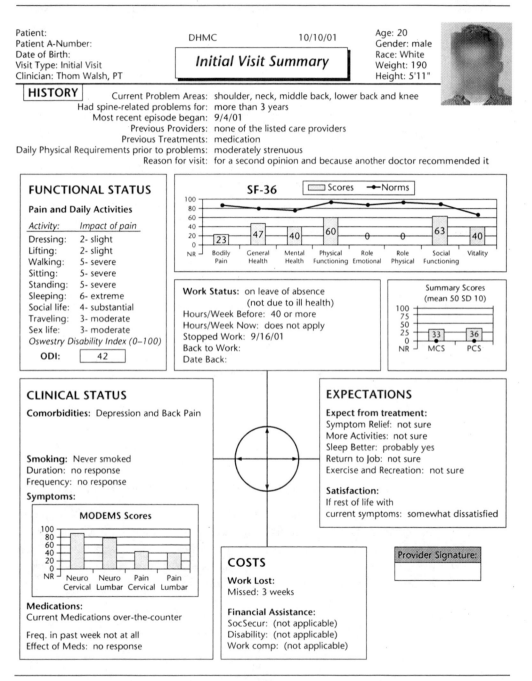

Patient:
Patient A-Number:
Date of Birth:
Visit Type: Initial Visit
Clinician: Thom Walsh, PT

DHMC   10/10/01

Initial Visit Summary

Age: 20
Gender: male
Race: White
Weight: 190
Height: 5'11"

HISTORY

Current Problem Areas: shoulder, neck, middle back, lower back and knee
Had spine-related problems for: more than 3 years
Most recent episode began: 9/4/01
Previous Providers: none of the listed care providers
Previous Treatments: medication
Daily Physical Requirements prior to problems: moderately strenuous
Reason for visit: for a second opinion and because another doctor recommended it

FUNCTIONAL STATUS

Pain and Daily Activities

Activity:	Impact of pain
Dressing:	2- slight
Lifting:	2- slight
Walking:	5- severe
Sitting:	5- severe
Standing:	5- severe
Sleeping:	6- extreme
Social life:	4- substantial
Traveling:	3- moderate
Sex life:	3- moderate

Oswestry Disability Index (0–100)

ODI: 42

SF-36   Scores   Norms

Bodily Pain 23, General Health 47, Mental Health 40, Physical Functioning 60, Role Emotional 0, Role Physical 0, Social Functioning 63, Vitality 40

Work Status: on leave of absence
(not due to ill health)
Hours/Week Before: 40 or more
Hours/Week Now: does not apply
Stopped Work: 9/16/01
Back to Work:
Date Back:

Summary Scores
(mean 50 SD 10)
MCS 33   PCS 36

CLINICAL STATUS

Comorbidities: Depression and Back Pain

Smoking: Never smoked
Duration: no response
Frequency: no response

Symptoms:

MODEMS Scores
Neuro Cervical, Neuro Lumbar, Pain Cervical, Pain Lumbar

Medications:
Current Medications over-the-counter

Freq. in past week not at all
Effect of Meds: no response

EXPECTATIONS

Expect from treatment:
Symptom Relief: not sure
More Activities: not sure
Sleep Better: probably yes
Return to Job: not sure
Exercise and Recreation: not sure

Satisfaction:
If rest of life with
current symptoms: somewhat dissatisfied

COSTS

Work Lost:
Missed: 3 weeks

Financial Assistance:
SocSecur: (not applicable)
Disability: (not applicable)
Work comp: (not applicable)

Provider Signature:

- The Spine Center creates an outcomes-based annual report and uses it as a key document during the center's all-staff annual retreat, where staff review improvements made and set up small teams to work on needed improvements for the coming year.
- The Spine Center contributes data to the National Spine Network, twenty-eight independent clinics that share outcomes data, enabling cross-site comparisons.
- The Spine Center is the lead organization for a $15 million, eleven-site, National Institutes of Health–sponsored, randomized clinical trial on the value of spine surgery for the three most common diagnoses for which spine surgery is performed.
- Many patients are delighted with the care they receive, but the Spine Center still has important improvements to make.
- The Spine Center has embraced the IOM's call for making quality data transparent and has started posting its outcomes and quality and cost data on the Dartmouth-Hitchcock Medical Center Web site (http://www.dhmc.org/qualityreports).

Case Study 2: Overlook Hospital Emergency Department

We have a culture of change right here that goes back many years to our first work with the reduction of thrombolytic cycle time. The ED moved to understanding how to use industrial quality improvement methods and microsystems thinking to be safer, more reliable, and better able to meet customer needs and expectations.

JAMES ESPINOSA, FORMER ED MEDICAL DIRECTOR

A Glimpse of the Uses of Data, Real-Time Flow Monitoring, and More

The Emergency Department of Overlook Hospital in Summit, New Jersey, has made data a critical part of its continuous improvement efforts, which began in 1994. Here are a few examples of the ways the ED uses data to create a rich, self-aware information environment that supports improved flow, quality, productivity, and patient and staff satisfaction:

- *Real-time process monitoring.* Real-time data on patient care cycle times are monitored and displayed continuously by special software to show whether the system's care for patients is flowing well or is experiencing bottlenecks. Measures tracked in real time include time to initial treatment, time to transfer to an inpatient unit, X-ray time, and cycle time for fast-track and routine patients.

- *Quality and productivity indicator tracking.* A system of process and outcome metrics is compiled and displayed using control charts and other graphical displays. Process indicators monitor trends in many areas, such as X-ray false-negative report rates, patient fall rates, and other indicators of growth and of safety.
- *Patient and customer satisfaction tracking.* The Overlook ED uses several formats to gain knowledge of its customers. It uses a national comparative database on patient satisfaction, in which it frequently scores at the 99th percentile, as well as locally developed customer satisfaction surveys for key internal customers (for example, residents in training and ED staff) and for peer microsystems (for example, the pediatric intensive care unit, radiology area, and emergency medical technician [EMT] squads).

These *data streams* create an information pool that is actively used in this ED microsystem—minute by minute, hourly, daily, weekly, and annually—to analyze performance patterns and to spot flaws that require action. Two regularly scheduled forums in which staff use the data for continual betterment are (1) the dynamic and energetic monthly microsystem meetings, chaired by the ED medical director, which are freewheeling exchanges of data, dialogue, and ideas, and (2) full-day annual retreats called *summits,* which look back to review progress and problems and forward to establish priorities and plans.

Other Facts About the Overlook ED

- The Overlook ED has implemented more than 80 percent of the ideas that have surfaced during the annual summits in the past several years.
- The Overlook ED has the highest staff satisfaction rating of any clinical unit in its four-hospital system.
- The Overlook ED has been recognized nationally—for example, the Centers for Medicare & Medicaid Services met CMS best-practice standards for *time to thrombolytics,* and it has received the American Hospital Association's Quality Quest Award.
- The Overlook ED has served as an important source of best-practice change concepts that the Institute for Healthcare Improvement has promoted in various programs and in its Breakthrough Collaboratives.

Case Study 3: Intermountain Health Care Shock Trauma Intensive Care Unit

> *The data system allows us to monitor the patient remotely and share information at any time in real time. I get to see and use data and information to help me take better care of the patient.*
>
> A STRICU CLINICIAN

Daily Work: The Wired Patient and Real-Time Monitoring

At the Shock Trauma Intensive Care Unit (STRICU) of Intermountain Health Care (IHC) in Salt Lake City, Utah, the data system is built around the patient and the clinical care team and is used every minute of every day with every patient. The injured patient is *wired* so staff can monitor clinical parameters, such as vital signs, intake and output, blood gases, and infusions, in real time. Each patient room has a bedside computer for entering all relevant information into the patient's electronic medical record (EMR). Every day starts with formal, interdisciplinary rounds, which take two or more hours to review and plan the care for the eight to twelve patients who are in the unit at any one time. During rounds the patient's clinical team—intensivist, nurse, technician, medical resident, primary physician, respiratory therapist, social worker, and family—reviews all aspects of the patient's status, with the assistance of the EMR projected on a large screen.

Using these data and a discussion of alternatives, the patient's team adjusts the care plan and then tracks the impact of the changes on the patient's clinical parameters. Despite the complexity of each patient's condition, the information technology environment makes it possible for staff to complete shift reports in ten minutes. Physicians can dial into the information system from home to monitor the patient remotely at any time of the day or night and can communicate with everyone on the care team any time, from any place. Current data, based on the local epidemiological profile, are available on the most common types of nosocomial infections, and decision support is built into the information system to guide the cost-effective selection of medications for patients who acquire infections.

Statistics that track trends over time are a way of life in the STRICU. Time-trended data on key performance indicators, such as medication error rates, protocol use rates, complication rates, and costs, are compiled and reviewed at monthly staff meetings by the unit's coordinating council and at annual all-staff retreats to monitor, manage, and improve performance.

Other Facts About the STRICU

- Protocols, which address topics such as heparin use, prevention of deep vein thrombosis, and pain relief, are developed and refined locally (by any member of the clinical team); each is typically less than one page long.
- Inflation-adjusted costs have been reduced over time and are currently at 82 percent of their 1991 levels.
- Safety is a primary concern; more than thirty types of errors are tracked.
- The EMR has been under development at IHC for decades, and the STRICU has a full-time staff member devoted to ongoing EMR and information system refinements.

Tips and Principles to Foster a Rich Information Environment

The three cases reviewed in the first half of this chapter give rise to a set of useful tips for leaders who are guiding microsystems, mesosystems, and macrosystems in quests to provide great care (that is, care that meets patients' needs) and to minimize delays and unnecessary costs. These tips are listed in Table 9.1.

In addition to the specific tips from the case studies, we have identified four principles concerning information, information technology, data, and performance results. These principles come from our detailed qualitative analysis of our twenty high-performing clinical microsystems (Nelson et al., 2002).

Principle 1: Design It—Provide Access to a Rich Information Environment. This is the primary principle among all these principles. Information guides intelligent action. Lack of information precludes the ability to take intelligent action. Processes that support Principle 1 are

- Designing the information environment to support and inform daily work and to promote core competencies and core processes essential for care delivery
- Establishing multiple formal and informal communication channels to keep all the microsystem players—patients, families, staff—informed in a timely way

Principle 2: Connect with It—Use Information to Connect Patients to Staff and Staff to Staff. The success of the clinical microsystem is contingent on the interactions between the players—patients, clinical staff, and support staff. The players must be connected for positive and productive interactions to take place and for the right things to be done in the right way at the right time. Processes that contribute to Principle 2 are

TABLE 9.1. TIPS FOR FOSTERING A RICH INFORMATION ENVIRONMENT.

Microsystem	Tips
Spine Center Specialty Practice	• Use full assessment of patient's health status to match the treatment plan to the patient's changing needs. • Integrate data collection and information technology into the flow of patient care delivery. • Use information technology to provide patients and staff with tailored health status data. • Use outcomes tracking over time to evaluate results of care for individual patients and for specific subpopulations of patients. • Build a clinical research infrastructure that can make use of structured data collection from patients and staff on top of a rich clinical information environment. • Use leadership, cultural patterns, and systems to make a firm foundation for technology.
Overlook Emergency Department	• Improve patient flow by visibly monitoring cycle times and key results in real time to promptly initiate needed actions. • Use comparative data to stimulate improvements in clinical processes and in patient satisfaction.
Shock Trauma Intensive Care Unit	• Use biomedical monitoring to provide ongoing information on the status of patients with complex, critical problems. • Use graphical and other visual data displays to connect staff to staff and staff to patients to develop optimal care plans. • Build local epidemiological knowledge, and use it to guide clinical decision making.

- Giving everyone the right information at the right time to do the work
- Investing in software, hardware, and expert staff to take full advantage of information technology to support medical care delivery
- Hearing everyone's ideas, and connecting them to benefit the patient and improve the actions that support servicing the patient
- Providing multiple channels for patients to interact with the microsystem and to receive information from the microsystem (for example, written materials, telephone calls, e-mails, Web-based information, shared medical appointments)

Principle 3: Measure It—Develop Performance Goals and Linked Measures That Reflect Primary Values and Core Competencies Essential for Providing Needed Patient Services. To improve performance or to maintain performance in the desired range of excellence, it is important to set goals that are aligned with critical values, competencies, and processes and to measure goal attainment over time. Processes that promote Principle 3 are

- Working with the microsystem team to set goals, and linking rewards and incentives to measured results
- Using measures to gauge performance, ideally in real time, in both *upstream* processes and *downstream* outcomes

Principle 4: Use It for Betterment—Measure Processes and Outcomes, Collect Feedback Data, and Redesign Continuously Based on Data. This last overarching principle completes the loop. It emphasizes using the information being gathered to provide insight to all the players, to instigate actions to improve or innovate, and to use the information streams to determine the impact of design changes. Processes that promote Principle 4 are

- Building data collection into the daily work of clinical staff and support staff
- Creating and using *self-coding* forms and checklists as part of work flow
- Turning the primary customer—the patient—into an information source, so that his or her interactions with the microsystem produce critical data elements in a standard or systematic manner
- Designing work processes and supporting technology to automatically *throw off,* or generate, important results that show how the system is working and the pattern of results that it is generating

Discussion

In this section we plunge deeper into the challenge of creating a rich information environment by discussing the central role information plays, by clarifying a fundamental informatics design principle, and by introducing three powerful frameworks for using and displaying vital data.

Information Is the Connector of All to All

As displayed in Figure 1.5 in Chapter One, information and information technology make up a feeder system that supports the four areas into which the key success characteristics are grouped—leadership, staff, patients, and performance. Information exchange is the interface that connects

- Member to member—staff to patients and staff to staff—within the microsystem
- Microsystem to microsystem
- Microsystem to mesosystem and macrosystem

Information technology facilitates effective communication. Multiple formal and informal channels are used to maintain accurate, honest, and timely dialogue among all parties.

Designing Information Flow to Support the Smallest Replicable Units of Activity

A rich information environment does not just happen, it must be designed and improved over time. It can be engineered to support the organization's ability to deliver high-quality services to patients at the level of the smallest replicable units (SRUs) of activity within a microsystem (Quinn, 1992). For example, gathering patient registration data, collecting patient health status data, arriving at a diagnosis based on the data, and assessing changes in patient outcomes over the course of treatment all represent SRUs of activity that are embedded in clinical microsystems. Each of these SRUs of activity can be supported by designing an information system—to capture, analyze, use, store, and reuse data—that fits well into the flow of work and supports doing the right work in the right way efficiently. Quinn (1992) makes the point that the leading service organizations in the world do exactly this and that to do so is a strategic advantage. To realize this advantage, however, requires (1) a fundamental understanding of the nature of frontline work and frontline processes and (2) building the information system from a core process base and capturing data in its most disaggregated form, that is, at the SRU level. This can be done, as demonstrated in each case study in this chapter, but doing so is extraordinary in today's health system. It needs to be ordinary in tomorrow's health system if we are to cross the *quality chasm* (Institute of Medicine. . . , 2001).

Making Progress by Building on Three Useful Frameworks

The path to the creation of a rich information environment can be made smoother and easier (though still not easy) by applying some useful frameworks:

- Feed forward and feedback
- The patient value compass
- The balanced scorecard

In the following sections we provide short introductions to each of these frameworks, using our case studies to illustrate how they can be adapted to the real world of clinical practice. When leaders apply these core ideas to specific clinical microsystems, they can create more powerful information environments.

Framework 1: Feed Forward and Feedback—Can We Use Data to Do the Right Thing Right the First Time and Every Time? Figure 9.2 portrays an information environment built by a microsystem in order to use both feed forward and feedback data to manage and improve care. The general idea involved in using feed forward is to collect data at an early stage in the process of delivering care, save it, and use it again at a later stage: that is, to manage and inform service delivery—to do the right thing, in the right way, the first time (in real time) for each patient. The general idea involved in using feedback is to gather data about what has happened to a patient, or a set of patients, and to use this information to improve care so that future patients will get the right thing, in the right way.

Both feed-forward and feedback methods are commonly used in care delivery. For example, many medical practices caring for patients with hypertension have a nurse or medical assistant measure the patient's blood pressure level and feed this information forward to the physician, who uses it to guide decision making concerning the treatment and the need for adjustments to the regimen. Likewise, many primary care practices show the level of control achieved by the panel of hypertensive patients under the care of each physician in the practice and will feed these comparative data back to identify the degree of success and to identify improvement opportunities.

The case studies presented at the beginning of this chapter offer examples of advanced uses of data feed forward:

- The Spine Center uses touch-screen computers to collect information on the patient's general and disease-specific health status; this database provides a well rounded basis for patient and clinician to engage in shared decision making to best match the patient's changing needs with the preferred treatment plan.
- The Overlook ED uses cycle time monitoring to determine if and when patient flow bottlenecks are occurring; this provides a basis for taking immediate corrective action before a slowdown degenerates into a meltdown.
- The IHC STRICU uses real-time monitoring of each patient's clinical parameters to feed forward into daily rounds; this provides full-bandwidth data for the multidisciplinary team to use to make sure the care plan matches the patient's acuity.

FIGURE 9.2. FEED FORWARD AND FEEDBACK IN A MICROSYSTEM: THE SPINE CENTER DESIGN FOR INFORMATION FLOW.

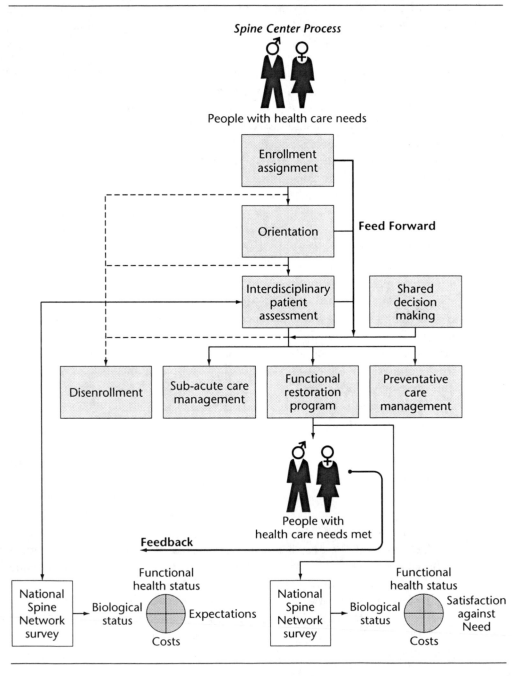

Each of these three clinical microsystems uses feed-forward data concepts to engineer timely data collection and interpretation into the microsystem and thus to enable staff to do the right thing at the right time. In addition, all three microsystems use a variety of data feedback methods (such as graphical data displays; statistical process control charts; data walls; and weekly, monthly, quarterly, and annual reports) to *aggregate up* performance measures and use the resulting information to manage and improve care. It is possible and desirable to use advanced process flow analysis methods, such as value stream mapping and other lean-thinking methods and tools, to specify the flow of information that should accompany the flow of health care service delivery (Rother & Shook, 1998).

Framework 2: Patient Value Compass—Can We Use Data to Measure and Improve the Quality and Value of Care?

Patient value compass (PVC) thinking can be used to determine whether the microsystem is providing care and services that meet patients' needs for high quality and high value (Nelson, Mohr, Batalden, & Plume, 1996; Nelson, Batalden, & Ryer, 1998; Splaine, Batalden, Nelson, Plume, & Wasson, 1998).

The PVC was designed to provide a balanced view of outcomes—health status, patient satisfaction, and patient care costs—for an individual patient or a defined population of patients. Like a conventional magnetic compass used for navigation, the PVC has four cardinal points that can be pursued in exploring answers to critical questions:

- West: What are the biological and clinical outcomes?
- North: What are the functional status and risk status outcomes?
- East: How do patients view the goodness of their care?—What is their level of satisfaction with services and perceived health benefit?
- South: What costs are incurred in the process of delivering care? What direct and indirect costs are incurred by the patient?

The PVC framework can be adapted to virtually any population of patients—such as outpatients, inpatients, home health clients, and community residents (Speroff, Miles, & Mathews, 1998). The model assumes that patient outcomes—health status, satisfaction, and costs—evolve over time and through illness episodes. For example, a person may be in generally good health at thirty-two years of age and then suffer a herniated disc, undergo short-term treatment for the disc problem, and regain full health. Then at age thirty-five he may reinjure his back, suffer from prolonged chronic back pain, lose his job, and become clinically depressed. At each point in the patient's illness journey it is possible, through data collection, to explore that individual patient's PVC for that point in time and compare it to his PVC readings at earlier points in time. PVC data can be collected and analyzed to answer the question, Is this patient improving or declining with respect to health status and satisfaction and in relation to his need for care, and at what cost?

The Spine Center case illustrates the use of the PVC framework to design the information environment. First, feed-forward data are used at each patient visit to create an up-to-date PVC, which is placed on the front of the patient's medical record and which launches the patient—clinician interaction (Figure 9.1). The individualized PVC puts the clinician in an excellent position to rapidly understand the patient's health strengths and health deficits and to codevelop a plan of care with the patient that best matches evidence-based medicine with the patient's own preferences and needs. Second, feedback data are used to evaluate the care for distinct subpopulations seen at the Spine Center, such as patients who underwent surgery for a herniated disk (Figure 9.3).

Many clinical microsystems and health systems in the United States and abroad use the PVC to manage and improve the quality and costs of care. Moreover, the PVC framework can be used to blend strategic thinking with specific objectives and target values for measurable results at the level of the system as a whole (the macrosystem) or at the level of clinical service lines (such as mesosystems for oncology care, cardiac care, and so forth) and frontline operating units within the system (that is, specific clinical microsystems).

Framework 3: Balanced Scorecard—Can We Use Data to Measure and Improve the Performance of the Microsystem? The balanced scorecard approach developed by Kaplan and Norton can be used to answer the question, Is the microsystem making progress in areas that contribute to operating excellence and strategic progress? It is a popular and powerful approach that has gained popularity during the past decade (Griffith, Alexander, & Jelinek, 2002; Kaplan & Norton, 1992, 1993, 2001, 2004; Oliveira, 2001). In contrast to the PVC, which uses the patient as the unit of analysis, the balanced scorecard model examines the organization or a smaller operational unit within the organization. Just as the PVC can work at multiple levels—the individual patient or a discrete subpopulation—the balanced scorecard can work at the level of the clinical microsystem, the mesosystem, or the macrosystem.

The balanced scorecard is designed to provide a well-rounded view, specifying and assessing an organization's strategic progress from four critical perspectives—learning and growth, core processes, customer viewpoint, and financial results. It can be used to answer fundamental questions such as these:

- Are we learning and growing in business-critical areas?
- How are our core processes performing?

FIGURE 9.3. PATIENT VALUE COMPASS: SPINE CENTER HERNIATED DISK PATIENTS.

Clinical Status

Common Health Problems

Comorbidities besides spine condition	57%
Depression	18%
Frequent headaches	18%
High blood pressure	14%
Osteoarthritis	11%
Heart disease	5%

Symptoms

Symptoms	Initial	Follow-Up	Improved
Oswestry Disability Index: How pain has affected your ability to perform activities	46	71	70%
MODEMS: Degree of suffering and bothersome			
Numbness, tingling, and/or weakness in *lower body*	41	70	69%
Numbness, tingling, and/or weakness in *upper body*	77	89	43%

Oswestry Disability Index (ODI): reported as low score is more disability.
Improved for ODI is a difference of 10 points or greater between Follow-up and Initial.
Improved for MODEMS is a difference of 5 points or greater between Follow-up and Initial.

Pain at Follow-Up

Experience pain in the neck, arms, lower back, and/or legs most or all of the time	33%
Medications at Follow-Up	
Taking medication(s)	61%

Functional Health Status

SF-36 Norm-Based (Mean 50 SD 10)	Initial	Follow-Up	Improved
Bodily pain	26	40	77%
Role physical	27	37	50%
Physical component summary	28	38	62%
Mental component summary	43	51	58%
General health			
Excellent & very good	40%	43%	26%

Improved for SF-36 is a difference of 5 points or greater between Follow-up and Initial.
Improved for General Health is a positive change in category from Initial to Follow-up.

Costs

Work Lost

Missed work (28 weeks average)	54%
On leave from work at follow-up	6%
Financial	
Receiving Worker's Compensation	17%
Litigation: legal action pending	6%

Charges: One-Year Episode Spine-Specific ICD-9 Codes

Spine Center		Outpatient		Inpatient	
Professional	$48,481	Diagnostic radiology	$63,498	Surgical	$1,525,132
Physical therapist	$71,032	Neurosurgery	$158,411	Inpatient	$2,810,156
		Orthopaedics	$160,987	Other	$737,737
		Pain clinic	$34,769		
		Office, urgent, other	$32,918		
Total	$119,513		$450,583		$5,073,025

$5,643,121

Patient Case Mix (July '98 to Mar. '02)

Patients (have follow-up survey)	170
Follow-up rate (N = 370)	46%
Average follow-up (SD) days	121 (47)
Average age (SD) years	44 (12)
Female	42%
Chronic greater than 3 years	35%
Prior surgery	14%

Hospital Surgery Indicators

One-day length of stay	69%
Discharged to home	91%
Average charges	$7,721

Satisfaction

Results of Treatment(s) Met Expectations

For ability to sleep	66%
For symptom relief	61%
For ability to do activities	55%
To return to work	54%

Satisfaction

Satisfied with treatment(s)	85%
Would choose same treatment(s)	85%

Median per patient: $13,330
Average: $15,995 (SD $10,818)
Range: $169 to $74,339

Note: SD = standard deviation.

- How do we look in the eyes of our customers?
- How are we doing at managing costs and making margins?

The balanced scorecard approach can be adapted to virtually any type of organization—a manufacturing plant, a service enterprise, or a health care system. Balanced scorecards offer a simple yet elegant way to link strategy and vision with

- Objectives for strategic progress
- Measures of objectives
- Target values for measures
- Initiatives to improve and innovate

Other positive features of the balanced scorecard framework are its capacity to (1) align different parts of a system toward common goals, (2) deploy high-level themes to ground-level operating units that directly serve the patient or customer, (3) establish a succinct method for communicating results and for holding operating units accountable for generating essential results.

Figure 9.4 shows a balanced scorecard for the Spine Center. The Spine Center examines its scorecard at its annual retreats in order to review its progress as revealed by measured results and to sharpen its strategic focus for the upcoming year through an analysis of improvement imperatives. Its balanced scorecard emphasizes top-priority objectives in each of the four dimensions. The figure shows, for example, that the Spine Center had yet to meet its goal of having 80 percent of patients participate by using the shared decision-making video. Patients having timely access to a provider are also targeted for improvement, and this is associated with the financial measure of utilization of clinic time for physicians.

Conclusion

These cases, principles, and frameworks can be used to create information-enriched health systems in which caring and skilled staff will find it easier to provide wanted and needed care. High-performing microsystems use data and other information to guide actions and improve performance. The intelligent design of the information environment and the regular use of information is essential for achieving excellence.

FIGURE 9.4. BALANCED SCORECARD FOR THE SPINE CENTER.

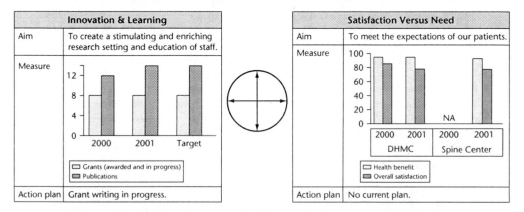

Key Processes	
Aim	To do the right things at the right time for the patients.
Measure	Shared decision making (SDM): Diagnosis-specific patients checked out either the Herniated Disc or Spinal Stenosis video. Access: Preferred appointment met for patients seeing a surgeon for the first time.
Action plan	SDM: No current plan to improve the process. Access: Scheduling/access workgroup formed in January 2002.

Innovation & Learning	
Aim	To create a stimulating and enriching research setting and education of staff.
Measure	
Action plan	Grant writing in progress.

Satisfaction Versus Need	
Aim	To meet the expectations of our patients.
Measure	
Action plan	No current plan.

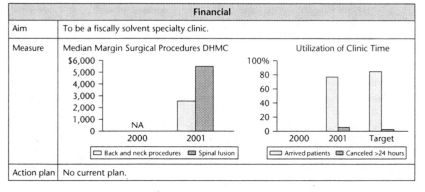

Financial	
Aim	To be a fiscally solvent specialty clinic.
Measure	
Action plan	No current plan.

References

Griffith, J., Alexander, J., & Jelinek, R. (2002). Measuring comparative hospital performance. *Journal of Healthcare Management, 47*(1), 41–57.

Institute of Medicine (U.S.), Committee on Quality of Health Care in America. (2001). *Crossing the quality chasm: A new health system for the 21st century.* Washington, DC: National Academies Press.

Kaplan, R. S., & Norton, D. P. (1992, January/February). The balanced scorecard: Measures that drive performance. *Harvard Business Review,* pp. 71–79.

Kaplan, R. S., & Norton, D. P. (1993, September/October). Putting the balanced scorecard to work. *Harvard Business Review,* 134–147.

Kaplan, R. S., & Norton, D. P. (2001). *The strategy focused organization.* Boston: Harvard Business School Press.

Kaplan, R. S., & Norton, D. P. (2004). *Strategy maps: Converting intangible assets into tangible outcomes.* Boston: Harvard Business School Press.

Nelson, E. C., Batalden, P. B., Huber, T. P., Mohr, J. J., Godfrey, M. M., Headrick, L. A., et al. (2002). Microsystems in health care: Part 1. Learning from high-performing front-line clinical units. *Joint Commission Journal on Quality Improvement, 28*(9), 472–493.

Nelson, E. C., Batalden, P. B., & Ryer, J. C. (Eds.). (1998). *Clinical improvement action guide.* Oakbrook Terrace, IL: Joint Commission on Accreditation of Healthcare Organizations.

Nelson, E., Mohr, J., Batalden, P., & Plume, S. (1996). Improving health care: Part 1. The clinical value compass. *Joint Commission Journal on Quality Improvement, 22*(4), 243–258.

Oliveira, J. (2001). The balanced scorecard: An integrative approach to performance evaluation. *Healthcare Financial Management, 55*(5), 42–46.

Quinn, J. B. (1992). *Intelligent enterprise: A knowledge and service based paradigm for industry.* New York: Free Press.

Rother, J., & Shook, J. (1998). *Learning to see.* Brookline, MA: Lean Enterprise Institute.

Speroff, T., Miles, P., & Mathews, B. (1998). Improving health care: Part 5. Applying the Dartmouth Clinical Improvement Model to community health. *Joint Commission Journal on Quality Improvement, 24*(12), 679–703.

Splaine, M., Batalden, P., Nelson, E., Plume, S. K., & Wasson J. H. (1998). Looking at care from the inside out. *Journal of Ambulatory Care Management, 21*(3), 1–9.

Weinstein, J., Brown, P. W., Hanscom, B., Walsh, T., & Nelson, E. C. (2000). Designing an ambulatory clinical practice for outcomes improvement: From vision to reality: The Spine Center at Dartmouth-Hitchcock, year one. *Quality Management in Healthcare, 8*(2), 1–20.

PART TWO

ACTIVATING THE ORGANIZATION AND THE DARTMOUTH MICROSYSTEM IMPROVEMENT CURRICULUM

CHAPTER TEN

OVERVIEW OF PATH FORWARD
AND INTRODUCTION TO PART TWO

Chapter Purpose

Aims. To promote organization-wide improvement through the introduction of an approach (the M3 Matrix) for building improvement capability at *all levels of a health system,* and to preview an action-learning program for frontline staff.

Objectives. At the completion of this unit, you will be able to

- Describe the current state of health care and the relevance of the Institute of Medicine's publication *Crossing the Quality Chasm* (Institute of Medicine [U.S.], Committee on Quality of Health Care in America, 2001).
- List specific, phased actions for leaders to take at the macrosystem, mesosystem, and microsystem levels

to create the conditions for performance improvement.

- Describe why a microsystem approach to improving performance is system based and engages the entire health system.
- State the value of using a story about a patient to engage staff at all levels of a health system.
- Outline the elements of an action-learning program for frontline staff.
- Identify the reasons why a lead improvement team (an interdisciplinary team representing all roles in a microsystem) makes an important contribution to anchoring improvement work in the real work of frontline microsystems.

This chapter traces the beginning of the improvement journey to build the capability of clinical microsystems to become high-performing frontline units.

Recap of Part One and Overview of Part Two

Part One of this book offers a way of thinking about improving care and leading the betterment of care. It describes some of the many facets and faces of microsystem thinking in health care. We introduced case studies, concepts, and principles to provide a broad and deep perspective on clinical microsystems. We described the pivotal role of microsystems in providing high-quality, high-value care that meets the need of patients to realize health benefits, and the need of staff to have meaningful work and to make a difference in the lives of patients and families.

Part Two of this book will focus on practical issues. It will deal with pragmatic issues—what to do and how to do it. The primary purpose of Part Two will be to describe an action-learning program for frontline microsystems. This program is the Dartmouth Microsystem Improvement Curriculum (DMIC), and it is grounded in the micro-meso-macrosystems matrix (M3 Matrix). This program has been under development for over a decade and has been used successfully by hundreds of microsystems in both North America and Western Europe.

Using Real Case Studies and Practical Applications of Microsystem Thinking, Methods, and Tools

Throughout Part Two of this book we will provide two case examples of microsystems using the tools and methods introduced in each chapter. These cases will present concrete examples of the Dartmouth Microsystem Improvement Curriculum in action. One case study looks at a hospital inpatient unit—an Intermediate Cardiac Care Unit—and the second case study examines a busy ambulatory practice—within a Section of Plastic Surgery. The progression of each group's lead improvement team through the tools and methods will be discussed throughout the text. (Other case studies can be found in the case study portfolio on http://www.clinicalmicrosystem.org. This collection of cases illustrates various applications of microsystem thinking across the health care continuum in North America and throughout Europe and the Middle East.)

The Intermediate Cardiac Care Unit (ICCU) we focus on in the inpatient unit case study is a thirty-seven-bed telemetry unit with medical and surgical cardiac patients at the Dartmouth-Hitchcock Medical Center. A dynamic and ever-changing census and fluctuating acuity of patients provide many challenges for this microsystem. The beginning of 2006 brought new leadership and a new direction for this highly stressed unit. A new nursing leader joined the staff of fifty; she began an intentional partnership with the ICCU physician medical director. Their intention to create world-class outcomes for patients and an improved workplace with high productivity caused them to start the unit on its developmental journey and to apply clinical microsystem thinking to make a clear and structured path for improvement.

The high-performing ambulatory unit in the Section of Plastic Surgery at Dartmouth-Hitchcock Medical Center, our second case study, began its microsystem development journey five years ago. It does outpatient minor surgical procedures as well as inpatient surgical procedures. The Plastic Surgery program learned it can only be the best it can be if it has deep knowledge of all aspects of its system.

Our hope is to help you weave together the Part Two chapters, the workbook materials in the Appendix to this book, the M3 Matrix, the DMIC, and the resources at http://www.clinicalmicrosystem.org so that you can build a customized strategy for the organization-wide improvement of your health system.

Before narrowing our focus to microsystems and the action-learning program, we first turn to the challenge that senior and midlevel leaders face—what can they do to create the conditions for frontline excellence? (Also see the discussion of leading meso- and macrosystems in Chapter Four.)

Working at All Levels of a Health System

At each level of a health care system, leaders can take actions that will create the conditions for quality and excellence in microsystems—the places where patients and families and health care teams meet.

Moving from Improvement Projects to Improving Systems

Donald Nielsen, a physician and expert on health care quality, has worked with many leading health care organizations and is a student of what works and what fails in transforming health systems to achieve high levels of performance. He uses the diagram shown in Figure 10.1 to explain what he sees happening (and what needs to happen) if health systems are to be successful in achieving and sustaining a culture of quality.

- *Project focus.* The first phase of improvement focuses on *projects*, as the health system seeks to improve quality by running a variety of projects in areas of high

FIGURE 10.1. EVOLUTION IN APPROACHES TO IMPROVING HEALTH SYSTEM QUALITY: FROM PROJECTS TO MESOSYSTEMS TO MACROSYSTEMS.

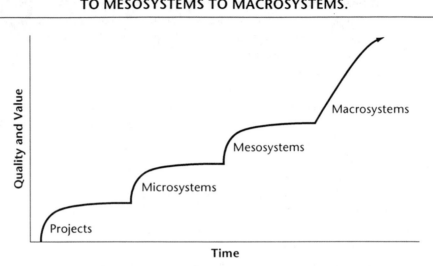

Source: Adapted from the work of Donald Nielsen.

interest. Many projects are successful, some fail, some are at first successful but fail to hold their gains. In this phase, quality work is viewed as special, ad hoc work by most staff members. The project participants often work extra hard, learn new skills, and take well-deserved pride in their accomplishments; usually they also know there is a clear start and a clear end to the project. Most health systems and provider organizations in the United States are in this phase. They will make real progress here and there, but it will be limited to whatever area was selected as the focus. Improvements arising from projects are sometimes difficult to sustain and are unlikely to spread and to transition on their own to the next challenge.

- *Microsystem focus.* The second phase of improvement focuses on microsystems, as the health system makes tactical use of microsystem thinking to build the habit for improvement into the fabric of some frontline systems. In this phase senior leaders promote improvement from the *inside out* in certain clinical microsystems. They encourage individual microsystems to develop their own capability to plan and make changes as part of their regular work routines. Frontline staff in the best-performing units have a sense that they work in a unique place with a wonderful group of people who care for a very special

EXHIBIT 10.1. LETTER TO THE EDITOR ABOUT A CLINICAL PROGRAM WITH A LOCAL AND NATIONAL REPUTATION.

To the Editor:

I have just completed treatment at a medical jewel more people in the Upper Valley should know about—the Spine Center at Dartmouth-Hitchcock Medical Center. In this innovative center, a team of world-class specialists in all aspects of back and spine care—from neurosurgery and orthopedics to psychology and physical therapy—assemble to review all aspects of any complex case. No more waiting and roaming from one source to another and obtaining conflicting views over a long period of time. Instead, different specialists exchange views face to face, backed by the most powerful diagnostic equipment and delivery techniques currently in use. All information is shared in a way that lets patients join appropriately in making the best decision.

I know of no other rural area that enjoys such capable specialists along with the most advanced technological and research facilities available anywhere. Just as important is the friendly and personal way the care is delivered. A small team knew my case intimately, provided the personal attention and follow-up associated with a small practice, and patiently responded to all the frightening questions—and analysis of alternatives—a person facing the possibility of back surgery wants answered.

All back sufferers in the Upper Valley are blessed to have this marvelous institution and its outstanding people.

James Brian Quinn
Hanover

Source: Quinn, 1999.

group of patients and families. These *breakaway* or *standout* microsystems might be considered *pockets of gold*. They have a good reputation, and stories are told and letters are written about the extraordinary care that this practice or that unit or clinical program provides (see, for example, Exhibit 10.1). There are some health systems in this phase of improvement, and their numbers are growing due to the attractive nature of the approach taken by these standout microsystems and the success they are achieving.

- *Mesosystem focus.* The third phase of improvement focuses on the mesosystem. At this stage, the good work done by individual microsystems to improve care begins to spread to other related microsystems. Mesosystems can be thought of as an interrelated set of "peer microsystems" that provide care to certain patient populations or support the care provided to these populations. Sometimes an individual microsystem that has made good progress on improving quality will start to "reach out" to other related microsystems to work on the way they connect with one another to transfer the patient from one microsystem to another or to work on the flow of supporting services and information. Another impetus for mesosystem development is for a health system to make it a priority to improve care for patients that "move through" many different but related microsystems. For example, patients with chronic problems—such as heart failure, or diabetes—or with serious acute problems—such as acute myocardial infarction or pneumonia—often receive care from many assorted outpatient and inpatient clinical units. Consequently, if every patient is to get the right care in the right place in the right time, then it is necessary to organize and improve care in the mesosystem that consists of all the different microsystems that contribute to the care of "this" kind of patient. Yet another trigger for mesosystem development is a decision to target particular "clinical service lines" such as cardiovascular care or spine care or women's health as strategic areas for growth and development. Creating a center of excellence for patient populations such as these requires extensive work to improve or redesign care within and between all the related microsystems and thereby calls for the development of a superior mesosystem.

- *Macrosystem focus.* The fourth phase of improvement focuses on the whole system, or *macrosystem,* as all parts of the system and all levels of the system *get it,* as they become aligned with the goal of organization-wide improvement. This whole-system approach is strategic and operational. In this phase leaders and staff are working to improve performance both within and between all the microsystems in the organization and to align all levels of the organization to improve quality, reduce real costs, and engage all staff members in both doing their work and improving their work. An important aspect of this leadership work is to focus on making smooth, safe, and effective connections between and across related microsystems and supporting systems; this involves improving and redesigning the functioning of mediating, midlevel systems, or *mesosystems,* such as clinical service lines, programs, or divisions. Horizontal and vertical alignment is essential.

The Baldrige National Quality Program (2006) framework provides one excellent approach for mobilizing the whole system to work on quality and performance and has been applied to health care. Chapter Four in Part One of this book discusses this approach at length and introduces the major leadership frameworks and specific suggestions for moving in this direction. A small number of health systems and frontline (microsystem) providers are in this phase of improvement, and there is much to learn from them.

We believe, fundamentally, that populations will have high-quality health care systems only when their health care delivery organizations take a systems-based approach to attaining and sustaining high-quality health care. We believe that macro-, meso-, and microsystem thinking can provide just such a systems-based approach for improving the quality of a whole health system with a vertical and horizontal alignment of strategy and actions. But to carry out such an approach requires synchronized action at all levels of a health care delivery organization. Improvement needs to be led from the *inside out* for microsystems and from the *outside in* for leaders creating the conditions for improvement. Paul Batalden reminds us that "every system is perfectly designed to get the results it gets" (personal communication to Donald Berwick, IHI president and CEO, 1996). Alignment of system levels with systems-based improvement offers the prospect of a better system and better results.

Using the M3 Matrix to Guide Actions at All Health System Levels

Figure 10.2 shows the M3 Matrix. It is called the M3 Matrix because it spells out actions that leaders can take at the three main levels of a health system:

- Macrosystem: actions taken by the senior leaders who are responsible for organization-wide performance
- Mesosystem: actions taken by the midlevel leaders who are responsible for large clinical programs, clinical support services, and administrative services
- Microsystem: actions taken by the leaders of frontline clinical systems who engage in direct patient care, provide ancillary services that interact with patient care, or provide administrative services that support patient care

The M3 Matrix displays actions not only according to the three system levels but also according to time frame, suggesting actions to consider taking immediately (within months one to six), in the short term (months seven to twelve), and in the long term (months thirteen to eighteen).

We believe that leaders of health care systems can use the M3 Matrix for developing a specific eighteen- to twenty-four-month action plan and for beginning to progress up "Nielsen's curve" (Figure 10.1) by making the transition from improvement based on projects to improvement based on microsystems to improvement based on mesosystems and the macrosystem—all the small systems coming together to make the whole system—and finally to the completion of a transformative journey.

Engaging the Whole Person in Doing the Work

Organizations cannot transform themselves without positive engagement of the workforce. The next two sections offer methods for (1) setting clear expectations on the need for everyone to take on improvement as part of daily work, and (2) making the need for dramatic improvements relevant and attractive by putting a specific human face on the imperative for change.

FIGURE 10.2. THE M3 MATRIX: SUGGESTIONS FOR LEADERSHIP ACTIONS AT THREE LEVELS OF A HEALTH SYSTEM.

Microsystems Developmental Journey: The Stages

1. Create awareness of our clinical unit as an interdependent group of people with the capacity to make change.
2. Connect our routine daily work to the high purpose of benefiting patients; see ourselves as a system.
3. Respond successfully to a strategic challenge.
4. Measure the performance of our system as a system.
5. Successfully juggle multiple improvements while taking care of patients, . . . and continue to develop our sense of ourselves as a system.

Microsystem Level	Mesosystem Level	Macrosystem Level
Inside Out 0–6 Months	*Creating the Conditions* 0–6 Months	*Outside In* 0–6 Months
Prework. At www.clinicalmicrosystem.org, read Parts 1, 8, 9 of series (click publications in left-hand menu, select readings from *Journal of Quality, Safety Improvement Microsystems in Healthcare;* watch Batalden streaming video • Form an interdisciplinary lead improvement team. • Begin the Dartmouth Microsystem Improvement Curriculum. • Learn to work together using effective meeting skills. • Rehearse within studio course format. • Practice in clinical practice. • Hold daily huddles, weekly lead improvement team meetings, monthly all-staff meetings. • Conduct learning sessions (monthly). • Hold conference calls (between sessions).	• Link strategy, operations, and people—*make it happen.* • Support and facilitate meso- and microsystem protected time to reflect and learn. • Identify resources to support meso- and microsystem development, including information technology and performance measure resources. • Develop measures of microsystem performance. • Address roadblocks and barriers to micro- and mesosystem improvements and progress. • Set goals and expectations.	• Develop clear visions and missions for meso- and microsystems. • Set goals for improvement. • Design meso- and microsystem manager and leadership professional development strategy. • Engage board of trustees with improvement strategies. • Expect all senior leaders to be familiar and involved with meso- and microsystem improvement. • Provide regular feedback and encouragement to meso- and microsystem staff. • Encourage patient and family involvement in improvement.

6–12 Months

- Reinforce staff by leadership.
- Engage in colleague reinforcement.
- Develop new habits through repetition.
- Put improvement science into action.
- Add more improvement cycles.
- Build measurement into practice.
- Increase use of measures, dashboards, and data walls.
- Use playbooks and storyboards.
- Understand and develop relationships (linkages) between microsystems.
- Improve use of PDSA and SDSA approaches.
- Incorporate best practices, using value stream mapping or lean design principles.

12–18 Months

- Continue "new way of providing care, continuously improving and working together."
- Actively engage more staff involvement.
- Ensure that multiple improvements are occurring.
- Network with other microsystems to support efforts.
- Coach network and development.
- Develop leadership.
- Conduct annual review, reflect, and plan retreats.
- Conduct quarterly system review and hold accountability meetings with meso- and macrosystem leadership.

6–12 Months

- Convene mesosystem and microsystems to work on linkages and handoffs.
- Facilitate system coordination.
- Link with electronic medical records.
- Link business initiatives or strategic plan to microsystem level.
- Attract cooperation across health professions, even if traditionally highly separate.
- Track and tell stories about improvement results and lessons learned at meso- and microsystem levels.
- Schedule rounds regularly at the microsystem level.
- Make improvement a regular agenda item.
- Inquire about results and data specifics to set goals and improvement.

12–18 Months

- Link performance management to daily work and results.
- Support and coach microsystem leadership development.
- Provide resources to support microsystem development.
- Provide feedback and encouragement to microsystems.
- Expect patient and family involvement in improvement.
- Encourage and support the search for best practices.

6–12 Months

- Expect improvement science and measured results from meso- and microsystems.
- Develop whole-system measures and targets or goals.
- Attract cooperation across health professions, even if traditionally highly separate.
- Design review and accountability quarterly meetings for senior leaders.
- Track and tell stories about improvement results and lessons learned at meso- and microlevels.
- Develop budgets to support and develop strategic improvement.
- Ensure resources (such as information technology) to support meso- and microsystems.
- Plan time in schedule to conduct rounds at meso- and microsystem levels to observe improvements and progress.

12–18 Months

- Develop professional development strategies across all professionals.
- Design HR selection and orientation process linked to identified needs of macro-, meso-, and microsystems.
- Consider incentive programs for reaching targets or goals.
- Create system to link measurement and accountability at the micro-, meso-, and macrolevel.
- Develop a Quality College for ongoing support and capability building throughout the organization.

(continued)

FIGURE 10.2. THE M3 MATRIX: SUGGESTIONS FOR LEADERSHIP ACTIONS AT THREE LEVELS OF A HEALTH SYSTEM. (Continued)

Some Questions for Leaders at All Levels to Consider

Microsystem Leader	Mesosystem Leader	Macrosystem Leader
• How does this microsystem work? Who does what to whom? What technology is part of what you regularly do?	• How do the *organization's messages* move?	• How does this work bring help or value to the patients? What stories illustrate that?
• What is the main or core process of the way work gets done here? How does it vary?	• How does the macrosystem strategy connect to the microsystems? What helps people adapt to and respond to it?	• What are the values that are part of the everyday work?
• What are some of the limitations you encounter as you try to do what you do for patients?	• How do the microsystems link strategy, operations, and people needed for successful execution?	• What helps people grow, develop, and become better professionals here?
• When you want to change the clinical care because of some new knowledge, how does that work?	• What is the process for identifying and orienting the microsystem leaders? For helping set their expectations? For reviewing their performance and for holding each clinical microsystem accountable for its performance?	• What helps people personally engage the never-ending safeguarding and improving of patient care?
• What are the helpful measures you regularly use here? How are those measures analyzed and displayed?	• What helps maintain a steadfast focus on "improved patient care outcomes by more reliable and more efficient systems that are regularly reflected on and redesigned?"	• What connects this whole place—from the patient and those working directly with the patient down to the macrosystem leaders?
• What are the things people honor as *traditions* around here? If you had to single out a few things that really contribute to and mark the identity of this clinical microsystem, what might you point to?	• What about your personal style of work speaks more convincingly than your words about the desired way of work in the organization?	• What helps the processes of inquiry, learning, and change within, between, and across microsystems and mesosystems?
• What do people ask questions about around here? Who asks? Who gets asked?	• How do you yourself facilitate improvement across microsystems and encourage patient and family focus?	• What helps people do their own work and improve patient outcomes, year after year?
• What does it take to make things happen around here? When did it work well? Who did what?	• What do you yourself regularly do to learn of improvements in the microsystems?	• What might be possible? What are some of the current limits the organization faces?
• How do information and information technology get integrated into the daily work and new initiatives around here?		• What are some of the most relevant external forces for this macrosystem and its micro- and mesosystems?
		• Do you have the measurements and feedback necessary to make it easy for you to monitor and improve the quality of your performance?

- When you add new people here, how do you go about it?
- How are things *noticed* around here?
- If you were to point to an example of *respect* among all staff here, what might you point to?
- How do the leaders get involved in change here?
- How are patients and families brought into the daily workings and improvement of the clinical microsystem?
- Do people have a good idea of each other's work? How is that brought about?
- Do you discuss the common patterns of the way you work? The ways you test changes in them?

- What can you yourself do to be present in microsystems?
- What are the cultural supports for measurably improving the quality, reliability, and value of care in the microsystems?
- What are the cultural changes required to measurably improve the quality, reliability, and value of care at the front lines?

- Are you treated with dignity and respect everyday by everyone you encounter, without any regard for hierarchy?
- Are you given the opportunity and tools that you need to make a contribution that gives meaning to your life?
- Does someone notice when you've done the job you do?
- As you think about what you do and your ability to change it—what gains have been made in the past 12 months?
- How do you actually do what you do? What changes have you been able to make? What changes are you working on now?
- What changes that you've tried haven't worked?
- Do people feel compelled to regularly justify or rationalize things that happen around here?

Go to www.clinicalmicrosystem.org, click on "streaming videos" on the left-hand menu bar of the home page, then select from the Clinical Microsystems streaming video series "A Microsystem's Self-Awareness Journey, Paul Batalden, MD." The videos are best viewed by RealOne Player.

Ask for Two Jobs: Providing Quality Services and Improving the Quality of Service. We all sense that people who enjoy their work, who are excited by and engaged in their work, are likely to do better work than others and to enjoy their work. We all know that staff satisfaction is related to patient satisfaction (Denove & Power, 2006; Nelson et al., 1992). We know that people who feel empowered and important in their work are more likely than others to find ways to improve their work and to take pride in their work (Buckingham & Clifton, 2001; Deming, 1986). We know that most people go into health care for one reason—they want to make a difference in the lives of people with real needs.

We know that leaders, at all levels of the organization, create the conditions for improvement to flourish and for excellence to emerge. The question, then, is, What might leaders do to engage staff and to bring forth the energy and creativity of the whole person in her or his everyday work? Of course there is no one simple answer; however, there are some things that leaders can do to fully engage staff. Here are two that are basic:

- *Set clear expectations.* Let everyone in your organization or area know that the mission is to deliver high-quality, high-value services and that the task is so big that everyone really has two jobs—to do the work and to improve the work. This goes to the heart of fostering a culture of quality, safety, and excellence. You are saying that everyday work involves both doing well what needs to be done and testing ways to improve the quality of what is done. Improvement is everyone's responsibility and needs to be a basic job expectation.
- *Foster relevant learning.* Improving work requires knowledge, skills, and effort, just as doing the work requires knowledge, skill, and effort. One way to make this expectation clear, and to promote the fundamental improvement of knowledge and skill, is to foster relevant learning. One way to accomplish this is to adapt the DMIC to fit into your health system's leadership and human resource development process.

The second section of the M3 Matrix (Figure 10.2) provides questions that leaders might ask themselves about each level of the health system (some of these questions might also be considered when engaging staff). Many leaders have found this starter list of questions and perspectives helpful for reframing their health care system and ensuring alignment for improvement.

Use Esther's Story: Engage the Head, the Hand, and the Heart. John Kotter is a noted authority on leading change. He has studied organizations that have succeeded and those that have failed at making transformational change. He teaches, consults, studies, and writes on this topic (Kotter, 1996; Kotter & Cohen, 2002).

Clearly, there is a great deal that goes into transforming an organization and creating the conditions for sustained excellent performance, but one aspect of success that stands out and is worth highlighting is this. *Organizations that succeed at mobilizing and engaging their staff succeed (in part) because they are able to engage the whole person—her or his intellect, efforts, and values. The successful organization finds ways to engage the head, the hands, and the heart.*

Paul Bate, chair of Health Services Management at University College London, in the United Kingdom, another authority on organizational change, and his colleagues at the Rand Corporation have studied high-performing health systems (at both the microsystem and macrosystem levels) in North America and the United Kingdom. This research has given Bate an understanding of the power of storytelling, and other methods of dramatization, to illuminate the patient's experience and to ignite improvement work in organizations that are achieving unprecedented levels of quality and safety (Bate, 1994).

One technique for engaging the energy and creativity of the whole person is to make use of stories and storytelling. In health care we believe that stories about patients that dramatize an individual's experiences and the person's and family's efforts to cope with the burden of illness can be a powerful source of insight and motivation. Because most health care professionals enter health care to make a difference, telling patient stories can even invite the reengagement of discouraged staff (Hurwitz, Greenhalgh, & Skultans, 2004).

One of the most rapidly improving health systems is the Jönköping County Council Health System (JCCHS) in Sweden. A large, vertically integrated health system, it has the best quality and lowest cost measures in Sweden. It has been a leading participant in the highly regarded Institute for Healthcare Improvement's Pursuing Perfection program (Institute for Healthcare Improvement [IHI], 2006). One thing that JCCHS leaders have done for more than five years is to tell and retell Esther's story (Exhibit 10.2). "Esther" is a fictional, but endearing and believable, elderly woman who lives alone and suffers from chronic obstructive pulmonary disease and other health problems. Whenever Esther's story is told, people immediately recognize the complexity of her care and her case. They see both the strengths and weaknesses in the way care is currently provided. Because Esther could be anyone's grandmother, mother, beloved aunt, or dear neighbor, everyone (physicians, nurses, secretaries, technicians, and administrators) can relate to her story. Having told Esther's story, JCCHS leaders ask a few powerful questions to invite staff to assess current care delivery and to generate ideas to improve and innovate. They ask such questions as these:

- What would Esther want?
- What does Esther need?

EXHIBIT 10.2. IMPROVING PATIENT FLOW:
THE ESTHER PROJECT IN SWEDEN.

"Esther" is not a real patient, but her persona as a gray-haired, ailing, but competent elderly Swedish woman with a chronic condition and occasional acute needs
has inspired impressive improvements in the ways patients flow through a complex
network of providers and care settings in Höglandet, Sweden.

Esther was invented by a team of physicians, nurses, and other providers
who joined together to improve patient flow and coordination of care for elderly
patients within a six-municipality region in Sweden. The productive work that has
been done on Esther's behalf led the Jönköping County Council, responsible for the
health care of 330,000 residents living around Höglandet, to become one of two
international teams participating in the Pursuing Perfection initiative. This program,
launched by the Robert Wood Johnson Foundation, is designed to help health care
organizations and hospitals dramatically improve patient outcomes by pursuing
perfection in all their major care processes. The Institute for Healthcare
Improvement (IHI) serves as the national program office for this initiative.

"I think it is very important that we call this work Esther," says Mats Bojestig,
chief of the Department of Medicine at Höglandet Hospital, Höglandet, Sweden,
one of the developers of the Esther Project and an Institute for Healthcare
Improvement (IHI) faculty member. "It helps us focus on the patient and her needs.
We can each imagine our own 'Esther.' And we can ask ourselves in our work,
'What's best for Esther?'"

Esther proved inspirational for the team. During the three-year project, they
were able to achieve the following improvements:

- Hospital admissions fell from approximately 9,300 in 1998 to 7,300 in 2003.
- Hospital days for heart failure patients decreased from approximately 3,500 in 1998
  to 2,500 in 2000.
- Waiting times for referral appointments with neurologists decreased from eighty-five
  days in 2000 to fourteen days in 2003.
- Waiting times for referral appointments with gastroenterologists fell from forty-eight
  days in 2000 to fourteen days in 2003.

The Esther Project grew from a need that many U.S. health systems share:
to improve the way patients flow through the system of care by strengthening
coordination and communication among providers.

Böjestig tells Esther's story this way: "Esther is eighty-eight and lives alone in a
small apartment. During the past few nights her breathing has become worse and
worse, and her legs have edema so severe that she cannot lie down but sits up all
night. She knows she needs health care. She phones her daughter in a nearby
town, who tells her to call her home nurse. The home nurse visits and says she
needs to see her general practitioner (GP). But Esther lives on the third floor
and can't manage the stairs.

"So the nurse calls an ambulance, and Esther goes to the doctor, who says
she needs to go to the hospital. Now three hours have passed. An ambulance
takes her to the emergency room (ER), where she meets an assistant nurse and
waits for three hours. She meets with a doctor, who examines her and orders an
X-ray and says she will have to be admitted. She comes to the ward and meets
more nurses."

EXHIBIT 10.2. (*Continued*)

Here Böjestig smiles. "Most days Esther is a little lonely, but today she is happy because she has already met 30 people!"

The Swedish health system is designed in a traditional, functional way: each link in the caregiving chain—the primary care physician (PCP), the hospital, the home care providers, the pharmacy—acts independently according to its function. "But Esther needs it to all fit together," says Böjestig. "It needs to flow like an organized process," he says, so each provider of care can take advantage of what others have done or will do.

Out of this need grew the Esther Project, which has six overall objectives:

1. Security for Esther
2. Better working relations throughout the entire care chain
3. Higher competence throughout the care chain
4. Shared medical documentation
5. Quality throughout the entire care chain
6. Documentation and communication of improvements

The Esther Project team consisted of physicians, nurses, social workers, and other providers representing the Höglandet Hospital and physician practices in each of the six municipalities. They were divided into two subgroups: the strategy group and the project management group.

To establish a clear picture of where the problems existed, team members conducted more than sixty interviews with patients and providers throughout the system. Together they analyzed the results, which included such statements as "patients in a nursing home rarely see their doctor" and "a patient getting palliative care at home was in contact with 30 different people during one week."

According to Böjestig the interviews also furnished providers with valuable realizations about the ways their individual work processes did or did not dovetail with the work of their colleagues in the care chain. Figuratively, if not literally, he says, interviewers would exclaim, "Are you doing that? I'm doing that too!"

The result of this lack of coordination, he says, is that even though Esther's social worker knows all about how Esther lives, for example, "still her GP asks her how she lives, and she tells it, and the hospital asks her, and she tells it again, and so on." Lack of coordination of information, particularly where medications are concerned, causes considerable redundancy and waste. In the worst case, it can lead to medical errors and avoidable illness.

The team devised an action plan that spelled out six main projects, designed to correspond to the six goals:

1. Develop flexible organization, with patient values in focus
2. Design more efficient and improved prescription and medication routines
3. Create ways in which documentation and communication of information can be adapted to the next link in the care chain
4. Develop efficient information technology support throughout the whole care chain
5. Develop and introduce a diagnosis system for community care
6. Develop a virtual competence center for better transfer and improvement of competence throughout the care chain

(*continued*)

EXHIBIT 10.2. IMPROVING PATIENT FLOW:
THE ESTHER PROJECT IN SWEDEN. (*Continued*)

Böjestig says that as part of its work, the team examined demand and capacity within the system and saw that the inadequate capacity for planned care was forcing patients to seek urgent care in inappropriate settings. "If Esther complains of headaches, and her GP says she should see a neurologist, in our system that referral would take three months. For Esther this is not acceptable. So she goes to the ER, and the doctor there knows that if he puts her in the hospital, the next day there will be a neurologist in to visit her."

Although it appeared that the demand was for inpatient admissions, it was really demand for better access to specialty care. So the team tested a process in which the queue for care was redesigned from two—one for acute care and one for planned care—into one. "Instead of having acute care go into the wards," says Böjestig, "it goes to the team."

This team, which includes the PCP, specialists as appropriate, nurses, and home nurses, has a collaborative relationship, through which team members decide together what's best for each patient. When a patient presents acute care needs, says Böjestig, the PCP can page a specialist on the team, who is expected to respond within two minutes. A telephone consultation may still result in an inpatient admission, but it allows the patient to be admitted directly to the ward without having to endure a visit to the ER, costly in both human and financial terms.

For their part the specialists began working toward open access scheduling, in which patients could be seen on the same day they call or their PCP calls. Closer cooperation among specialists and other providers meant that PCPs and home care nurses were able to do for patients some of the things specialists had been doing.

Additionally, patient education was recognized as a critical element in keeping patients out of the hospital. Nurses were trained to educate heart failure patients, for example, about how to take vital measurements at home and tweak their medication accordingly.

Böjestig says that all 250 providers in the network received training in the project's goals and processes. And the investment paid off. "We have closed about 20 percent of our bed capacity," he says, "and moved that capacity to where the need is bigger."

The continuing focus of the project team's work, says Böjestig, is "how to create value for Esther." He says that the project changed the attitudes among those who work for Esther, because "the focus is on her now."

"The important things for us to ask as leaders or workers in the health care system," says Böjestig, "is can we still continue to work in systems that are not integrated? Is it fair to our knowledge? Is it what we want to do? Is it best for Esther?"

- Why can't we do this for Esther?
- Can we find a way to just try to do this for Esther?

These simple questions dramatize a recognizable person's health and health care experiences. They serve as an open invitation to become curious about what might be done (the head), to engender the will and energy to get it done (the heart), and to call forth the skill to do what has never been done before (the hand).

Focusing on the Microsystem Level

When people are sick or injured or have a health condition that they cannot manage on their own, they often seek health care from educated and trained professionals. They wish to have a healing relationship or a relationship that protects or promotes their health. Patients and families invite these health professionals—physicians, nurses, clinicians—into their lives to provide needed assistance. When and where a person with a health need interacts with a health care professional and supporting staff, a clinical microsystem is at work.

Microsystems are the places where patients and families and health care teams meet. Microsystems are the unit of action—the *sharp end* of the health care system. It follows then, that if a health care wishes to produce high-quality health care, care that meets the needs of the individual, then it must have high-quality microsystems that are always *on*—perpetually able to discern what a person wants and needs and able to design and deliver the care that best matches that person's needs. This relationship is shown in Figure 1.1 in Chapter One. Donald Berwick and the Institute of Medicine (IOM) subcommittee responsible for the report *Crossing the Quality Chasm* depicted the pivotal and determinate position of the microsystem when they made the health care "chain of effect" diagram (Institute of Medicine. . . , 2001).

All large health systems (macroorganizations) have microsystems as their basic building blocks. These microsystems make health care *real*, and they vary widely in their ability to do the job—to give all patients what they want and need exactly when they want and need it (Institute for Healthcare Improvement, 2000). Improving requires learning grounded in the experience and daily reality of the work of health care in that frontline context.

So we focus on frontline systems because the only way to design and deliver care that consistently and efficiently meets people's needs is to grow the capability of the microsystems to realize their mission by providing high quality to each person they serve. Excellent service and care every time for every . . . patient—if this is the aim, new learning and new ways of thinking and acting and interacting are required to achieve it. If the aim has merit and is fundamentally in line with people's needs for health care, then most people in most microsystems will need to embark on a developmental journey to build their capability.

We have seen that scores of clinical microsystems have found it possible to set out on their own developmental journeys and to make great progress in improving their ability to provide highly reliable, high-quality, high-value care. This journey toward peak performance is challenging, enjoyable, engaging, empowering, and transformational. Its chief hallmarks are action learning and discovery and also the emergence of inside-out motivation and action to make a superior thing.

Understanding the Role of Experiential Learning in the Improvement of Care

Jerome Bruner (1960), a famous educator, believed that more people act their way into believing than believe their way into acting. He was a proponent of using *action learning* to advance education. David Kolb (1984) has advanced and popularized the idea of action learning; his model of the experiential learning cycle is shown in Figure 10.3. He believes that the way most people learn most things is by running through a cycle (or ascending spiral) made up of the interplay of four things—concrete experience, reflective observation, abstract conceptualization, and active experimentation:

1. A person experiences something, and
2. Reflects on what he has experienced and on what he or she has observed and tries to make sense out of it, and
3. Turns this sense-making activity into an abstract concept that might be used to guide future action, and

FIGURE 10.3. EXPERIENTIAL LEARNING MODEL.

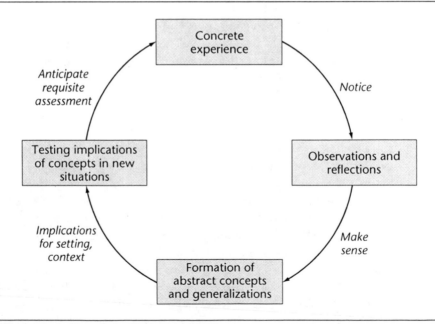

Source: Adapted from Kolb, 1984; Weick, 2000.

4. When circumstances arise in the future, he or she tests out the abstract concept on a particular case in point, which leads once again to a new experience and the start of a new cycle.

We can further enrich our understanding of this learning by studying how professionals such as airplane pilots, physicians, nurses, and architects learn. Donald Schön, an authority on adult learning and the ways that professionals learn, has used the architectural studio course to demonstrate the most effective means for helping professionals move towards mastery of their field (Schön, 1983).

Architectural students gain knowledge, insight, and skill in powerful learning environments called *studio courses;* these courses are at the core of the students' professional education experience. Studio courses challenge architects-in-training to design a project, such as a town hall, a cathedral, an elementary school, or a fire station. By the end of the term most students have succeeded at doing something they were not capable of doing earlier. They have met the design challenge, usually more or less successfully, because the conditions for learning have been well designed. The conditions for learning in a studio course consist of a rich mix of ingredients:

- A specific goal set for the learner that becomes a worthwhile challenge that engages the learner's creativity
- An informal learning place to interact with faculty and other students
- A studio course master who can guide and challenge the learner
- The development of blueprints and models to graphically illustrate plans and ideas
- Open and honest critique of the learner's work by faculty and fellow learners
- The learner's effort to design a superior thing by drawing on his or her own insights and reflection, past and present learning, creativity, and intelligence

In this environment, over time, the architectural students increase their capability to design a superior building that meets the needs of their clients, fits into the local context and culture, and can be built at an affordable cost.

We have designed a learning program for members of clinical microsystems—the Dartmouth Microsystem Improvement Curriculum (DMIC)—that builds on the ideas of leading educators such as Bruner, Kolb, Schön, and others. This learning program aims to do for microsystem members what a studio course does for architectural students. The curriculum invites microsystem members—health professionals, administrative and support staff, patients, and families—into shared experiences that challenge them to make a superior thing (high-quality and high-value health care). Together they increase their capability to improve performance by acquiring knowledge, skills, principles, and concepts that they adapt to their own unique microsystems. The curriculum and structure also provide a setting for busy microsystem members to learn to work together in new and different ways. They use this learning to understand and to test new ways to provide care and services that can better meet people's needs for high-quality, affordable health care.

Using Experiential Learning to Advance the Developmental Journey of Microsystems

Whether they have recognized it or not, all microsystems are on a developmental journey. It is the nature of clinical microsystems, as "living, adaptive" systems (one form of complex, adaptive systems) (Zimmerman, Lindberg, & Plsek, 1999) to be constantly changing and adjusting to internal forces and external conditions. Old patterns of thinking and acting evolve over time, and new patterns emerge (slowly or rapidly, depending on the conditions) as a microsystem attempts to adjust to changing conditions in an ever-changing world.

The goal of the DMIC is to expedite and to guide a clinical microsystem's developmental journey toward peak performance. We have deliberately modeled the DMIC on Kolb's, Bruner's, and Schön's ideas about how professionals learn. We try to create rich conditions for learning by setting up a studio course for clinical teams that include interdisciplinary members of microsystems.

A brief description of the DMIC learning process follows:

Preparation: Getting Ready

- Secure macro- and mesosystem senior leader support and encouragement at macrosystem and mesosystem levels.
- Define the microsystem that is ready to begin its developmental journey, and its members. Identify the different member roles (patient, family, physician, nurse, technician, receptionist, transport staff, social worker, and so forth).
- Assemble a *lead improvement team* that represents all the member roles. It is highly desirable to have at least one person to represent each role that plays a part in the microsystem.
- Begin the learning by providing a common frame of reference and introducing microsystem thinking. Lead improvement team members may do some reading before the first session.
- Determine a clear multimedia communication plan that describes how lead improvement team members are to reach the other members of the microsystem.

Baseline Assessment: Discovering the Microsystem

- Discover your microsystem. See what you have never seen before by viewing the clinical program as a small system that can be understood by studying its 5 P's—purpose, patients, professionals, processes, and patterns—and the ways in which its *parts* interact with one another.
- Use the 5 P's framework for assessing the clinical setting as a small system. Just as you can assess, diagnose, and treat a patient, you can assess, diagnose, and treat your microsystem.
- Make a wall poster to summarize the 5 P's assessment and to illustrate the gross anatomy of the microsystem and some of the detail that is embedded—the *fine structures* and *key processes* and *vital patterns* and *core outcomes*.
- Review *metrics that matter* (Figure A.14 in the Appendix) specific to your population of patients.

Primary Diagnosis: Selecting a Worthwhile Challenge for Improvement

- Following the assessment, you have an invitation to make a diagnosis.
  Identify the strengths of your microsystem, and celebrate them.
  Identify improvement opportunities revealed by your assessment.
  Determine what the organization's strategic needs are that your microsystem could or should address.
  Determine national professional group recommendations.
  Review the Institute of Medicine's six quality aims—safe, timely, effective, efficient, equitable, and patient-centered.
- In light of the previous steps, make your primary diagnosis.
  Although there may be multiple worthy themes that identify areas for improvement, select a single, important, and worthwhile theme to focus your (first or next) improvement work on for the next six to twelve months.
  This theme becomes the focus for the shared learning. This represents your studio course programmatic challenge.

Primary Treatment: Using the Scientific Method to Make and Sustain Improvements

- Now that the assessment and diagnosis have been made, it is time to take action and to move into the improvement work.
- In this phase of the learning the members of the lead improvement team learn how to work together effectively as an interdisciplinary team and to
  Establish clear, measurable aims that are aligned with the overall theme for improvement.

Analyze the current process using flowcharts.

Use cause and effect thinking by making a fishbone diagram.

Develop promising change concepts.

Use the scientific method to rapidly test changes (plan-do-study-act) and to maintain gains once the aim has been reached (standardize-do-study-act).

Build data collection and practical methods for measuring and monitoring into daily work.

- As this action learning progresses, fundamental principles and basic improvement techniques are introduced to help all involved make the journey of building improvement capability smooth and successful.

Reflection and Celebration

- At the conclusion of this initial cycle of learning, the members of the microsystem's lead improvement team

Reflect on what they have achieved and on what they have learned along the way.

Celebrate their successes.

Begin making plans to tackle a new theme and to extend improvement knowledge and skills to all the members of their microsystem.

Review the M3 Matrix to make a detailed plan for the next six to twelve months in order to continue the developmental journey and to further increase their capability to do their work, improve their work, and take pride in their work.

For convenience, we divide the learning into several modules that have a logical order and flow one into another. The remaining chapters in Part Two of this book provide details on the Dartmouth Microsystem Improvement Curriculum that we have just described. Table 10.1 outlines each chapter: the topic, aim, and learning objectives and the between-sessions work.

Adapting DMIC to Different Settings and Conditions

The DMIC has been used by many leaders in varying settings. It works best when it is adapted to fit local conditions and each system's unique requirements. Some of these different approaches to using DMIC to build capability in frontline, interdisciplinary microsystem teams are described next.

The formal DMIC learning sessions are often attended by six to twelve microsystem lead improvement teams. These sessions are also usually attended by the mesosystem leaders who supervise the leaders of the participating

TABLE 10.1. DARTMOUTH MICROSYSTEM IMPROVEMENT CURRICULUM.

Chapter and Purpose	Objectives	Between Learning Sessions Work
Chapter 10: To promote organization-wide improvement, through the introduction of an approach the (M3 Matrix) for building improvement capability at all levels of a health system, and to preview an action-learning program for frontline staff	1. Describe the current state of health care and the relevance of the Institute of Medicine's publication *Crossing the Quality Chasm*. 2. List specific, phased actions for leaders to take at the macrosystem, mesosystem, and microsystem levels to create the conditions for performance improvement. 3. Describe why a microsystem approach to improving performance is system based and engages the entire health system. 4. State the value of using a story about a patient to engage staff at all levels of a health system. 5. Outline the elements of an action-learning program for frontline staff. 6. Identify the reasons why a lead improvement team (an interdisciplinary team representing all roles in a microsystem) makes an important contribution to anchoring improvement work in the real work of frontline microsystems.	1. Review the M3 Matrix and develop an organized, specific strategy for the three levels of your system. 2. Specify the frontline microsystem development strategy. 3. Identify lead improvement teams for microsystem development. 4. Select a patient population for a primary focus, and write your own "Esther" story.
Chapter 11: To describe the origin of clinical microsystem thinking and the research on it, and to identify microsystems in your health care system	1. Define and identify the clinical microsystems in your health care system. 2. Describe how systems thinking is connected to microsystems. 3. Link systems thinking with the microsystem.	1. Begin to develop a microsystem wall graphic that models your own system and also offers the physical space to display what people are learning, additional information, and results of the improvement work and the efforts to change.

(continued)

TABLE 10.1. DARTMOUTH MICROSYSTEM IMPROVEMENT CURRICULUM. *(Continued)*

Chapter and Purpose	Objectives	Between Learning Sessions Work
	4. Describe the microsystem connections to research from the service industry and the Institute of Medicine.	2. Identify a communication strategy.
Chapter 12: To identify concepts and methods for holding effective and productive meetings with a lead improvement team	1. List the four common roles and functions for effective meetings. 2. Describe the meeting process and the seven steps in the agenda template. 3. List the work to be done before meetings. 4. List the processes to be followed during meetings. 5. Create a draft list of ground rules for your lead improvement team members to use when learning how to work together in a meeting. 6. Describe the steps for maintaining the rhythm of improvement.	1. Conduct sixty-minute meetings with an interdisciplinary lead team using effective meeting skills. 2. Use an agenda to hold a meeting to brainstorm a draft set of ground rules. 3. Identify a place and time to hold weekly lead improvement team meetings.
Chapter 13: To do an assessment of your clinical microsystem using the 5 P's framework, a tested analytical method that focuses on purpose, patients, professionals, processes, and patterns	1. Organize your microsystem assessment so it is systematic. 2. Describe your deeper knowledge of your microsystem purpose, patients, professionals, processes, and patterns. 3. Identify key tools and methods for gaining deeper knowledge. 4. Engage all members of your clinical microsystem in the process of assessment and awareness building. 5. Review, analyze, and draw conclusions about the relationships among the 5 P's. 6. Identify strengths and opportunities for improvements based on the 5 P's assessment.	1. Review the 5 P's, and determine which data and information can be obtained from your organization and which data and information will be collected through other means, such as the microsystem workbook, tools, and forms. 2. Identify who will collect which data and information. 3. Create a timeline for collecting data and reporting on the assessment work.

Chapter 14: To understand and apply the model for improvement, in conducting disciplined, sequential tests of change for the purpose of making measurable improvements that can be sustained

1. Define the model for improvement.
2. Describe the two components of the model for improvement.
3. List the detailed steps of PDSA.
4. Develop a clear *plan* to test a change.
5. Describe the point at which a PDSA cycle becomes a SDSA cycle.
6. State where PDSA↔SDSA cycles fit in the improvement process.
7. Use the PDSA↔SDSA worksheet to guide actions.

1. Review and discuss the model for improvement, to clarify the path forward for the lead improvement team.
2. Review the PDSA↔SDSA worksheet to gain insight into the next steps.

Chapter 15: To select a worthy theme on which to focus improvement actions, based on assessments made using the 5 P's, on organizational strategy, and on consideration of national or professional guidelines and recommendations

1. Define a theme for improvement.
2. Describe the benefit of identifying a theme for improvement.
3. Describe what to consider when selecting a theme for improvement.
4. Describe how theme selection is connected to assessment information and data.
5. Identify where theme selection fits in the overall improvement process.
6. Describe the process of identifying and selecting a theme for improvement.

Select a theme to focus your improvement work; base your choice on
1. Your 5 P's assessment data and information.
2. A review of information from external forces such as the Institute of Medicine, Institute for Healthcare Improvement, and Joint Commission for Accreditation of Healthcare Organizations (JCAHO).
3. A review of your own organization's strategic priorities.

Chapter 16: To create a global aim statement to focus the improvement work based on the theme the lead improvement team selected

1. Define a global aim.
2. Identify the importance of the relationship between the global aim, the improvement process flow, and theme selection.
3. Describe how to manage new ideas and topics within the context of writing a global aim.
4. Write a global aim statement using a template.

1. Write a global aim for improvement based on your theme selection
2. Share all global aim progress and drafts with all members of the microsystem.

(continued)

TABLE 10.1. DARTMOUTH MICROSYSTEM IMPROVEMENT CURRICULUM. (*Continued*)

Chapter and Purpose	Objectives	Between Learning Sessions Work
Chapter 17: To define process-mapping techniques, with a specific focus on high-level flowcharts and deployment flowcharts	1. Define process mapping. 2. Describe the differences between high-level flowcharts and deployment flowcharts. 3. Describe the relationship between the global aim statement for improvement and the flowcharting process. 4. Create a high-level flowchart or deployment flowchart using several techniques. 5. Develop a process to engage all members of the microsystem in the creation and modification of the flowchart.	1. Draft a flowchart of the process identified in your global aim statement. 2. Display the flowchart draft for all the staff to review and add to. 3. Modify the flowchart based on feedback.
Chapter 18: To create a detailed specific aim statement based on the selected theme and the global aim statement to further guide and focus improvement activities	1. Define what a specific aim is. 2. Describe the connections between specific aim, process flow, global aim selection, and theme. 3. Use the specific aim template. 4. Describe the *improvement ramp* that leads microsystem members to meet overall improvement aims.	1. Create your specific aim, based on your flowchart.
Chapter 19: To define cause and effect diagrams and the process of creating them to gain deeper knowledge of the factors that contribute to end results	1. Define cause and effect diagrams (fishbone diagrams). 2. Describe the principle of the web of causation in relation to a fishbone diagram. 3. Create a cause and effect diagram specific to the outcome you are studying. 4. Describe the function of cause and effect diagrams in the big picture of improvement.	1. Create a fishbone diagram to show the causes that contribute to your specific aim. 2. Display the draft fishbone diagram for all to review and modify. 3. Make the modifications to the fishbone based on feedback.

Chapter 20: To define the process that a lead improvement team can use to develop a large list of ideas for improving a process and then to systematically reduce the number to the very best ideas

1. Define the methods and describe the steps in the process of brainstorming and multi-voting.
2. Describe the differences between interactive brainstorming, silent brainstorming, and nominal group techniques.
3. Apply brainstorming and multi-voting to a topic in order to select a specific change idea to test.
4. Develop a process to engage all staff in the review and consideration of the results of the brainstorming and multi-voting session.
5. Develop a process to engage all staff in the creation and modification of a fishbone diagram.

1. Brainstorm and multi-vote to choose a change idea to test that is related to your specific aim statement.
2. Develop a process to engage all staff in the review and consideration of the results of the brainstorming and multi-voting work.
3. Develop a clear plan to test a change idea.
4. Review the plan with all staff.
5. Determine dates and preparation needed to test the change idea quickly.
6. Use the PDSA↔SDSA worksheet to guide actions.

Chapter 21: To understand how change concepts can contribute to developing new change ideas for improvement

1. Define a change concept.
2. List common change concept categories.
3. Identify when change concepts enter the overall improvement process.
4. Describe how a change concept can lead to specific change ideas.
5. Describe a clinical example of a change concept applied to a change idea.

1. Review the change concept list, and use it to stimulate thinking about ways to redesign your process.
2. Research the best-known change ideas for the process you aim to improve.

Chapter 22: To understand how to make and interpret run charts and control charts, two methods for measuring and displaying data trends over time

1. Describe how plotting data over time and using run charts and control charts fit into the improvement process.
2. Make and interpret a run chart.

1. Create a run, or control chart specific to your PDSA cycle.
2. Display "the chart on a data wall" for all staff to see real-time progress.

(continued)

TABLE 10.1. DARTMOUTH MICROSYSTEM IMPROVEMENT CURRICULUM. (Continued)

Chapter and Purpose	Objectives	Between Learning Sessions Work
	3. Make and interpret one type of control chart.	3. Build measurement into every microsystem member's activities.
Chapter 23: To create a clear action plan of next steps for planning and monitoring improvement activities and progress made	1. Describe the importance of an action plan. 2. Differentiate between an action plan and a Gantt chart. 3. Explain the connections among the action plan, the Gantt chart, and your improvement work. 4. Describe how to manage improvement activities over time. 5. Write an action plan or a Gantt chart, or both.	1. Write a Gantt chart specific to your long-term improvement plan. 2. Write an action plan each week, to promote between-meeting completion of tasks.
Chapter 24: To make plans to tell the improvement story, measure progress over time, and sustain improvement using standard processes	1. Describe the improvement fundamentals needed to maintain and sustain improvement. 2. Identify where improvement data can be posted for viewing by all microsystem members to increase their knowledge about purpose, progress, and priorities. 3. Design a microsystem playbook that documents standard ways of performing processes and that can be used in orientation, performance appraisals, and daily improvement work. 4. Develop a storyboard to document your microsystem's improvement journey and progress made over time.	1. Create a storyboard showing your microsystem's current state. 2. Start and maintain a data wall of results, achievements, and processes to be monitored. 3. Create and actively manage your microsystem playbook.

microsystems. The sessions might be held monthly, weekly, or biweekly or be grouped together over the course of a single week. Here are some of the patterns we have seen:

- Monthly sessions bring microsystem lead improvement teams together, under the sponsorship of senior and midlevel leaders, for one full day or one or two half days once a month for six to nine months.
- Weekly or biweekly sessions bring microsystem lead improvement teams together, under the sponsorship of senior and midlevel leaders, for one to two hours once a week or once every two weeks for six to nine months.
- An intensive weeklong workout session brings microsystem lead improvement teams together, under the sponsorship of senior and midlevel leaders, for six to eight hours per day for five consecutive days.

Each of the remaining chapters in Part Two provides topic-specific knowledge from the DMIC. The best format and the most practical pace for teaching this knowledge within the context of an interdisciplinary lead improvement team are determined by the local conditions. Health care systems might also take advantage of *toolkits*, specially packaged learning materials that target particular kinds of health care organizations, or they might try an applied learning approach.

- Toolkit method. Use a microsystem-based toolkit to guide action learning: for example, *Clinical Microsystems: A Path to Healthcare Excellence* (Godfrey, Nelson, & Batalden, 2005) is a guide for improving care in hospitals and is sponsored by the Dartmouth Medical School, the American Hospital Association, the Institute for Healthcare Improvement, Premier, Inc., and VHA, Inc. Other toolkits are available on the Web site http://www.clinicalmicrosystem.org. Toolkits can also be used within an academic program to educate health care professional students (physicians, nurses, and administrators).
- Applied microsystem education. Have health professional students work in small groups with the staff of an actual clinical microsystem to go through the 5 P's assessment process or through the diagnosis and treatment process described earlier in the descriptions of the DMIC learning process. This can be done in multiple sessions over the course of an academic term or as an intensive workout.

The DMIC approach for health professional education in academic settings and for leadership and staff development in delivery systems is being used in a variety of health systems worldwide. The Web site http://www.clinicalmicrosystem. org offers more ideas and resources on ways to adapt this way of learning to your own setting.

Understanding the Value and Composition
of a Lead Improvement Team

In several places we have suggested establishing a lead improvement team to guide the microsystem's participation in the DMIC. The idea behind this is to make sure that your microsystem education considers all the roles held by all the system's essential members. Every member of a microsystem has an important role to play and offers a unique perspective. Just as you would not wish to coach a baseball team without having all the players present, you should not choose to mentor microsystem team learning without having all the members either present or represented. In health care organizations it is often impossible to have all the members present for action learning, but it is usually possible to have all member roles represented (including current or former patients and families).

Review Questions

1. How will real case studies support your improvement journey?
2. What are the levels of the organization that should be considered when strategically planning improvement?
3. What is the importance of "Esther"?
4. What specific activities contribute to system improvement (beyond improvement projects)?
5. How does the *studio course* format support learning and practical application?

Prework

1. Review the M3 Matrix, and develop an organized, specific strategy for the three levels of your system.
2. Specify the frontline microsystem development strategy.
3. Identify lead improvement teams for microsystem development.
4. Select a patient population for a primary focus, and write your own "Esther" story.

References

Baldrige National Quality Program. (2006). *Health Care Criteria for Performance Excellence.* Retrieved September 1, 2006, from http://www.quality.nist.gov./PDF_files/2006_ HealthCare_Criteria.pdf.

Batalden, P. B., Nelson, E. C., Gardent, P. B., & Godfrey, M. M. (2005). Leading the macrosystem and mesosystem for microsystem peak performance. In S. Berman (Ed.),

From front office to front line: Essential issues for health care leaders (pp. 1–40). Oakbrook Terrace, IL: Joint Commission Resources.

Bate, P. (1994). *Strategies for cultural change.* Boston: Butterworth-Heinemann.

Bruner, J. S. (1960). *The process of education.* New York: Random House.

Buckingham, M., & Clifton, D. O. (2001). *Now, discover your strengths.* New York: Free Press.

Deming, W. E. (1986). *Out of the crisis.* Cambridge, MA: MIT Center for Advanced Engineering Study.

Denove, C., & Power, J. (2006). *Satisfaction: How every great company listens to the voice of the customer.* New York: Penguin Group.

Godfrey, M., Nelson, E., & Batalden, P. (2005). *Clinical microsystems: A path to healthcare excellence. Toolkit.* Hanover, NH: Dartmouth College.

Hurwitz, B., Greenhalgh, T., & Skultans, V. (2004). *Narrative research in health and illness.* Malden, MA: BMJ Books.

Institute for Healthcare Improvement. (2000). *Idealized design of clinical office practices.* Boston: Author.

Institute for Healthcare Improvement. (2006). *Pursuing perfection: Raising the bar for health care performance.* Retrieved June 1, 2006, from http://www.ihi.org/IHI/Programs/ PursuingPerfection.

Institute of Medicine (U.S.), Committee on Quality of Health Care in America. (2001). *Crossing the quality chasm: A new health system for the 21st century.* Washington, DC: National Academies Press.

Kolb, D. A. (1984). *Experiential learning: Experience as the source of learning and development.* Upper Saddle River, NJ: Prentice Hall.

Kotter, J. P. (1996). *Leading change.* Boston: Harvard Business School Press.

Kotter, J. P., & Cohen, D. S. (2002). *The heart of change: Real-life stories of how people change their organizations.* Boston: Harvard Business School Press.

Nelson, E. C., Rust, R. T., Zahorik, A., Rose, R. L., Batalden, P., & Siemanski, B. A. (1992). Do patient perceptions of quality relate to hospital financial performance? *Journal of Health Care Marketing, 12*(4), 6–13.

Quinn, J. B. (September 9, 1999). Letter to the editor. *Valley News* (Lebanon, NH), p. 7.

Schön, D. A. (1983). *The reflective practitioner: How professionals think in action.* New York: Basic Books.

Weick, K. E. (2000). Emergent change as a universal in organizations. In M. Beer & N. Nohria (Eds.), *Breaking the code of change* (pp. 223–241). Boston: Harvard Business School Press.

Zimmerman, B., Lindberg, C., & Plsek, P. (1999). *Edgeware: Insights from complexity science for health care leaders.* Irving, TX: VHA.

CHAPTER ELEVEN

INTRODUCTION TO MICROSYSTEM THINKING

Chapter Purpose

Aim. To describe the origin of clinical microsystem thinking, and the research on it, and to identify microsystems in your health care system.

    Objectives. At the completion of this unit, you will be able to

- Define and identify the clinical microsystems in your health care system.

- Describe how systems thinking is connected to microsystems.
- Link systems thinking with the microsystem.
- Describe the microsystem connections to research from the service industry and the Institute of Medicine.

T his chapter will assist you and your interdisciplinary lead improvement team to gain insight about the origins and significance of clinical microsystems in your health care system.

What Is a System in Health Care?

Building on Deming's *systems thinking*, health care is viewed as a system in Figure 11.1. A *system* is defined as a network of interdependent components that work together to try to accomplish a specific aim (Deming, 1986). A system possesses flow,

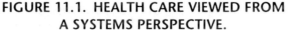

FIGURE 11.1. HEALTH CARE VIEWED FROM A SYSTEMS PERSPECTIVE.

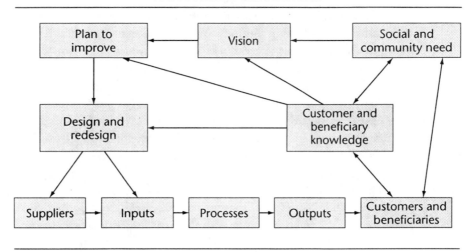

Source: Adapted from Deming, 1986, by P. B. Batalden.

FIGURE 11.2. HEALTH CARE IS AN OPEN SYSTEM, CAPABLE OF CONTINUAL IMPROVEMENT.

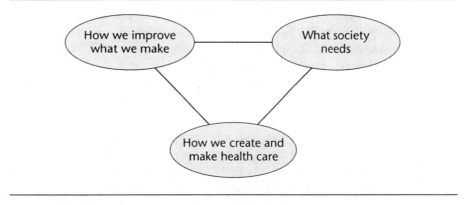

constraints, sequence, and context. A system has an aim; absent an aim there is no system. In general, health care systems exist to meet the needs of patients, families, and communities. Further, health care can be viewed as an *open* system, one capable of continual improvement, as shown in Figure 11.2.

How Did Clinical Microsystem Knowledge Evolve?

In the last decade of the twentieth century J. Brian Quinn, professor emeritus of the Amos Tuck School of Business Administration at Dartmouth College, spent years studying the most successful service companies in the world. He observed that the world's fastest-growing, most profitable, and most successful companies—such as SAS, Nordstrom, Wal-Mart, McDonald's, and Intel—progressively learned to focus on the frontline work in their service organizations and their smallest replicable units (SRUs). Quinn's observations showed that all these top-performing organizations comprised small replicable units that connected the *core competence* of the enterprise to the customers of that enterprise. His findings were published in an extraordinary book titled *Intelligent Enterprise* (Quinn, 1992). He reported that the leading service organizations organized around, and continually engineered, the frontline interface relationships that connected the organization's core competence with the needs of individual customers. It was this frontline interface that was referred to as the *smallest replicable unit*, or the *minimum replicable unit*.

During the 1980s and early 1990s, Paul Batalden and Gene Nelson, considering the work of W. Edwards Deming, Joseph Juran, Avedis Donabedian, and others, adapted these thinkers' modern improvement concepts and methods to health care. Batalden and Nelson studied patient outcomes and researched ways to improve the design of health care systems. During this time, Nelson and Batalden also developed the clinical value compass framework to measure and improve the quality and cost of health care (Batalden, Nelson, & Roberts, 1994; Nelson et al., 1995; Nelson, Mohr, Batalden, & Plume, 1996).

Using their research findings, Batalden and Nelson began teaching what became known as the "microsystem course" in the graduate program at the Center for the Evaluative Clinical Sciences at Dartmouth Medical School. They also continued to study how clinical teams can design and manage small systems of care to provide services for specific patient populations. When they read *Intelligent Enterprise* and learned about Quinn's research and identification of the SRU, Batalden and Nelson realized that their work on "panels of patients" and Quinn's research on the smallest replicable units within the world's foremost service companies were closely related. They translated the smallest replicable unit (SRU) concept into health care, determining that—a clinical microsystem could be thought of as health care's SRU.

We described the continued development of clinical microsystem thinking in Chapter Two, which presented the clinical research we conducted to explore high-performing microsystems in health care.

What Is a Clinical Microsystem?

A clinical microsystem is the place where patients, families, care teams, and information come together. Whenever and wherever there is a patient who is being cared for by a clinician or a clinical team, there is a microsystem with that patient at its center. It is the place where quality, safety, outcomes, satisfaction, and staff morale are created. You know it as a primary care practice, an emergency department, an inpatient unit, or an extended care facility. A microsystem also exists where care for heart failure or diabetes or breast cancer is given and where patients, families, and visiting nurses come together in a home. A clinical microsystem is a system. It is, technically speaking, a complex, adaptive system. Our formal definition states:

> A *clinical microsystem* can be defined as the combination of a small group of people who work together on a regular basis to provide care and the subpopulation of patients who receive that care.
>
> It has clinical and business aims, linked processes, and a shared information environment, and it produces services and care that can be measured as performance outcomes. These systems evolve over time and are often embedded in larger systems or organizations.
>
> Like any living, adaptive system, the microsystem must (1) do the work, (2) meet staff needs, and (3) maintain itself as a clinical unit.

In short, a clinical microsystem consists of a small group of doctors, nurses, and other clinicians; some administrative support; some information and information technology; and a small population of patients, all of which are interdependent and work together toward a common aim.

Where Do Clinical Microsystems Fit in the Health Care Delivery System?

It is the nature of systems to contain systems and to be embedded inside systems. The living cell is a system, and together with other cells it forms organs, and organs form the human body, and humans form families, and families form communities—all systems. Figure 11.3 shows how it is possible to view the health care system as a set of concentric circles, with smaller systems embedded in larger systems.

The individual patient's self-care system is the innermost system. The patient is literally at the center of the health care system. The next system level is the patient and individual caregiver. The microsystem is next, with the patient, family,

FIGURE 11.3. THE EMBEDDED SYSTEMS OF HEALTH CARE.

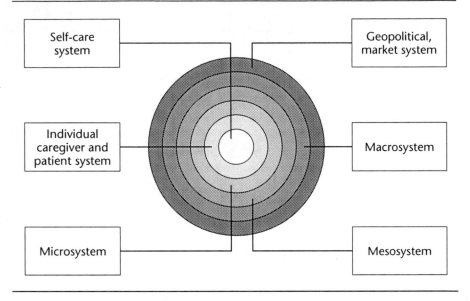

physicians, nurses, technicians, nurse practitioners, physician assistants, nursing assistants, and other professionals working with the patient. The microsystem is nested within the mesosystem of health care, which often takes the form of service lines (such as cardiac care) or departments (such as surgery or nursing). All of this fits within the larger organization, or macrosystem. The outer layer of these embedded health systems consists of the environment—the community, health care market, and health policy and regulatory milieu. This general structure—of small health systems embedded in larger health systems—applies to most health care systems in the developed world.

What Does a Clinical Microsystem Look Like?

Clinical microsystems are omnipresent throughout health care systems. They are the building blocks of health care systems. They exist in various states—some being intentionally designed and well developed and others not being purposefully designed nor fully developed.

One typical example of a clinical microsystem is a pediatric practice with 2 physicians, 1 nurse practitioner, 1 medical assistant, and 1 secretary. This practice is part of (nests within) a department of 36 pediatricians, which is part of a large medical center with 280 MDs and 1,200 staff, which is part of an integrated delivery system that serves a region.

Figure 1.3 (in Chapter One) shows the *anatomy* of a clinical microsystem. This anatomy includes the microsystem's purpose, patients, professionals, processes, and patterns.

The functioning, or *physiology*, of a microsystem (Figure 11.4) can be studied using process and systems thinking. The *inputs* are patients and families with health care needs; they enter a system of care and then emerge as *outputs*, with the hoped-for results being health care needs being met. The balanced measures on each side of the system of care show before and after measures of the goodness of the care system.

Why Focus on the Clinical Microsystem?

Wheatley and Kellner-Rogers (1996) state, "If we want to work with a system to influence its direction . . . a normal desire as we work with human organizations . . . the place for us to work is deep in the dynamics of the system where [its] identity is taking form" (p. 100). The clinical microsystem is the basic building block of any health care delivery system. It is where professional identity is formed and is transformed. It is the unit in which espoused clinical policy is put into practice (clinical policy-in-use). It is the place where *good value* and *safe care* are made. Most variables relevant to patient satisfaction are controlled here, and this is where most health professional formation occurs after initial professional preparation. The microsystem is where workplace motivators reside. The larger organization can be no better than the sum of its frontline units, or microsystems.

How Do Clinical Microsystems Link to *Crossing the Quality Chasm?*

The first clinical microsystem research was completed by Julie Mohr and Molla Donaldson in 2000 (Donaldson & Mohr, 2000). In this research the success characteristics of high-performing microsystems were first identified. The significance of the microsystem for improving the U.S. health system was called out by Berwick in the chain of effect for improving health care (Figure 1.1, in Chapter One), and this thinking lies behind the Institute of Medicine (IOM) report *Crossing The Quality Chasm* (Institute of Medicine [U.S.], Committee on Quality of Health Care in America, 2001).

FIGURE 11.4. THE PHYSIOLOGY OF A MICROSYSTEM: A GENERIC MODEL.

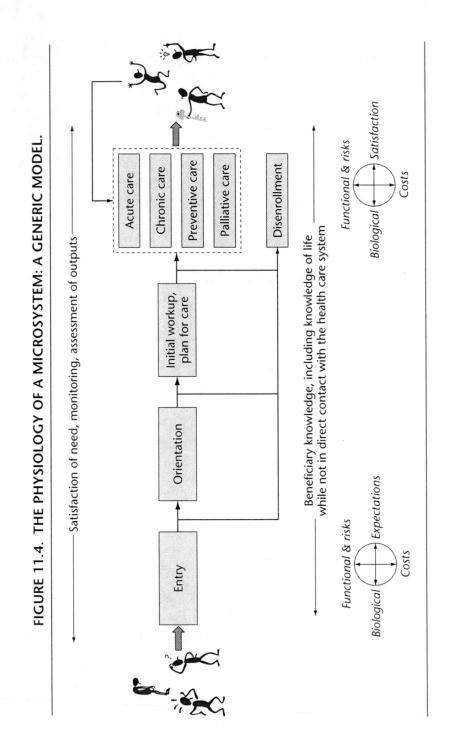

What Were the Findings of the Dartmouth Clinical Microsystem Research?

Research conducted in 2001, funded by the Robert Wood Johnson Foundation, resulted in the identification of primary success characteristics that built on the IOM research. Figure 1.5 (in Chapter One) shows these primary success characteristics: leadership, microsystem support, staff focus, interdependence of care team, performance results, process improvement, patient focus, and information and information technology. This research also identified the important, if not primary, characteristics of education and training, community and market focus, and patient safety.

Working to develop these success characteristics guides microsystems into the improvements that will make them into high-performing frontline units (see Chapter One).

What Does a Microsystem's Developmental Journey Look Like?

Microsystems evolve over time. Some move from a relatively low level of self-awareness to a high level of awareness and functional capability by taking several steps that can be thought of as a journey (as represented graphically in Figure 11.5).

A frontline unit's awareness that it is a microsystem often begins with an external provocation. Someone might ask a staff member, "Could you draw me a picture of how your microsystem works," or, "Could you help me understand the flow of daily activities from the perspective of the patient and family?" This picture is often the beginning of awareness of how people work together. It also often reveals some *foolishness*, things that people are not very proud of or things they recognize as not very dependable. With that recognition of some foolishness they might take action to minimize its impact in the microsystem. If they are successful in eliminating the foolishness, they often experience a sense of self and self-awareness that leads in turn to an understanding that the microsystem can improve itself and that change is possible without permission from anybody else.

This new sense of responsibility and awareness often gives staff important insights into the daily workings of the microsystem and the recognition that it is possible to change one's own work environment and that things are going along better than before. Eventually, someone will ask, "Why do we do what we do," and, "What is our purpose?"

A conversation begins about the patients who benefit from the microsystem's work. The microsystem staff begin to explore their own purpose in relation to the

FIGURE 11.5. A MICROSYSTEM'S SELF-AWARENESS JOURNEY.

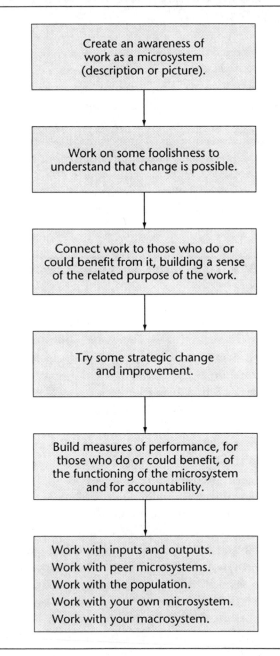

needs of patients. Making the purpose of the microsystem explicit is an important developmental step on the journey toward awareness of the microsystem as a system. The purpose, the interdependent members, the information and technology—all contribute to the functioning of this microsystem. This awareness then becomes people's basis for understanding the usual work of the microsystem when strategic improvement is introduced; the members of the microsystem can now begin to process the improvement against their knowledge of their own microsystem and the patients it serves. The path to systematic, sustained improvement is more than a recipe with steps to be followed. Microsystem members can complete the steps for short-term change but often cannot sustain the new way of doing things if they are not aware of themselves as making up a functioning system—a system now changed in a way that makes sense. Conversely, gains from change efforts are often sustained and further explored by the self-aware microsystem. The microsystem members become increasingly curious about the functioning of their microsystem and the ways they might change it. They often want to measure performance and understand who benefits and how much change is actually occurring. The process of change also feeds people's curiosity about the daily work in microsystems that understand their work as a system, particularly the work in other clinical units that they engage with to provide patients with all needed care. This curiosity leads a microsystem to interactions with peer microsystems and to explore the inputs it receives; staff work further to discover the expectations of the populations they care for and these populations' needs. These self-aware microsystems begin to work much more consciously on the relationship of their microsystem to its larger context, the mesosystems and macrosystem that contribute to its identity.

It's important to note that the steps and events just described may not happen in this order. They may not happen within any particular time period. However, these events, however ordered and timed, do often happen in microsystems that begin to get a sense of themselves and to build their own capability to improve themselves and to become better and better at self-organizing and self-improving.

Conclusion

Now you have a better understanding of how microsystem thinking evolved, the importance of the systems approach to improvement, and how microsystems can develop over time. The chapters that follow will support your efforts to increase self-awareness in microsystems to foster ongoing improvement, and they will provide detailed information about the Dartmouth Microsystem Improvement Curriculum (DMIC). The big DMIC picture is shown in Figure 11.6. Each

FIGURE 11.6. IMPROVEMENT RAMP.

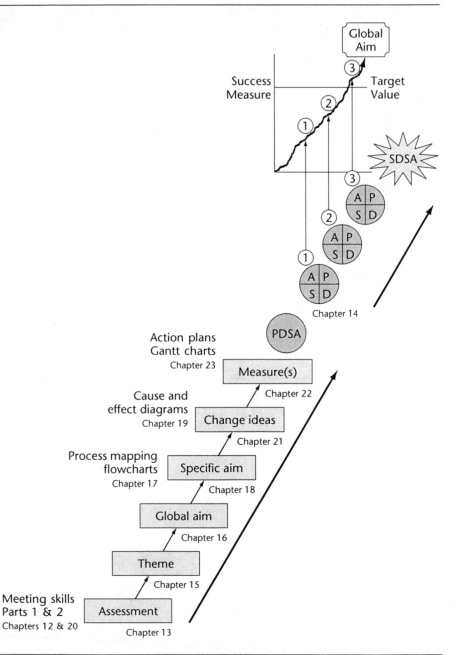

subsequent chapter will focus on one aspect of this big picture, which takes the form of an *improvement ramp*.

Case Studies

Intermediate Cardiac Care Unit (ICCU)

The ICCU's lead improvement team attended a three-day educational program to learn about the fundamentals of microsystem improvement; the curriculum introduced general microsystem knowledge, tools for understanding the process of designing change, and improvement methods that could be built into the ICCU's daily routines. The program finished with drafting an action plan for the future. The lead improvement team consisted of the medical director, nursing director, cardiac fellow, nurses, a multifunctional patient care unit technician, and a social worker who functioned as a discharge coordinator. During each of the three days, they practiced new meeting skills and were coached by experts to encourage and guide them as they, together, discovered their work as a system. The vice president of Patient Services attended the opening and closing of the program to clarify expectations, to offer support, and to encourage them to begin and to continue their journey of improvement using microsystem methods. On the last day the vice president stated clearly her expectations for measurable improvements and told the staff that she would regularly visit the ICCU to witness and observe improvements and measured results.

Plastic Surgery Section

With the leadership of the lead physician, the practice manager, lead nurse, and lead administrative secretary, an interdisciplinary lead improvement team was convened to participate in a ten-week course to learn improvement application within the context of plastic surgery. The team held one-hour weekly improvement meetings to learn and apply improvement tools and methods.

Review Questions

1. What does a clinical microsystem consist of?
2. What is the connection between systems thinking and microsystems?
3. What research has been conducted specific to microsystems?
4. What are the success characteristics of a high-performing clinical microsystem?

Between Sessions Work

1. Begin to develop a microsystem wall graphic that models your own system and also offers physical space to display what people are learning, additional information, and results of the improvement work and the efforts to change.
2. Identify a communication strategy.

References

Batalden, P. B., Nelson, E. C., & Roberts, J. S. (1994). Linking outcomes measurement to continual improvement: The serial "V" way of thinking about improving clinical care. *Joint Commission Journal on Quality Improvement, 20*(4), 167–180.

Deming, W. E. (1986). *Out of the crisis.* Cambridge, MA: MIT Center for Advanced Engineering Study.

Donaldson, M. S., & Mohr, J. J. (2000). *Exploring innovation and quality improvement in health care microsystems: A cross-case analysis.* Technical Report for the Institute of Medicine Committee on the Quality of Health Care in America. Washington, DC: Institute of Medicine.

Institute of Medicine (U.S.), Committee on Quality of Health Care in America. (2001). *Crossing the quality chasm: A new health system for the 21st century.* Washington, DC: National Academies Press.

Nelson, E. C., Greenfield, S., Hays, R. D., Larson C., Leopold, B., & Batalden, P. B. (1995). Comparing outcomes and charges for patients with acute myocardial infarction in three community hospitals: An approach for assessing "value." *International Journal for Quality in Health Care, 7*(2), 95–108.

Nelson, E. C., Mohr, J. J., Batalden, P. B., & Plume, S. K. (1996). Improving health care: Part 1. The clinical value compass. *Joint Commission Journal on Quality Improvement, 22*(4), 243–258.

Quinn, J. B. (1992). *Intelligent enterprise: A knowledge and service based paradigm for industry.* New York: Free Press.

Wheatley, M. J., & Kellner-Rogers, M. (1996). *A simpler way.* San Francisco: Berrett-Koehler.

CHAPTER TWELVE

EFFECTIVE MEETING SKILLS I

Chapter Purpose

Aim. To identify concepts and methods for holding effective and productive meetings with a lead improvement team.

  Objectives. At the completion of this unit, you will be able to

- List the four common roles and functions for effective meetings.
- Describe the meeting process and the seven steps in the agenda template.

- List the work to be done before meetings.
- List the processes to be followed during meetings.
- Create a draft list of ground rules for your lead improvement team members to use when learning how to work together in a meeting.
- Describe the steps for maintaining the rhythm of improvement.

Before your microsystem starts its improvement journey, fundamental organizing should occur to ensure that the interdisciplinary lead improvement team can use disciplined meeting skills and members can succeed in their work together. This chapter addresses an initial set of these skills; later, Chapter Twenty will examine some additional specific useful techniques. (See Figure 12.1.)

FIGURE 12.1. IMPROVEMENT RAMP: MEETING SKILLS.

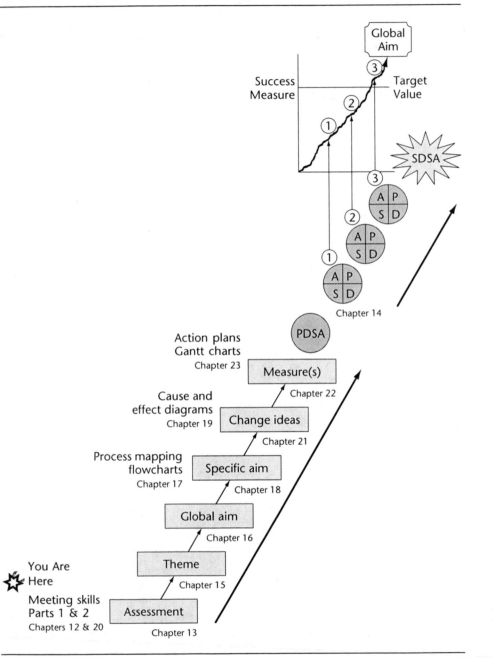

Once you identify the members of your lead improvement team, they need to begin using effective meeting skills. A key to successful improvement efforts is developing an improvement discipline with rhythm and pace and with actions that recur daily, weekly, monthly, and yearly—and that make local *sense*. Learning to hold productive and effective meetings is a key part of developing improvement discipline.

What Is a Productive and Effective Meeting?

A *productive and effective meeting* is one that is conducted in a disciplined manner, with active participation from all microsystem role representatives, resulting in clear action items, an evaluation of the meeting, an agenda for the next meeting, and a sense among the members that their time was well-spent. Meeting actions are clearly documented in meeting notes, usually placed on large flipcharts. The meeting is usually conducted with attention to good time management and often is completed within an hour's time, from start to finish.

Why Use Meeting Skills and Roles?

Time is precious. Members of a frontline clinical unit have limited amounts of time for holding meetings and being involved in the improvement of their microsystem. Without discipline, meetings can be disorganized, have limited member participation, end without having set clear next steps, and be perceived as a "waste of time."

Identifying common meeting roles helps members of the interdisciplinary team become more aware of their work together and more skilled in essential meeting tasks. It is helpful to rotate the meeting roles so that each team member can gain insight into the importance of each role and practice the skills of each role.

What Are Effective Meeting Roles?

The four essential meeting roles are

- Leader
- Timekeeper
- Recorder
- Facilitator

The *leader* of the meeting prepares the agenda, helps the group move through the agenda, and elicits participation from all members. The team's formal leader does not necessarily hold this role all the time because the real purpose of the role is to guide the team through a planned agenda. The meeting leader is also a group member and contributes ideas, interprets data, and participates with other members in making team decisions.

The *timekeeper* works to keep group members aware of their use of time, to help them keep themselves on a schedule with an agreed-on time allotment for each agenda item. If the group makes a prior agreement to it, the timekeeper can verbally announce such markers as the amount of time remaining for each individual agenda item, the halfway point, or when the allotted time for an item is up. The fact that allotted time is up does not mean the work is over, and the group may wish to add time for further consideration of the item while also agreeing on a time adjustment for the other items. The timekeeper role can be intimidating for some team members, due to the sense that announcing how much time is left or that the allotted time has been reached is a controlling function, so it is helpful to make it clear that time management is a shared responsibility—not the SOLE responsibility of the timekeeper.

The *recorder* is responsible for the meeting record, noting the progress of the meeting and listing *next step* items along with their owners and timelines, and so on. The recorder is encouraged to make a visible record, using one or more flipcharts and writing with markers so the whole group can follow the written documentation of the meeting and simultaneously ensure the accuracy of the note taking. It is helpful for the recorder to clearly note next steps, step owners, and timelines as the meeting progresses so that at the end of the meeting the team can quickly review what these steps are and who is responsible for doing what by when. It is also helpful for the recorder to keep a *parking lot,* a list of ideas not related to the current agenda but worth remembering and perhaps addressing in future agendas.

Although not a necessary role for every meeting, a *facilitator* can monitor the group process in order to allow the group to benefit from the contributions of all its members. In high-energy meetings it is easy for some members to dominate or for the group to unintentionally stray from the meeting agenda and to discuss other subjects. If the leader needs help, the facilitator can comment on the group processes at work, pointing out, for example, that a few members of the group are engaged in a tangential or paired conversation or that the discussion is not on track with the meeting agenda, and can encourage the group to stay focused. The facilitator can also note when it is clear that all members of the group are not engaged in the meeting and can suggest ways for the group to get itself back on track. The facilitator needs to concentrate on the meeting process and social dynamics; for this reason it may be difficult for the person taking this role to get deeply involved in the topic being discussed.

Can the Leader and Facilitator Roles Be Combined?

Experienced leaders are often able to combine the two roles of leader and facilitator, keeping the agenda moving and on track and also engaging everyone's full participation. However, keeping the roles separate when a group first begins to hold effective meetings helps everyone—especially the facilitator—to understand the benefits of a disciplined group process.

Can the Leader and Recorder Roles Be Combined?

Depending on the aim of the meeting it may be useful to combine the leader and recorder roles. In meetings where processes such as brainstorming or multi-voting are the central activity, the leader and recorder roles can often be combined. Again, this might make most sense when the team has gained experience in using these methods and is comfortable with the roles. Recording is hard work because it involves such careful listening.

Should the Facilitator Be an Outsider?

Not usually; however, there are times when the facilitator should be a professional and separate from the group. This approach may be useful, for example, when the topic evokes a lot of tension or has high conflict potential. Under these circumstances the team might benefit from having an outsider take on the task of balancing the conversation and keeping everyone on track. When team members assume meeting roles, they practice new skills and new ways of working together within an interdisciplinary group. New experiences create new learning that helps produce a new local culture. All too often a clinical team will defer to the traditional leader—usually a physician or nurse; this is especially likely when group members represent a clear hierarchy of roles and jobs. Practicing within a structure of tools and techniques for effective meetings can be important in learning to work together in new and positive ways. For example, when a senior physician is the leader at one meeting and a clinical secretary is the leader at the next meeting, the switch in roles contributes to group members' sense of interdependence and adds to each member's perceived value, regardless of salary or experience.

What Are the Phases of an Effective Meeting?

Think of a meeting as a process consisting of three steps. First, there is a *premeeting phase* in which the meeting date, time, and place are organized. The aims for the meeting and its agenda are also established in this phase, and the next steps assigned during the previous meeting are reviewed.

The second phase of an effective meeting is the *in-meeting phase*, the actual meeting at which the team focuses on and works on the aims. During this phase the team determines the next actions that need to occur, who will *own* these next steps, and what the timeline is for completion.

The third and final phase of an effective meeting is the *postmeeting phase*, in which team members follow through on meeting decisions. The action steps that have been assigned are taken, monitored, and reviewed. Talking with the person assigned to the action step (perhaps during daily huddles), and assessing the process of completing the work, will help the group or microsystem leader keep the overall agenda on track. At times it may be discovered that the next step cannot be completed before the next meeting. At this point the leader of the meeting makes adjustments to the agenda and puts the follow-through action on a subsequent agenda.

What Processes Are Evident in an Effective Meeting?

During the meeting the group engages in the following processes to move through the agenda and to achieve the meeting aims:

- Makes decisions
- Manages time
- Shares leadership
- Listens and contributes
- Manages conflict
- Gives feedback
- Learns new things
- Has fun

What Is the Seven-Step Meeting Process?

Using the seven-step meeting process (Executive Learning, 1993) ensures a disciplined meeting held in an efficient and productive manner. This process spells out how to move through an agenda in an efficient and productive manner. It also takes full advantage of the meeting roles previously discussed. Many groups find this disciplined style of conducting meetings restrictive and uncomfortable *at first*. But groups that work through their initial discomfort and persist often cannot then imagine holding meetings using their previous methods because of the tremendous gains in efficiency and productivity stemming from the new methods. Here are the seven steps:

1. *Clarify the aims of the meeting and what the team will get done during the meeting.* Reviewing the aims gives you the opportunity to set reasonable number of topics to be discussed in the time available. Meetings frequently try to discuss and make decisions on too many topics within the allotted time, often only sixty minutes.

2. *Review or assign the meeting roles: leader, recorder, timekeeper, and facilitator.* Many clinical teams have found it beneficial to take the time to determine the leader, recorder, timekeeper, and facilitator for the next meeting, both to save time and to ensure that the premeeting work is monitored and the current meeting's agenda gets set up in advance. Some clinical teams find that selecting a meeting leader for a set period of time helps to ensure the organization of and follow-through on meeting topics. For example, some groups designate a person to be the leader for a month, or another period of time, and then rotate the leader role to another person for a month, and so on.

3. *Review the agenda, and determine how much time to spend on each item.* This helps the group to identify a reasonable number of items for the agenda. With the group present, the leader reviews the items of the agenda and the allotted times for each item. While assigning a designated time to each agenda item, the group may determine it does not have enough time to cover all the items. When this happens, the group may want to move an item to the next meeting's agenda.

4. *Work through the agenda items by discussing and reviewing data and information.* The leader should consciously move through the agenda items one by one and keep the group on track. The facilitator should watch that all members of the group are participating and that appropriate and helpful meeting techniques are being used as needed throughout the meeting. This is especially important for new groups learning new habits for effective meetings. It is easy to revert to old behaviors, such as not taking turns for talking, interrupting, and not inviting participation by all members. The facilitator should alert the group when the discussion is straying from the stated meeting aims.

5. *Review the meeting actions by reading through the (flipchart) record, making changes or additions, and deciding what to keep for the formal meeting record.* The recorder should be tracking agenda items and next steps throughout the meeting. Putting the

notes on a flipchart encourages members of the group to actively review the meeting record throughout the meeting and to ensure that group decisions are being accurately documented. After all the agenda items have been addressed, the recorder should briefly review the meeting record with the team to validate and clarify the documentation.

6. *Plan the next actions, and determine who will do what in the postmeeting phase.* Determine the aims and plan the agenda for the next meeting. This step is essential in staying disciplined and avoiding ending up with too much work for the next meeting. This step also provides the group with clear agenda items in advance of the next meeting and helps establish a visible path forward.

7. *Evaluate the meeting; determine what went well and what could be improved in the future.* This is the most frequently skipped step in the seven-step meeting process. Groups are eager to end the meeting and sometimes will not take a few minutes at the end to evaluate how well the meeting went. However, it is important for group development to take the time to assess how well the group performed the meeting roles and followed the seven-step meeting process. Congratulating the group on following the agenda and times, acknowledging personal improvements that will contribute to future meetings, and offering encouragement to members assuming new meeting roles will all contribute to the growth of the team and its ability to hold effective meetings. Some lead improvement teams use a 10-point perception scale (in which 1 = "poor" and 10 = "best meeting ever") to rate their meetings. At a minimum, feedback from each member about "what went well" in the meeting and "what could be improved" for future meetings is essential. This evaluation process takes less than five minutes.

What Does a Meeting Agenda Template Look Like?

A sample of a meeting template that you could adapt to your own situation is shown in Figure 12.2. Notice that the roles and meeting steps are listed on the agenda. Many groups complete this template for each meeting to remind themselves of appropriate meeting discipline. With repeated use of this template the meeting roles and process become a habit for the group. Interdisciplinary groups often report that using the meeting template feels awkward for the first few meetings but that with practice the meeting roles and process become the norm for the group, making it easier for team members to work together in an enjoyable and efficient way.

FIGURE 12.2. SAMPLE MEETING AGENDA TEMPLATE.

<table>
<tr><td colspan="4">

Meeting Agenda

Department name: _____

Day, date: _____

Time of meeting: _____

Meeting location: _____

</td></tr>
<tr><td colspan="4">

Aim of our microsystem:

</td></tr>
<tr><td colspan="4">

Leader:
Recorder:
Timekeeper:
Facilitator:
Participants:

</td></tr>
<tr><th>Time</th><th>Method</th><th>Item</th><th>Aim or Action</th></tr>
<tr><td></td><td></td><td>

1. Clarify objectives of this meeting
  A.
  B.

</td><td></td></tr>
<tr><td></td><td></td><td>

2. Review Roles
  Leader:
  Recorder:
  Timekeeper:
  Facilitator or adviser:

</td><td></td></tr>
<tr><td></td><td></td><td>

3. Review agenda and assign times

</td><td></td></tr>
<tr><td></td><td></td><td>

4. Work through agenda items
  A.
  B.
  C.
  D.

</td><td></td></tr>
<tr><td></td><td></td><td>

5. Review meeting record

</td><td></td></tr>
<tr><td></td><td></td><td>

6. Plan next agenda

</td><td></td></tr>
<tr><td></td><td></td><td>

7. Evaluate meeting

</td><td></td></tr>
</table>

Source: Adapted from Executive Learning, 1993.

What Are the Ground Rules for Meetings?

In one of your early group meetings, put time on the agenda to draft meeting ground rules. As members of an interdisciplinary group planning to meet regularly to discuss and improve processes, it is important for all of you to agree on how you will work with each other within the meeting. Determining how the group members will encourage participation by everyone, learn to listen to one another, and change how they interact with one another contributes to a positive flow and sets helpful guidelines that generate effective meetings.

Groups usually allow thirty minutes or less to brainstorm a list of ideas specifying how members will act during the meetings. Here are some examples of ground rules that teams have adopted:

- Practice not interrupting each other.
- Work to include others' ideas.
- Treat other team members the way you would like to be treated.
- Try not to repeat the same point—even if you did not get the response you hoped for the first time you said it.
- Practice not defending previously held viewpoints—suspend them for a while; you might learn something new.
- Try not to be too nice at the expense of rigor—help the group progress in its thinking.
- Practice forgiveness for new ideas and ways of learning that do not seem to work as well as they might eventually.
- Laugh a little.

Some additional ground rules to consider come from Nabil Musallam (personal communication, 2003) at the University of California's Davis Medical Center:

- Participate in the meeting and not in the hall.
- Speak to the agenda item being discussed.
- Plan your words to conserve time.
- Clearly state opinion or fact—if it is a fact, give the references.
- For opinions, use only "I" statements, unless you have permission to speak for the "we."
- If you oppose, you must propose.

Many groups have found these examples helpful in drafting their own ground rules. Once a team has established ground rules, it is helpful to display them during every meeting to remind members of what they all have agreed to. It is also helpful to periodically assess how well meetings are following the ground rules.

Note that it is the responsibility of all the members to hold each other accountable for the agreed-upon behaviors.

What Are Some Tips for Getting Started with Productive Meetings?

Once an interdisciplinary lead improvement team is identified, it is important to contact the members and determine a *regular* day, time, and place to meet. Having a regular schedule and logistics eliminates confusion and uncertainty about when and where each meeting will be held. The meeting becomes part of people's regular routine. Because of the importance of the work the group is trying to improve, meetings should be held weekly or every other week. There will always be action items to follow up on as well and next steps to be identified.

Create a method for keeping members who cannot be present at a meeting informed and up to date. Some groups, for example, use the *buddy system* to ensure that information and decisions are shared with everyone. Other suggestions include making a speaker phone and conference line available for group members to call in to the meeting to save travel time.

The tools and supplies that support effective meetings can be organized and made readily available by maintaining a *goodie bag*, or *meeting toolkit*. Many groups have found the following list helpful; it indicates the materials and supplies that should be readily available to accomplish various meeting processes:

- Large markers to use on flipcharts
- Pads of flipchart paper (the self-adhesive type is very useful)
- Masking tape to post flipchart sheets that are not self-adhesive
- Post-it Notes (large and small)
- Small markers, such as Sharpies, to write on Post-it Notes so they can be read from a distance
- Graph paper to chart data
- Tacks to post flipcharts on bulletin boards
- Stopwatch to measure time
- Fun items like play dough, Koosh balls, and other hand toys that group members find helpful for restless hands

To set the scene for a successful meeting, arrive early and set up the flipcharts and materials for the meeting. Always strive to start and end on time. This courtesy demonstrates respect for the group members.

The combination of using effective meeting skills and roles and starting and ending on time will help your team hold successful meetings. At the same time, members of the group will be developing new skills and discipline in holding meetings and learning to work together in more productive ways than they did formerly.

How Do You Keep a Rhythm of Improvement?

The rhythm of improvement can be maintained through various types of regularly planned events so that staff develop the discipline and pace of improving daily, weekly, monthly, and yearly, with a focus on providing care while improving the care (see Figure 12.3). These events include

- *Daily* five- to seven-minute huddles to convene the clinical team and to make operational and improvement plans for the day
- *Weekly* sixty-minute lead improvement team meetings
- *Monthly* all-staff meetings to share improvement activities and discuss processes of care, outcomes, and improvements
- *Yearly* all-staff retreats to reflect on the past year and plan operations and improvements for the future year

FIGURE 12.3. RHYTHM OF IMPROVEMENT.

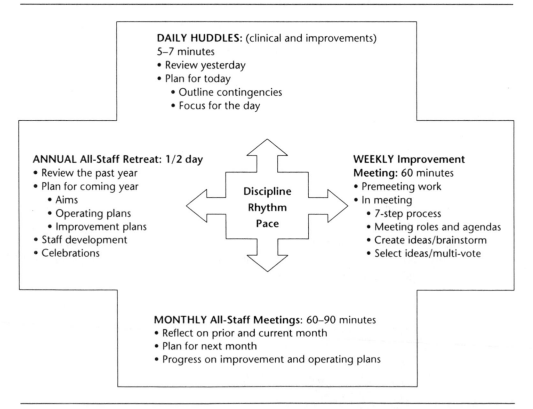

Case Studies

Intermediate Cardiac Care Unit (ICCU)

During the three-day microsystem learning program, the ICCU's lead improvement team decided to hold its weekly improvement meetings on Wednesdays, from 1:30 to 2:30 P.M., in the ICCU conference room. Team members made a commitment to use the new meeting skills and improvement tools on their path forward and established these ground rules:

- Standard set meeting time.
- Honor the time.
- Start and end on time.
- Be prepared.
- Turn cell phones and pagers off.
- No interruptions.
- Stick to the agenda and issues.
- No sidebars or social conversations.
- If you oppose, you must propose.
- Everyone participates.
- Come to the meeting with an open mind.
- Respect everyone's ideas.

Figure 12.4 displays a sample ICCU meeting agenda.

Plastic Surgery Section

The weekly lead team meetings are held on Wednesdays from 11 A.M. to noon in the outpatient clinic's conference room. The team has held its meetings faithfully since 2003, whether all members are present or not. Team members have found they always have improvement data and processes to review, and because the meeting leader role rotates among them, the meetings just naturally flow as part of their work. When the Plastic Surgery lead improvement team started its improvement journey, members agreed on these ground rules:

- Consistently hold weekly meetings on Wednesdays at same time.
- Practice effective meeting skills, including roles and timed agendas.
- Work to be inclusive during the meeting.
- Interdisciplinary involvement is key to successful improvements.

FIGURE 12.4. SAMPLE ICCU MEETING AGENDA.

ICCU Redesign Agenda—ICCU Conf. Room
1:30–2:30 P.M.

DATE: Wed., March 22

TIME	OUTCOME	MEETING PROCESS
2 min.		**A. Identify meeting roles:** Leader: Shelly Facilitator: Margie Time Keeper: Jean Recorder: Ed Guests: Melanie, Dave
5 min.		**B. Work through agenda items:** 1. Attending debrief rounding process week 4—Dr. Dave: What's going well?
5 min.		Other staff input: What's going well? What could be improved? (attending and group)
5 min.		What is the role of the facilitator?
5 min.		2. Review PDSA 3b: ran the post-call patients first (facilitator represents the RN) to get them out on time, then POD to POD with the RN.
10 min.		4 P.M. "run the list" global rounds: Who's going home tomorrow? What is our goal? What do we want to measure?
5 min.		3. Summary of what we have learned to date.
10 min.		4. Create PDSA 4??
5 min.		5. How best to communicate to staff.
5 min.		6. Global aim statement–finalize!!
5 min.		**C. Review meeting record and plan next agenda—evaluate meeting:** **Assign roles:** 1. 2. 3. Future agenda items: Mission statement

Note: POD = a geographical place in the ICCU consisting of a group of patient rooms.

Review Questions

1. What roles support effective meetings?
2. What is the seven-step meeting process?
3. How can ground rules support effective meeting skills?
4. What materials are likely to be needed for team meetings?
5. What can you do daily, weekly, monthly, and annually to establish improvement rhythm?

Between Sessions Work

1. Conduct sixty-minute meetings with an interdisciplinary lead team using effective meeting skills.
2. Use an agenda to hold a meeting to brainstorm a draft set of ground rules.
3. Identify a place and time to hold weekly lead improvement team meetings.

Reference

Executive Learning. (1993). *Continual improvement handbook: A quick reference guide for tools and concepts*. Healthcare Version. Brentwood, TN: Author.

CHAPTER THIRTEEN

ASSESSING YOUR MICROSYSTEM WITH THE 5 P'S

Chapter Purpose

Aim. To do an assessment of your clinical microsystem using the 5 P's framework, a tested analytical method that focuses on *purpose, patients, professionals, processes,* and *patterns.*

　　Objectives. At the completion of this unit, you will be able to

- Organize your microsystem assessment so it is systematic.
- Describe your deeper knowledge of your microsystem's purpose, patients, professionals, processes, and patterns.

- Identify key tools and methods for gaining deeper knowledge.
- Engage all members of your clinical microsystem in the process of assessment and awareness building.
- Review, analyze, and draw conclusions about the relationships among the 5 P's.
- Identify strengths and opportunities for improvement based on the 5 P's assessment.

　　The assessment of your clinical microsystem is the beginning of that system's improvement journey. Through the assessment described in this chapter, the interdisciplinary lead improvement team will learn new information and data about the microsystem and use that material to inform their selection of improvement themes and aims. (See Figure 13.1.)

FIGURE 13.1. IMPROVEMENT RAMP: ASSESSMENT.

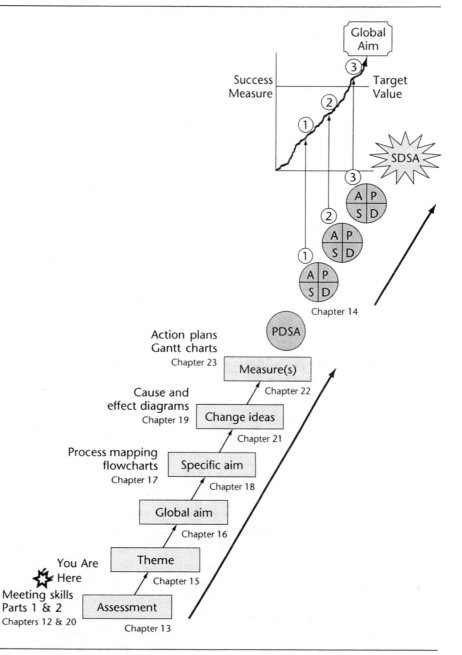

How Does an Interdisciplinary Lead Improvement Team Begin to Assess and Improve a Clinical Microsystem?

Think patient care. To improve a patient's health status you assess, diagnose, treat, and conduct follow-up based on biomedical and clinical care science. This process includes the patient and the family.

To improve a microsystem's "health" status—you assess, diagnose, treat, and follow-up—just as with patients—based on improvement science and the science of clinical practice. This process should include all members of the clinical microsystem. The main idea is for the microsystem to build understanding and to discover its capability from the *inside out.*

Using effective meeting skills (Chapters Twelve and Twenty) you convene the lead improvement team, representing all microsystem members' roles, to begin to review data and information about the microsystem.

The 5 P's framework is a tested and useful method for microsystem members to begin to see their microsystem in a new way and to begin to ask new questions. John Kelsch (1990), formerly the corporate director of quality for Xerox Corporation, once observed that "to do things differently, we must see things differently. When we see things we haven't noticed before, we can ask questions we didn't know to ask before."

Moreover, doing a 5 P's assessment does not mean that improvement activities need to be postponed. Many clinical teams do their assessment before starting to make improvements, but some begin organizing improvement efforts and learning about their system's 5 P's simultaneously. The discoveries that occur in the 5 P's diagnostic process often make the needed improvements clear, and ultimately, the 5 P's inform improvement activities and planning now and in the future.

What Does the 5 P's Framework Look Like?

The 5 P's framework can be thought of as a structured method of inquiring into the *anatomy* of a clinical microsystem (see Figure 1.3). Every complex, adaptive system has structure, process, patterns, and outcomes (Zimmerman, Lindberg, & Plsek, 1999), and you can make these features explicit and analyze them by using the 5 P's framework in your microsystem.

It is often useful to create a poster-sized version of the 5 P's diagram to visually display your microsystem's 5 P's facts for all staff to review and understand. A template for such a poster can be found and downloaded at http://www. clinicalmicrosystem.org (click on Tools) (also see Figure 13.2 in the ICCU case study at the end of this chapter).

What Resources Are Available to Guide the 5 P's Assessment?

The Primary Care Workbook in the Appendix contains a tested and helpful collection of tools to help you assess your microsystem and by so doing to build the knowledge base and system awareness of your interdisciplinary lead improvement team. In addition, the Dartmouth Clinical Microsystem Toolkit (Godfrey, Nelson, & Batalden, 2005a) includes two workbooks that focus on hospital microsystems: *Improving Care Within Your Inpatient Units and Emergency Department* (Godfrey et al., 2005c) and *Improving Care Between Your Clinical Units* (Godfrey et al., 2005b). More outpatient and specialty workbooks can be found at http://www.clinicalmicrosystem.org, along with full-page worksheets and tools.

What Is a Helpful Way to Introduce Your Team to the Assessment Process?

Lead improvement teams have gained deeper insight into and knowledge of their microsystems in various ways. Each microsystem is unique, and the group should determine the best method and pace for conducting their assessment. An important consideration is the amount of data and information that is, or is not, readily available. Use the workbook in the Appendix or on the Web site to preview what you might do and how you might make a strategy for forward progress. After you have previewed all the suggested data and information, you can formulate a plan to collect the data and information you need. One example of such a plan is Figure A.1 in the Appendix. Completing the data organization table in this figure will give you an outline of the material that need to be reviewed and descriptions of where current data are available. The *practice profile* worksheet in Figure A.2 will also guide you in obtaining the needed data and information.

What Are the 5 P's?

The following description of the 5 P's is essential information for microsystem leaders. Moreover, by sharing this information with everyone in the microsystem, leaders can promote learning, understanding, and awareness that is broad and deep; this improves the functioning of your microsystem.

Purpose

The purpose of your microsystem may go beyond the microsystem's mission statement. If a mission statement is available, then consider having an active discussion among all the microsystem members to enable each person to make a connection between himself or herself and his or her values on the one hand and the microsystem's purpose on the other.

High-performing microsystems have a clearly stated purpose and mission. All too often, busy interdisciplinary lead improvement teams have not taken the time to discuss and agree on the purpose of the microsystem. Every member of the microsystem should have the opportunity to contribute to the purpose statement. This active discussion aims to connect individual members with the microsystem's purpose. It reveals each member's view of the microsystem purpose. Clarifying the purpose statement also establishes a guiding light for setting priorities and making decisions in the microsystem.

Patients

Individual members of the microsystem have knowledge about the patients they provide care and services to. This knowledge usually concerns individual patients or what happens on certain days of the week or during specific shifts. General population knowledge and general facts about the microsystem are not usually shared by all members of the microsystem. Gaining deeper knowledge about the patients and subpopulations of patients that the microsystem serves can enrich all members' decision making and their design of care and services. This knowledge can help microsystem members become better informed about how to take good care of patients and how to improve their delivery system.

Professionals

Every member of the clinical microsystem who provides and contributes to the care of patients should be thought of as a professional. If every person, in every role, is respected for what he or she contributes to the smooth functioning of the microsystem, then individual self-esteem, morale, and engagement all rise. Charles Mayo, one of the Mayo Clinic's founders, reminds us, "There are no inferior jobs in any organization. No matter what the assigned task, if it is done well and with dignity, it contributes to the function of everything around it and should be valued accordingly by all" (Mayo, n.d.). Learning more about all the microsystem's professionals and what they do, what hours they work, what they wish to learn, and how they rate their workplace increases awareness for future improvement.

Processes

The interdisciplinary members of a microsystem participate in various processes, systems, and steps to care for patients. Their tasks are interrelated and should complement one another. Often microsystem members have never taken the time to meet to review specific processes of care that are repeated regularly in the system. The different views and perspectives of each member are revealed when the lead improvement team is asked to create a flowchart to show how routine care is delivered or how a patient enters the microsystem. This lack of knowledge about how the current process actually works and how it varies underlies and contributes to much of the waste and poor reliability within a microsystem. Identifying core processes and engaging all members in flowcharting the current state is a way to begin to design more efficient and effective processes. It gives the microsystem members insight about the contributions that each person makes to the process (see Figure A.11, in the Appendix). This often works best when one or two members construct the initial flow diagram and then others are asked to improve upon this draft. Eventually, the flowchart can be posted for all to review and edit.

Observing and measuring *cycle times* in processes of care can also help a microsystem group identify waste in daily work. Viewing the process of care through "the eyes of the patient" (see Figure A.5, in the Appendix) is a powerful tool for gaining important insight into that process from the patient perspective.

Patterns

Patterns exist in every microsystem but often go unnoticed, unacknowledged, or unleveraged. Does everyone in your microsystem meet regularly to discuss what patients want and need or to talk about care or the microsystem's quality, cost, and safety outcomes? Who talks to whom? Who never talks to whom? What are the *metrics that matter* for the microsystem (see Figure A.14 in the Appendix and Godfrey et al., 2005c, p. 22)? Do all members know about, review, and discuss these metrics and causal systems? What has the microsystem improved, and what makes the members most proud? What does the microsystem celebrate? All of these patterns and more can be acknowledged and taken into consideration when increasing member's awareness about a microsystem and when taking action to improve that microsystem.

After making a plan and beginning to obtain the data and information, the lead improvement team is ready to review the microsystem's current state. Collecting a sample of information about each of the 5 P's is a good way to begin.

It requires that you identify the sources for the data. (The materials in the Appendix of this book can facilitate the collection, display, and assessment of the information about each of the 5 P's.) The resulting characterization of the system's current state can be very helpful as the microsystem members continue to gain deeper knowledge about its work.

A helpful five-step exercise follows. Remember, this exercise is best done by your interdisciplinary lead improvement team. It can be done in multiple sessions, to give the team time to review and discuss and to determine next steps and gain more information. For example, you could plan five sequential meetings, with a focus on one P at each meeting. Useful materials are (1) a microsystem wall poster, (2) five envelopes, each with preliminary information for one of the P's, and (3) tape. Here's how it works:

1. Assign a meeting leader, facilitator, timekeeper, and recorder prior to starting. Develop an agenda and timeline to cover all five steps in this exercise. Be sure to assign enough time for the team to cover each of the exercise steps. Plan enough time at the end of all the sessions to synthesize the information and prepare a report.

2. Prepare five envelopes that contain preliminary information from your microsystem about the 5 P's (purpose, patients, professionals, processes, patterns), one P per envelope. Some important information will be available and some will not. Use the workbook in the Appendix and the Web site to help you identify the data needed to assess and diagnose your microsystem. Focus on one P at a time. It is important to review the data, determine what additional information is needed and where it may be obtained, and then move to the next P.

3. Use the microsystem workbook to determine which tools will help the lead improvement team to gain deeper insight into the microsystem. Some of the needed microsystem information is in each of the envelopes that you prepared; the microsystem workbook can help you to assess and diagnose your microsystem, and it provides additional tools for collecting desired information.

4. When reviewing each P, some of the questions that follow this exercise may facilitate the team discussion.

5. At the end of the 5 P's series the lead improvement team will have a deeper awareness of its microsystem and can report back to all the microsystem members and summarize the learning and conclusions. The lead improvement team will also know what additional information it needs to deepen its own knowledge about its microsystem.

Review the following discussion questions when performing each section of this exercise:

1. Purpose
   a. What do you think about your organization's mission statement and the microsystem's mission statement?
   b. How are these two statements aligned with each other?
   c. How could your microsystem's purpose statement be improved?
2. Patients, professionals, processes, patterns
   a. What do you see after reviewing the information?
   b. What other information do you need, and how can you obtain it?
   c. Can you begin to make any initial assessments?
   d. How can the microsystem workbook help you with the assessment?
3. Prepare a report on your findings (in the form of wall poster) for all the members of your microsystem.
   a. Post graphical displays and tables under each of the 5 P's on the microsystem wall poster, displaying the information for all staff to review.
   b. Make intentional plans for team members to identify microsystem members to review the microsystem wall poster findings, to increase awareness and to stimulate further discussions.

What Should You Do with the Assessment Findings?

The 5 P's findings should be posted for all staff members in the clinical microsystem to review and comment on. It is important to identify a common area for posting the ongoing assessments, data, and information of the lead improvement team so as to invite all microsystem members to become interested and informed. The microsystem wall poster is a helpful model. Encourage all members of your microsystem to explore the relationships among the 5 P's to begin to see the different connections, draw new conclusions, and identify new system processes and designs that can be developed with this new, deeper knowledge.

Case Studies

Intermediate Cardiac Care Unit (ICCU)

To better inform the team improvement activities, the ICCU lead improvement team began the assessment of the system's 5 P's at its first microsystem learning sessions. Team members reviewed available data, determined they needed to gather more information on the ICCU, and developed a plan to evaluate staff satisfaction in the workplace and to collect staff assessments of core and supporting processes. The team actively reviewed and adapted the many forms and methods in the *Improving Care Within Your Inpatient Units* workbook (Godfrey et al., 2005c) to inform their work. They put up a large poster containing the core and supporting processes assessment tool so all staff could rank how well the various ICCU processes were working. After much discussion among team members and with the broader ICCU staff, the team drafted this purpose statement for the ICCU:

> The ICCU will create an environment in which cardiac patients and their families can receive excellent, comprehensive, specialized state of the art quality care. This will be accomplished by caring, competent professional staff that has the support and resources to do their best work to promote the emotional, physical and intellectual well-being of patients, families and caregivers.

Figure 13.2 is an example of the microsystem wall poster the ICCU lead improvement team used after initiating its 5 P's assessment.

Plastic Surgery Section

Through the ten-week course the lead improvement team was able to gain deeper insight into its microsystem's 5 P's. Team members created a microsystem wall poster to display their findings and engage other staff members' interest and curiosity. They discussed and identified their *purpose:* "Partner with our customers to improve form and function for better living."

They became more mindful of their *patients* and patient populations: pediatric, cosmetic, and reconstructive. A patient satisfaction survey revealed low patient satisfaction scores in the following areas:

- Ease of coordinating care
- Wait in waiting or exam room
- Wait for appointment

The section's *professionals* included six surgeons, three residents, three registered nurses, one registered nurse first assistant, one licensed practical nurse, two licensed nurse assistants, one physician assistant, two certified medical assistant, five secretaries, a half-time practice manager, a lead registered nurse, and an administrative supervisor. Through their improvement journey team members realized there were many opportunities to optimize the roles of their professionals

FIGURE 13.2. ICCU WALL POSTER FOR THE 5 P'S MICROSYSTEM ASSESSMENT.

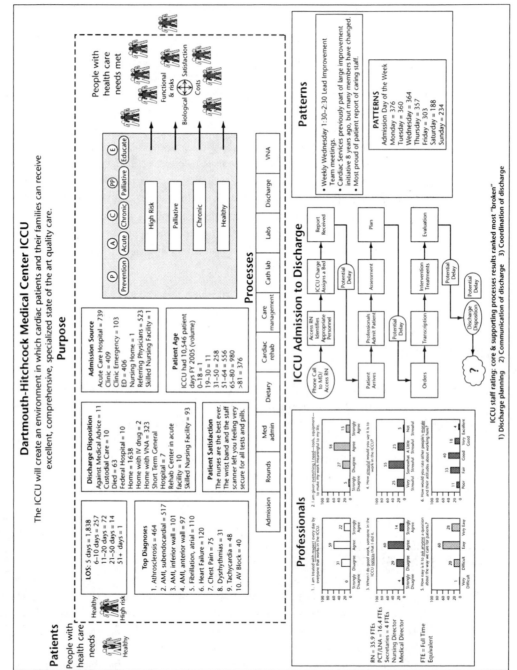

and increase staff morale. The initial staff satisfaction survey showed a high level of work unhappiness.

The *processes* they gained insight into included the scheduling systems for outpatient appointments and inpatient surgeries. They realized the system of care extended beyond their four walls. They measured cycle time in the clinic for new patient visits and minor surgical procedures and uncovered a great deal of variation in practice.

The lead improvement team members also realized there were *patterns* of access within their plastic surgery system that they needed to know more about before they could improve total system access to care, including outpatient visits, minor surgeries, and inpatient surgical procedures; this is shown in Figure 13.3. Team members began to discuss and observe the patterns in their practice. They uncovered measures specific to appointment scheduling, including poor access to appointments for new patients. A pattern of undesired variation was discovered in the way physicians scheduled follow-up visits for patients. Follow-up volumes varied significantly across the physicians.

Review Questions

1. How can you use a systematic method to assess your microsystem?
2. What are the 5 P's of a microsystem?
3. What tools and methods in the workbook in the Appendix can be used to make your assessment?
4. Who should be involved in assessing and improving your microsystem?
5. What are the next steps in your microsystem's improvement journey?

Between Sessions Work

1. Review the 5 P's and determine which data and information can be obtained from your organization and which data and information will be collected through other means, such as the microsystem workbook, tools, and forms.
2. Identify who will collect which data and information.
3. Create a timeline for collecting data and reporting on the assessment work.

FIGURE 13.3. PLASTIC SURGERY SECTION ACCESS PATTERNS.

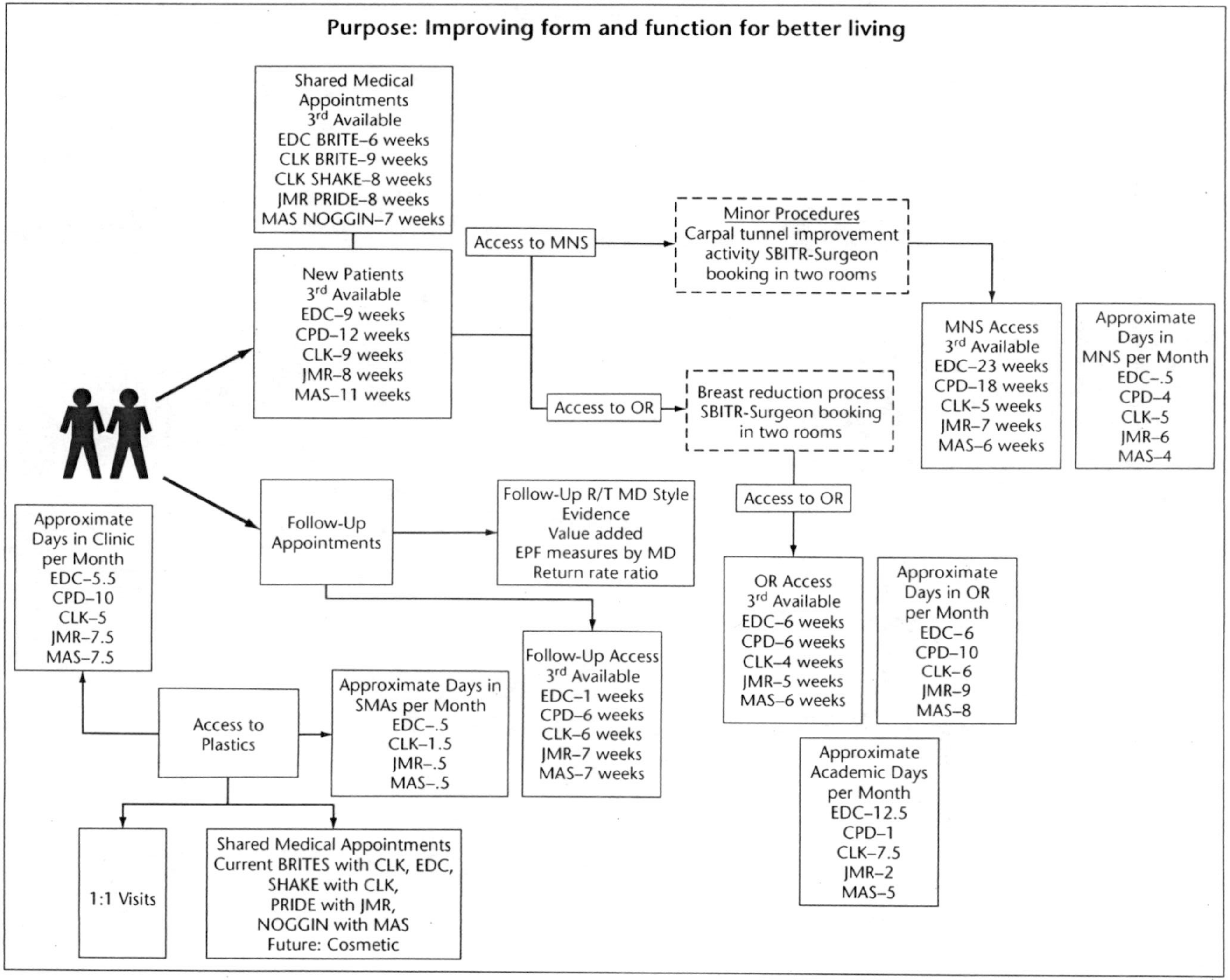

Purpose: Improving form and function for better living

Note: MNS = minor surgery; OR = operating room; RT = return visit

References

Godfrey, M., Nelson, E., & Batalden, P. (2005a). *Clinical microsystems: A path to healthcare excellence.* Toolkit. Hanover, NH: Dartmouth College.

Godfrey, M., Nelson, E., & Batalden, P. (2005b). *Clinical Microsystems: A path to healthcare excellence: Improving care between your clinical units.* Workbook. Hanover, NH: Dartmouth College. Available http://www.jcrine.com.

Godfrey, M., Nelson, E., & Batalden, P. (2005c). *Clinical Microsystems: A path to healthcare excellence: Improving care within your inpatient units and emergency department.* Workbook. Hanover, NH: Dartmouth College.

Kelsch, J. (1990). Continuous quality improvement: The Xerox way. Presented at a meeting of the West Paces Ferry Hospital Association, Atlanta, GA.

Mayo, C. (n.d.). Quoted on the Web page *Jobs at Mayo Clinic.* Retrieved June 27, 2006, from http://www.mayoclinic.org/jobs.

Zimmerman, B., Lindberg, C., & Plsek, P. (1999). *Edgeware: Insights from complexity science for health care leaders.* Irving, TX: VHA.

CHAPTER FOURTEEN

THE MODEL FOR IMPROVEMENT

PDSA ↔ SDSA

Chapter Purpose

Aim. To understand and apply the model for improvement in conducting disciplined, sequential tests of change for the purpose of making measurable improvements that can be sustained.

    Objectives. At the completion of this unit, you will be able to

- Define the model for improvement.
- Describe the two components of the model for improvement.

- List the detailed steps of PDSA model.
- Develop a clear *plan* to test a change.
- Describe the point at which a PDSA cycle becomes a SDSA cycle.
- State where PDSA ↔ SDSA cycles fit in the improvement process.
- Use the PDSA ↔ SDSA worksheet to guide actions.

It is important for all microsystem members to see the road ahead in the improvement journey. The improvement model discussed in this chapter is the method of choice for testing ideas for change leading to improvement. Figure 14.1 shows where you are now in the Dartmouth Microsystem Improvement Curriculum. With this focus on the model for improvement, we bring the scientific method explicitly into the improvement process.

FIGURE 14.1. IMPROVEMENT RAMP: MODEL FOR IMPROVEMENT.

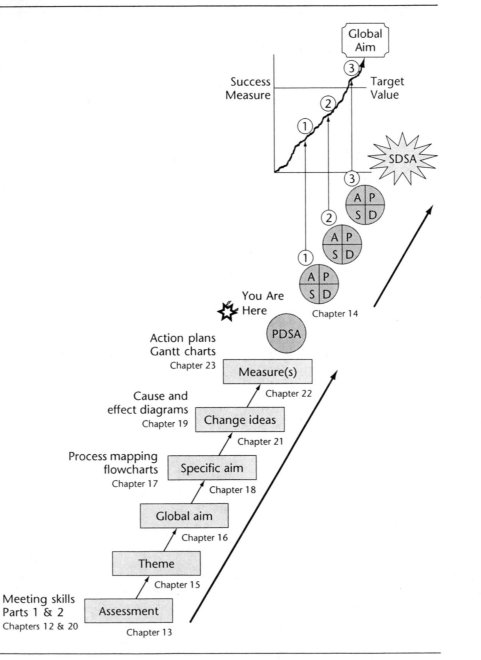

Tom Nolan and his colleagues at Associates in Process Improvement and the Institute for Healthcare Improvement have popularized the model for improvement (Langley, Nolan, Norman, Provost, & Nolan, 1996). This model, by incorporating the PDSA model, uses the scientific method for disciplined improvement. It also reminds improvement teams of the questions they should answer before starting their tests of change (Langley et al., 1996).

What Is the Model for Improvement?

The *model for improvement* (diagrammed in Figure 14.2) provides an overarching framework for testing change ideas that are expected to make improvements. The model has two parts. It starts with three questions to focus your improvement work, and then it leads you to run tests of change using the scientific method, or plan-do-study-act (PDSA) method. This process is shown in more detail in the following list:

1. Fundamental questions come first and clarify the improvement to be tested.
   - *Aim. What are we trying to accomplish?* Setting a clear aim with specific measurable targets.
   - *Measures. How will we know that a change is an improvement?* Qualitative and quantitative measures support real improvement and inform the progress of the change toward the stated aim.
   - *Changes. What changes can we make that will result in an improvement?* We need to create a statement of what we believe we can change to effect improvement. This change idea reflects our hypothesis about causes and effects.
2. Next, the changes are tested using the four steps known as plan, do, study, and act.

FIGURE 14.2. MODEL FOR IMPROVEMENT.

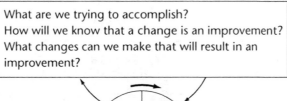

What are we trying to accomplish?
How will we know that a change is an improvement?
What changes can we make that will result in an improvement?

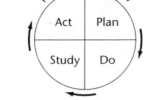

Act | Plan
Study | Do

Source: Langley et al., 1996. Used with permission.

Why Use the Model for Improvement?

The model for improvement provides a clear path forward for testing ideas that are likely to lead to successful improvements. The three questions elicit answers that specify the aim of the test, how improvement will be recognized, and what each specific change is. Addressing these questions helps organizations to avoid starting change without thoughtful planning that has identified the causal systems at work and ways to measure the results. The model for improvement also offers the PDSA method, a scientific approach for testing change and for making improvements.

How Does the Model Fit into the Improvement Process?

The model for improvement, in theory, comes into the improvement process after you have completed your assessments, selected a theme, and developed a global aim. The reality is that it starts when you are able to define a specific aim and when you are getting ready to test some changes. Another way to depict this sequence of moving from theme to global aim to specific aim to testing changes is shown in Figure 14.3. As you can see, a theme may have multiple global aims and specific aims with attached PDSA cycles, and all are connected back to the theme.

FIGURE 14.3. THEMES, AIMS, PROCESSES, AND PDSA CYCLES.

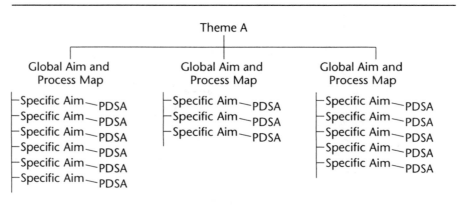

What Is the PDSA Part of the Model?

As mentioned earlier, PDSA stands for plan, do, study, and act. This model is commonly used to conduct tests of change in a disciplined and rapid fashion (see Figure 14.4). This structured, continuous quality improvement method has four steps that are used repetitively to test changes; it provides a clear path forward for testing ideas, learning from the testing, and moving ahead with better-informed actions to make improvements.

Walter A. Shewhart described a four-step improvement process in his 1939 book *Statistical Method from the Viewpoint of Quality Control.* W. E. Deming, a student of Shewhart, encouraged a systematic approach to problem solving and promoted this four-step process for use in continual improvement. Deming first referred to it as the Shewhart cycle. Others have called it the Deming cycle or the Deming wheel or the PDCA (plan, do, check, act) cycle (Deming, 1986).

FIGURE 14.4. THE COMPLETE PDSA CYCLE.

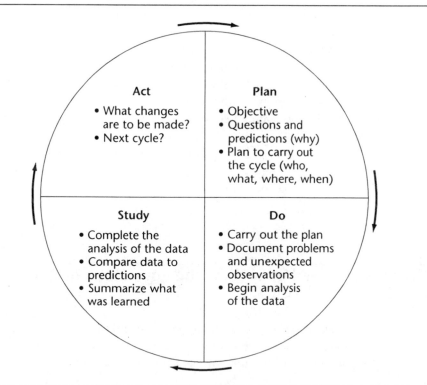

What Are the Benefits of Using PDSA?

The focus of PDSA is *experimentation*—such as testing out new change ideas to see if you can get better results.

- PDSA offers a disciplined model for testing improvements based on four steps: plan, do, study, act. All too often ideas for change are acted on without detailed planning and organization. There is a saying, "The devil is in the details." The discipline of PDSA will help you think through and plan for the "devilish" details of the idea you wish to test. Using this approach will increase your chances of successfully and rapidly reaching your aim.
- PDSA calls for small-scale testing and focuses attention on the theme and aims of improvement. It can lead to early, measured successes and increased staff enthusiasm.
- PDSA can be completed quickly, with minimal expenditure of resources and without taking great risks or using large amounts of time.
- PDSA invites clarity about *who* does *what, when,* and with what materials and supplies to ensure that those involved in the test are clear on roles and functions.
- PDSA makes it clear to all involved in the microsystem that the test is a pilot; to be conducted in a small way over a short period of time. This often diminishes anxiety and resistance to trying out a change idea. Once everyone in the microsystem realizes that the test will inform future activities and improvements, many people will support the test and be interested in the findings.
- PDSA helps staff gain new knowledge and fresh experience. This enables the lead improvement team to improve on the original change idea and thereby increase the likelihood of success.

What Is Involved in Each of the Four Steps of Plan, Do, Study, and Act?

In the *plan* phase you describe the objective and the specific change to be tested. This step clarifies the preparation that must be completed before the test is carried out, and considers the possible *upstream* and *downstream* impacts.

The plan includes clarification of

- The *hunch* that is being tested
- People's roles and functions during the test (planned actions)
- When the test will occur
- The education and training to be conducted before the test
- The data to be collected to determine if the test has been a success
- Who will observe and collect data during the test
- How long the test will be conducted (short period of time)
- What you expect to happen

The *do* phase of PDSA occurs when the pilot test is actually carried out, based on the preparations in the planning step. During the do phase, it is essential to have an identified member of the lead improvement team assigned to oversee the pilot and to collect qualitative and quantitative data and information about the test of change, data and information that will inform the next PDSA cycle. This individual should be ready to

- Document unexpected events
- Hear member feedback about the pilot test
- Have an eye for measured results
- Provide an open ear to listen to the pilot participants' feedback as they run the pilot

The individual overseeing the pilot can hold a *huddle* right before starting it, to ensure that everyone is clear on roles, functions, and processes and to plan time to debrief the participants periodically during the pilot.

The *study* phase occurs after the do phase. It is the period of time that is used to analyze the data, to reflect on results, and to debrief microsystem members about the pilot test experience. Be sure to plan time for reflection. Use the data and information collected during the pilot to evaluate what happened. Your team members should compare what they expected to happen with what actually happened and summarize lessons learned. They should identify any unexpected positive or negative results and determine what could be improved next.

The *act* phase occurs when you and your team are ready to determine whether or not the idea being tested should be modified or abandoned in light of the results achieved. Given what was learned during the test, what is the next step? The team should use what it has learned to improve its next test of change as it moves up the improvement ramp (Langley et al., 1996). Once the team has determined the next step—to refine, abandon, or try on a larger scale—it should start its next PDSA cycle.

What Is the SDSA Cycle?

Whereas the focus of the PDSA cycle is experimentation, the focus of the SDSA cycle is *standardization*. The idea behind this is simple and powerful. You run experiments (PDSA tests of change) until you reach your measured aim. Then, once you are able to achieve the desired level of performance, you want to maintain these gains by continuing to do the right things the right way. This calls for the adoption of a standard method and its continued use until the time comes to make new improvements.

The SDSA (standardize-do-study-act) cycle is the approach you take once you have successfully done one or more PDSA cycles and have enough experience and measured outcomes to determine that you have reached your original aim. The purpose of using the SDSA approach is to hold the gains that were made using PDSA cycles and to standardize the process in daily work.

Once you have reached the point where you should switch from the PDSA cycle to the SDSA cycle, that is not the end of the story. As new technologies arrive, and as your microsystem gains additional process practice and insight, you may need to move from SDSA back to PDSA again, to learn additional information and to test new ideas and processes. This back-and-forth process—between experimentation and standardizing—will result in higher levels of efficiency and an ability to hold your gains. Never think that once a process is in the SDSA cycle it will stay constant. Ongoing review and evaluation will tell you whether the best-known practice is in place and may reveal that you need to move back to PDSA, as shown in Figure 14.5.

FIGURE 14.5. THE BACK-AND-FORTH RELATIONSHIP OF PDSA AND SDSA.

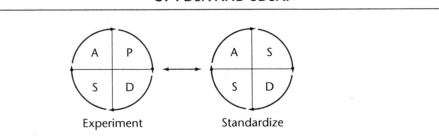

What Is Involved in Each of the Four Steps of Standardize, Do, Study, and Act?

The first SDSA step is to standardize. Standardized tasks are fundamental for continuous improvement and employee empowerment. Through repeatedly performing a task in a standardized manner, people gain new knowledge and insights for further improvement activities.

Liker (2004) has reminded us that American industrialist Henry Ford, pioneer of the assembly-line production method, once stated, "Today's standardization . . . is the necessary foundation on which tomorrow's improvement will be based. If you think of 'standardization' as the best you know today, but which is to be improved tomorrow-you get somewhere. But if you think of standards as confining, then progress stops" (p. 141). In a similar vein Brent James, a vice president for medical research and executive direction at Intermountain Health Center, Salt Lake City, Utah, often suggests it's more important to do something the same way than to do it the right way, because if you do it the same way you can learn from the results and then discover the best way (personal communication to E. C. Nelson, 1995).

This is the important assumption that supports SDSA thinking: it couples standardization with learning. It is through standardizing and stabilizing the process that learning and deeper insight occurs and processes and outcomes can be continuously improved.

The *standardize* phase in the SDSA cycle starts with determining how the current best process will be standardized in your daily work (Figure 14.6). A good first step toward standardization is to make a deployment flowchart to show who should do what and in what order. Also consider how you can shape the environment to help the process unfold reliably and consistently. Think about new habits your microsystem has adopted successfully. What helped it to maintain them? How will new employees be oriented to them? This can help you and your team gain insight into how to successfully maintain this new improvement, by making the new standard method a habit.

What are you learning in the *do* phase about the standardization within daily work? As you perform the new standardized process, what helps to ensure that it is done in a standardized way? What inhibits it from being done consistently?

As you *study* the standard process, what measures let you know whether the process is being done consistently? How many times does the process not get completed in a standard way? When you talk with those involved in the new process, what can you learn about the reasons the process is or is not consistent? Based on the lessons from the field, are there signs that SDSA should move back to PDSA? What are the indications for change?

FIGURE 14.6. THE COMPLETE SDSA CYCLE.

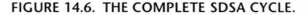

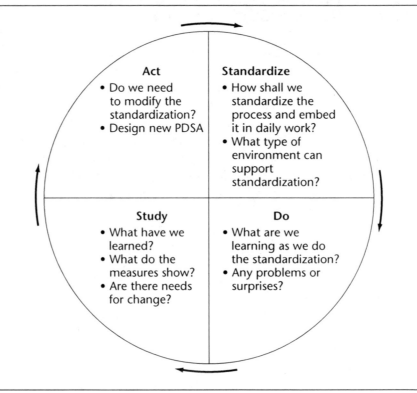

To *act,* consider what changes need to occur and be tested. Review the PDSA cycle and design a new pilot based on the knowledge you have obtained using the standard process. Once you have conducted the new PDSA cycle, be prepared to move back to SDSA after you have tested and refined the new improved process, and once again consider making a deployment flowchart to make the standard process clear to all.

What Tools Can Assist Your PDSA Cycle ↔ SDSA Implementation?

The PDSA ↔ SDSA worksheet shown in Figure A.15 in the Appendix is a helpful tool. It provides a map and reminders for conducting PDSA ↔ SDSA work. Many frontline teams use this worksheet to guide and record progress. (You can also find this worksheet at http://www.clinicalmicrosystem.org.)

What Are Some Tips for Using the PDSA ↔ SDSA Method?

- Always start with a specific aim statement.
- Answer the question, What are we trying to accomplish?
- The question, How will we know if this is an improvement? can only be answered with data.
- Small tests of change done in short periods of time accelerate learning and pave the way to rapid improvement. For example:
    Start with six patients
    Test for three shifts
    Test for two days
    Start with one to two providers
    Sample every other patient or process
- Designate someone to *oversee* the test and be the ears, eyes, and support to those engaged in it.
- Offer participants the opportunity to debrief *frequently* during the pilot.
- Have fun with special food or materials during the pilot.
- Celebrate completion of the first pilot, to encourage staff to continue.
- Post results in your microsystem space for all to see.
- When going to SDSA, use a deployment flowchart to provide a clear picture of who does what and in what order.
- When doing SDSA, schedule regular reviews to reflect on the process, monitor results, and avoid *slippage*.
- Sustain the effort by having a clearly designated work process *owner* who leads the SDSA phase of the process change.
- Alert senior leaders to the fact that PDSA ↔ SDSA is being used to make improvement.

Case Studies

Intermediate Cardiac Care Unit (ICCU)

The ICCU lead improvement team members reviewed the model for improvement to become aware of the path ahead of them and to become more knowledgeable about the discipline of improvement. They believed this would support their becoming a community of scientists. Figure 14.7 shows how the ICCU team used multiple PDSA cycles within the improvement model to reach its aim of improved communication.

FIGURE 14.7. THE ICCU'S PDSA RAMP OF TESTS.

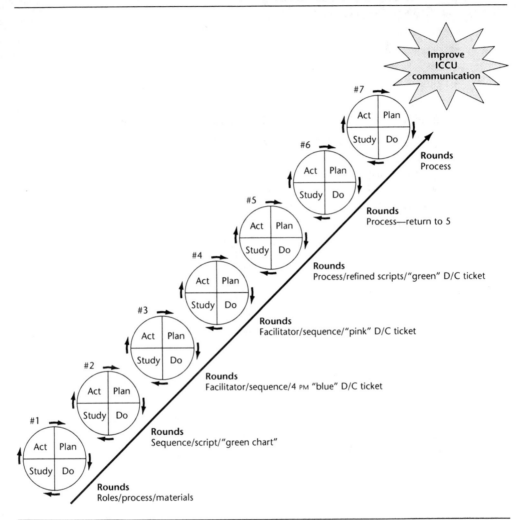

Improve
ICCU
communication

#7

| Act | Plan |
| Study | Do |

Rounds
Process

#6

| Act | Plan |
| Study | Do |

Rounds
Process—return to 5

#5

| Act | Plan |
| Study | Do |

Rounds
Process/refined scripts/"green" D/C ticket

#4

| Act | Plan |
| Study | Do |

Rounds
Facilitator/sequence/"pink" D/C ticket

#3

| Act | Plan |
| Study | Do |

Rounds
Facilitator/sequence/4 PM "blue" D/C ticket

#2

| Act | Plan |
| Study | Do |

Rounds
Sequence/script/"green chart"

#1

| Act | Plan |
| Study | Do |

Rounds
Roles/process/materials

Note: D/C = discharge.

Plastic Surgery Section

Review of the improvement model by the section's interdisciplinary lead improvement team provided the structure and discipline of improvement. The team members were eager to have successful improvements, and the model gave them a path forward to follow and a way to measure progress. With all that the lead improvement team was learning about the processes to be improved, the improvement model provided a paced, disciplined way to move through improvement activities without being overwhelmed.

Review Questions

1. What is the model for improvement?
2. What is a PDSA cycle, and how does it differ from a SDSA cycle?
3. Can an improved process move between PDSA and SDSA cycles?
4. What are the key elements of each phase of PDSA and SDSA?
5. When does an improved process move from SDSA to PDSA?

Between Sessions Work

1. Review and discuss the model for improvement, to clarify the path forward for the lead improvement team.
2. Review the PDSA ↔ SDSA worksheet (Figure A.15) to gain insight into the next steps.

References

Deming, W. E. (1986). *Out of the crisis.* Cambridge, MA: MIT Center for Advanced Engineering Study.

Langley, G. J., Nolan, K. M., Norman, C. L., Provost, L. P., & Nolan, T. W. (1996). *The improvement guide: A practical approach to enhancing organizational performance.* San Francisco: Jossey-Bass.

Liker, J. K. (2004). *The Toyota way: 14 management principles from the world's greatest manufacturer.* New York: McGraw-Hill.

Shewhart, W. A., with Deming, W. E. (1939). *Statistical method from the viewpoint of quality control.* Washington, DC: The Graduate School, Department of Agriculture.

CHAPTER FIFTEEN

SELECTING THEMES FOR IMPROVEMENT

Chapter Purpose

Aim. To select a worthy theme on which to focus improvement actions based on assessments made using the 5 P's, on organizational strategy, and on consideration of national or professional guidelines and recommendations.

    Objectives. At the completion of this unit, you will be able to

- Define a theme for improvement.
- Describe the benefit of identifying a theme for improvement.

- Describe what to consider when selecting a theme for improvement.
- Describe how theme selection is connected to assessment information and data.
- Identify where theme selection fits in the overall improvement process.
- Describe the process of identifying and selecting a theme for improvement.

After assessing the microsystem and considering organizational strategies and priorities along with external recommendations, your lead improvement team should choose one theme to focus improvement activities on (see Figure 15.1). Other themes can be identified and addressed later.

FIGURE 15.1. IMPROVEMENT RAMP: THEME.

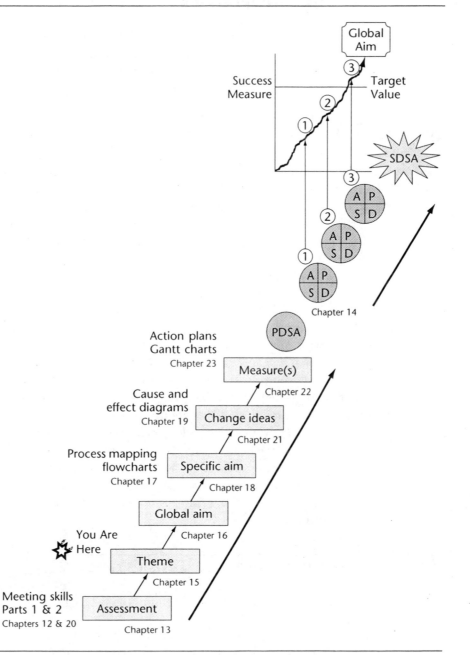

What Is a Theme for Improvement?

A *theme for improvement* is a broad and worthwhile area in which to begin your improvement work. You choose it by looking at assessment information and by considering such other factors as strategic priorities that come from senior leaders. The theme gives your microsystem a major focus to guide its improvement activity.

Why Use a Theme?

Kerr White, a notable figure in the field of health services research, often asked, "How do you eat an elephant?" Then he would answer his own question: "One bite at a time" (personal communication to E. C. Nelson, 1982). Selecting a single worthy theme to focus improvement on is a one-bite-at-a-time approach to change, allowing you to change one part of a system at a time while still recognizing that much more improvement, perhaps even whole microsystem improvement, may really be needed.

Many of us would often like to change everything at once, but this is only rarely possible. Usually, we are better off trying to make improvements on a vital part of our system and thereby fit improvement work into ongoing clinical or operational work. Once you review your 5 P's data and information, personal experiences, what you and the members of the microsystem know intuitively, what you know from your engagement with the relevant scientific literature, and what the larger system is asking your microsystem to do, you will find there are many broad areas that could benefit from improvement.

A good way to start the theme selection process is to create a list of themes. When you do this, it is wise to engage everyone, seeking all members' ideas and interpretations of the assessment data and information. Then, after considering many themes, it is best to select one theme for an exclusive initial improvement focus and thus avoid the distraction arising from an awareness of the enormity of the improvement possibilities.

What Are the Theme Selection Considerations?

To develop ideas for worthy themes, take into consideration

- Your 5 P's assessment data and information
- Your performance metrics and gaps between your results and best-practice results

- Your staff views of what is "intolerable" in daily practice
- Your patient and family views of what is delightful and what is unacceptable in the delivery of care and services
- Your organization's strategic goals and priorities

Aligning your microsystem's improvement themes with the macrosystem's strategic priorities will attract helpful resources for the changes you seek, while also supporting the entity-wide achievement of important goals and the improved performance of your microsystem.

The Institute of Medicine (IOM) report *Crossing the Quality Chasm* (Institute of Medicine [U.S.], Committee on Quality of Health Care in America, 2001) recommends examining six quality dimensions when working to improve health care: (1) safety, (2) effectiveness, (3) patient-centeredness, (4) timeliness, (5) efficiency, and (6) equity. These dimensions offer important starting places as you focus and choose where to begin.

Many professional groups have adopted important visionary goals that can also serve as microsystem improvement themes. For example, the Cystic Fibrosis Foundation (2005, p. 4) has created these "seven worthy goals" to guide improvements at Cystic Fibrosis Centers:

1. Patients and families are full partners with the Cystic Fibrosis care team. Care will be respectful of individual patient preferences, needs, and values.
2. Children and adolescents will have normal growth and nutrition. Adults' nutrition will be maintained as near normal as possible.
3. All patients will receive appropriate therapies for maintaining lung function and reducing acute episodes of infection.
4. Clinicians and patients will be well-informed partners in reducing acquisition of respiratory pathogens, particularly P. aeruginosa and B. cepacia.
5. Patients will be screened and managed aggressively for complications of CF, particularly CF-related diabetes.
6. Severely affected patients will be well supported by their CF team in facing decisions about transplantation and end-of-life care.
7. Patients will have access to appropriate therapies, treatments, and supports regardless of race, age, education, or ability to pay.

Another useful model for theme selection comes from the Institute for Healthcare Improvement's Idealized Design of Clinical Office Practice (IDCOP) program, which revolves around four broad themes: access, interaction, reliability, and vitality. The model displays these key themes and their relationship to ideal

FIGURE 15.2. KEY THEMES AND COMPONENTS
OF IDEAL PRACTICES.

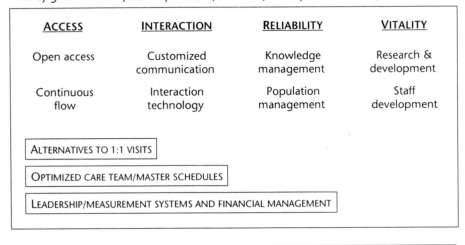

"They give me exactly the help I want (and need) exactly when I want (and need) it."

ACCESS	INTERACTION	RELIABILITY	VITALITY
Open access	Customized communication	Knowledge management	Research & development
Continuous flow	Interaction technology	Population management	Staff development

ALTERNATIVES TO 1:1 VISITS

OPTIMIZED CARE TEAM/MASTER SCHEDULES

LEADERSHIP/MEASUREMENT SYSTEMS AND FINANCIAL MANAGEMENT

Source: Institute for Healthcare Improvement, 2000. Used with permission.

practices (Figure 15.2). It may be helpful for initiating your lead improvement team's thinking about a theme to select as its starting point. Use a theme that helps everyone realize the importance and *sensibility* of his or her work on improving care.

What Process Can You Use to Generate Theme Ideas and Select a First Theme?

Once you have gathered all the information and data from assessing your microsystem and have taken into consideration the additional perspectives mentioned previously, your team can generate an inclusive list of possibilities by conducting a brainstorming session. It can then select a theme from the brainstorming results by following a multi-voting process (see Chapter Twenty for details on both these techniques). Brainstorming can engage all members of your team in discussing and buying into the improvement focus. Be sure to keep the list of brainstormed ideas for future reference and consideration.

What Are the Next Steps?

After selecting a theme for improvement, you will want to further define the particular starting point for your change efforts. You can do this by developing a global aim and related specific aims as targets for your improvement work.

Case Studies

Intermediate Cardiac Care Unit (ICCU)

After analyzing their 5 P's assessment and considering their new observations and views about the ICCU, the ICCU lead improvement team members selected the theme of communication in the ICCU for their initial improvement work. Communication is a very broad theme that influences many things, such as safety, relationships with patients and families, interactions between professionals, and work that goes between the ICCU and departments such as admitting and the catheterization laboratory. Communication was selected because it has a profound effect on the flow of patients into and out of the ICCU and also on the flow of daily care.

Plastic Surgery Section

After reviewing their 5 P's, the metrics that matter, and other assessment tools, the Plastic Surgery Section's lead improvement team members identified the following broad themes for potential improvement:

- Understanding each other's work: optimization of roles
- Understanding core and supporting processes
- Professional development and growth: for all on the team
- Building and maintaining safety and trust
- Timely access for our patients: understanding and balancing the schedule of outpatient appointments, minor surgery cases, and main operating room cases

Through discussions and identification of important linkages to the organization's strategic plans, the lead improvement team members chose the theme of *access* to work on first. They kept their original list to use when considering future improvement themes.

Review Questions

1. What is a theme for improvement, and why have one?
2. What should you consider when selecting a theme for improvement?
3. Where does theme selection fit in the overall improvement process?
4. How might you select a theme for improvement?
5. What are the next steps after you have selected a theme?

Between Sessions Work

Select a theme to focus your improvement work; base your choice on

1. Your 5 P's assessment data and information
2. A review of information from external forces, such as the Institute of Medicine, the Institute for Healthcare Improvement, and the Joint Commission on Accreditation of Healthcare Organizations
3. A review of your own organization's strategic priorities

References

Cystic Fibrosis Foundation. (2005, June). *Cystic Fibrosis Foundation opportunity statement.* Bethesda, MD: Author.

Institute for Healthcare Improvement. (2000). *Idealized design of clinical office practices.* Boston: Author.

Institute of Medicine (U.S.), Committee on Quality of Health Care in America. (2001). *Crossing the quality chasm: A new health system for the 21st century.* Washington, DC: National Academies Press.

CHAPTER SIXTEEN

IMPROVEMENT GLOBAL AIM

Chapter Purpose

Aim. To create a global aim statement to focus the improvement work based on the theme the lead improvement team selected.

Objectives. At the completion of this unit, you will be able to

- Define a global aim.
- Identify the importance of the relationship between the global aim, the improvement process flow, and theme selection.
- Describe how to manage new ideas and topics within the context of writing a global aim.
- Write a global aim statement using a template.

After assessing your microsystem and selecting a theme, it is useful to write out a global aim. As this chapter explains, the global aim helps you become more detailed and specific about what you intend to improve (see Figure 16.1).

What Is a Global Aim?

A *global aim* is a statement about your improvement theme. It clarifies, bounds, and connects the improvement theme to your daily work processes. It points to an essential, theme-related process that is critical to patients and staff.

FIGURE 16.1. IMPROVEMENT RAMP: GLOBAL AIM.

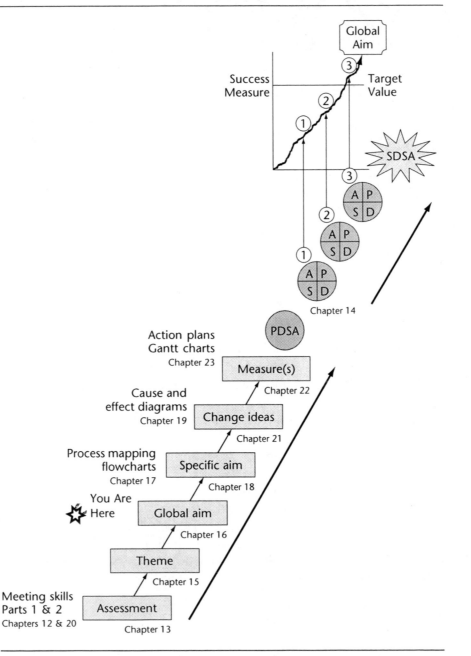

Why Use a Global Aim?

The global aim puts your theme into context and is a great place from which to start your improvement work. The global aim states clearly what you intend to improve and may also state numerical goals and dates that will define improvement achievement.

It is often helpful to create *stretch goals* to strive for when setting out to make an improvement. Setting goals that are very easy to attain may not result in substantial improvement. Achievable stretch goals provide a high-bar aim to strive for. The scientific literature can sometimes help you identify a level of performance achieved by others that may be seen as a stretch target in your microsystem.

The global aim also helps you to operationalize and focus the improvement theme. It is easy to get excited and start tangential conversations when working on improvement. When topics not related to the global aim come up in conversations about improvement, it is often a good idea to write them down in a *parking lot* list that can be used to identify possible improvement efforts in the future. The global aim statement can keep you focused on the current theme.

How Do You Write a Global Aim?

The template in Figure 16.2 helps lead improvement team members write a clear global aim statement that is detailed and specific.

As you use this template, notice the increasing clarity of focus. The name of the process to be improved and the clinical location of that process are clearly identified, along with the points where the process begins and ends. This is an important step because health care staff are often not in the habit of identifying work processes, and many health care processes can be long and detailed. Identifying where you want to focus limits the general scope of the effort. For example, a microsystem might work to improve the access process beginning with the patient's entry into the clinical practice for a medical visit and ending after the physician sees the patient. This is taking a somewhat smaller "bite" of the "elephant" than the team would if it looked at a larger process that starts before the visit and extends until some time after the patient exits the clinic.

What Are the Next Steps?

Once the statement of the global aim for improvement is written and you have checked that it aligns with the selected improvement theme, you and your team should create a high-level flowchart of the process you wish to improve. Be

FIGURE 16.2. TEMPLATE FOR WRITING A GLOBAL AIM STATEMENT.

Theme for Improvement _____

Global Aim Statement

Create your aim statement that will help keep your focus clear and your work productive.

We aim to improve _____
(Name the process)

in_____
(Clinical location in which process is embedded)

The process begins with _____
(Name where the process begins)

The process ends with _____
(Name the ending point of the process)

By working on the process, we expect _____
(List benefits)

_____

It is important to work on this now because _____
(List imperatives)

_____

prepared to revisit, adjust, and fine-tune the statement of global aim after the flow-chart has helped you and your microsystem members "see" the work more clearly. For example, you may decide to change the start point or end point, or you may modify the process stated in your theme, based on additional information and understanding.

Case Studies

Intermediate Cardiac Care Unit (ICCU)

Having selected the theme of communication, the ICCU lead improvement team used the template in Figure 16.2 to develop a global aim statement. It states:

We aim to improve the *process of communication* in the ICCU. The *process begins* with the initial notification of the need for patient admission. The *process ends* with the appropriate discharge disposition of the patient.

By working on this process we expect (1) improved patient care and efficiency, (2) improved flow of consistent information between patients, providers, and families, (3) improved communication along the health care continuum, (4) a reduction in readmissions, and (5) a reduction in stress. *It is important to work on this now because* we have identified the need to improve (1) satisfaction of patients, families, and care professionals, (2) prevention of near misses and errors, and (3) preparation to care for patients.

Plastic Surgery Section

The global aim statement for the access theme identified by the lead improvement team of the Plastic Surgery Section reads as follows:

We aim to *improve the patient appointment access process* to plastic surgery. The *process begins* with the patient phone call for an appointment. The *process ends* with the initial evaluation of the patient in the clinic. *By working on this process we expect* (1) improved patient satisfaction with appointment scheduling, (2) decreased appointment backlog (currently 99 days until appt.), (3) improved staff satisfaction, with a decrease in workplace toxicity, and (4) increased productivity. *It is important to work on this now because* we have identified the need to improve (1) patient satisfaction, (2) staff satisfaction, (3) scheduling variations, (4) productivity.

Review Questions

1. Where does the global aim fit in the overall improvement process?
2. How does the selected theme inform the global aim?
3. What should you do when new topics and themes not related to the global aim arise out of conversations about improvement?
4. What does the global aim template ask you to do?

Between Sessions Work

1. Write a global aim for improvement based on your theme selection.
2. Share all global aim progress and drafts with all members of the microsystem.

CHAPTER SEVENTEEN

PROCESS MAPPING

Chapter Purpose

Aim. To define process-mapping techniques, with a specific focus on high-level flowcharts and deployment flowcharts.

   Objectives. At the completion of this unit, you will be able to

- Define process mapping.
- Describe the differences between high-level flowcharts and deployment flowcharts.

- Describe the relationship between the global aim statement for improvement and the flowcharting process.
- Create a high-level flowchart or deployment flowchart using several techniques.
- Develop a process to engage all members of the microsystem in the creation and modification of the flowchart.

Process mapping follows creation of a global aim (see Figure 17.1). A good global aim states where the process begins and where it ends, and therefore points out where the process map should start and where it should finish. This chapter will guide you in creating a process map that is based on the global aim and that will provide insight for the lead improvement team as it determines a more specific aim.

FIGURE 17.1. IMPROVEMENT RAMP: PROCESS MAPPING.

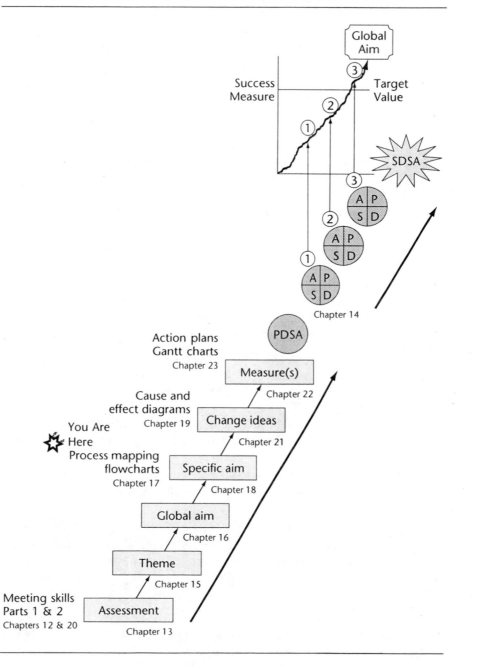

What Is Process Mapping?

Process mapping is a method for creating a diagram that uses graphic symbols to show the steps and the flow of a process. Other commonly used names for a process map are *flow diagram* and *flowchart*.

Why Use Process Mapping?

Most health care professionals know their part of each process they are involved in, but they do not know, and do not take the time to know, how the rest of the process works. This can lead to confusion, mistakes, needless complexity, undesired variation, and a general lack of agreement on how care and services are actually processed and delivered. Unwanted variation, waste, delays, and rework exist within the processes of care. This is the result of a lack of thoughtful design and of common agreement on how the process currently works.

The benefits of creating a flowchart for a process include

- Engaging interdisciplinary members in the creation of a process map
- Gaining agreement about the sequence of steps in the process
- Correcting misunderstandings about how the process works
- Spotting places where the same things are done differently for no rational reason
- Explaining the steps pictorially to promote better understanding than written procedures give
- Replacing pages of words with a picture of a process
- Identifying problem areas based on an understanding of variation, waste, delays, and rework
- Identifying supplier-customer relationships in a process (for example, who provides what to whom as the process rolls forward)

Before improvements can be identified for a process, the process's *anatomy*, or steps, must be understood. Gene Nelson (2006) points out that "just like you should know anatomy before you do surgery, you should know the detailed steps of a process before improving it."

Definition of a Process

A *process* is a series of related work activities that together transform *inputs* into *outputs* for the benefit of someone. In mainstream health care the inputs are the needs of a patient, a family, or a population of patients, and the processes we wish to have deeper understanding of are the processes of health care service delivery. The outputs are the outcomes of the health care delivered: clinical results, functional outcomes, patient satisfaction, and costs. Keep in mind that "every system is perfectly designed to get the results it gets" (personal communication to Donald Berwick, IHI president and CEO, 1996). To stimulate our thinking and to get better results, we need to design processes and systems with the desired results in mind.

Definition of a Flowchart

A *flowchart* is a picture of the sequential steps and the directional flow of those steps in a process. The different types of steps and events are represented by various symbols. This step-by-step picture can be used to describe a current process, depict an improved process, document a standard method for doing a process, or specify an ideal process. It can even be used to make a plan for a project. It is important for improvement work to begin with a representation of the current process—the way the process actually works now.

What Are the Commonly Used Flowchart Symbols?

Many of the symbols commonly used to make flowcharts are shown in Figure 17.2.

- The *oval* indicates the beginning point and the ending point of the process you are mapping. When you first start to make a flowchart of a process, it becomes very obvious why having a global aim statement with a clearly stated start point

FIGURE 17.2. FLOWCHART SYMBOLS.

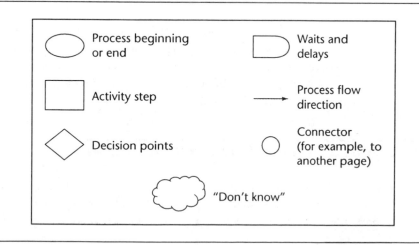

and end point is fundamental to process improvement work. The beginning and the end of the process, as specified in this statement, define the boundaries of the flowchart you will create.

- The *box* represents an activity step.
- The *diamond* shows a decision point in the process, where one must respond *yes* or *no*. A yes or no decision point leads to a distinct flow for each of its two options.
- The *elongated D* depicts delays in the process. This symbol should alert you to further evaluate this step to understand the sources of waits and delays.
- The *arrow* shows the directional flow of the process.
- The *circle* indicates that the steps continue on another page or on another part of a larger flowchart. A letter placed in the circle tells you where to pick up the process on the next page.
- The *cloud* represents *don't know;* what happens in this step is not known or understood. When an interdisciplinary team cannot describe a step, it is a signal that one or more people who are part of the process are not contributing to the discussion. Further discussion should follow with those involved in this step. You may wish to add people to the lead improvement team to ensure that all who have a role in the current process are involved in flowcharting that process. Alternatively, you may simply need to review the flowchart with others to get all parts of the process mapped correctly and accurately. Note also that differing views about a process are normal and reflect the differing ways that the various health professions do their work. It is helpful to reconcile those differences from the viewpoint of the patient and family whenever possible.

What Does a High-Level Flowchart Look Like?

A *high-level flowchart* is used to show the "big picture," the view from 30,000 feet. Making a high-level flowchart is a good place to start mapping a process, and then you can proceed to determine what steps need detailed descriptions and need to be shown on a more detailed flowchart. Figure 17.3 shows a simple, high-level flowchart of a medical office visit.

What Does a Detailed Flowchart Look Like?

A *detailed flowchart* provides a more refined picture of a high-level flowchart step, breaking that step into smaller steps or smaller clusters of actions. Detailed flowcharts are usually necessary to support improvement work in moving forward to

FIGURE 17.3. HIGH-LEVEL FLOWCHART OF A MEDICAL OFFICE VISIT.

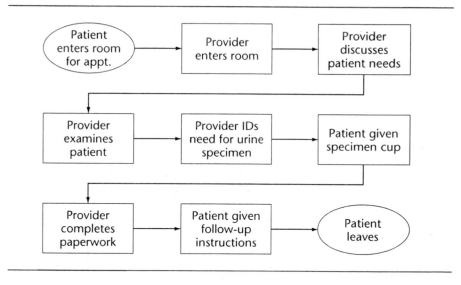

meet sharp, specific aims and to run useful tests of change. Figure 17.4 shows a detailed flowchart of a treatment process.

What Are Some Tips for Creating a Flowchart?

Begin with the global aim statement to determine where the process starts and where the process ends. This determines the boundaries of the flowchart. It is important to have the flowchart boundaries align with the aim statement and to have the aim align with the selected improvement theme in your domain of responsibility.

Also remember that you are creating a flowchart of the *current* process. Oftentimes people will create a flowchart that mixes reality with wishful thinking and guesses. To avoid this trap, frequently remind everyone of the need to understand the current state of the process in order to properly identify improvement opportunities.

A good way to start listing the steps is to ask what happens *first*, then what happens *next*, then what happens *next*, and so on. When the next step "depends" (if this happens, then that happens), pick the most common next step and follow what happens after it, and then go back to follow the other next step. Keep it simple when you first start. Finally, turn the list of steps into a flowchart, using the

FIGURE 17.4. DETAILED FLOWCHART OF TREATMENT PROCESS FOR CYSTIC FIBROSIS–RELATED DIABETES (CFRD).

Goal: Early detection of CFRD and excellent treatment

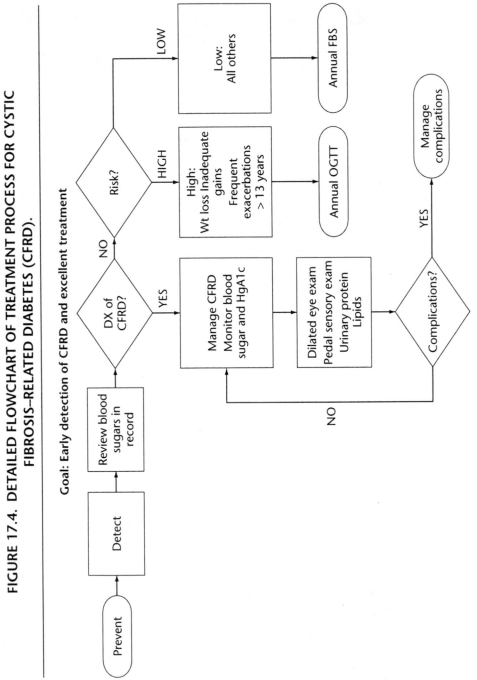

basic symbols. The flowchart can be drawn on a flipchart so the entire team can see the process unfold as described.

Some teams find Post-it Notes helpful for creating a process flow diagram. Post-its eliminate the need to erase and redraw steps as you work out the process because you can simply move the Post-its as needed.

It is always helpful to observe the current process after you complete the first draft of your high-level flowchart of that process. You can modify the flowchart as you *observe the current state* and as you talk to others involved in the process who understand the details, nuances, exceptions, conditional branch points, and sources of variation that are desired or undesired.

After finishing the high-level flowchart, display it in the relevant clinical area and invite other staff members to review and modify. This step is a good way to engage staff in improvement activities and to expand everyone's overall knowledge of the process.

What Does a Deployment Flowchart Look Like?

A *deployment flowchart* shows the process flow in relation to the people or groups involved in each step (see Figure 17.5). This type of flowchart shows how people fit into the process sequence and how they relate to one another. Deployment flowcharts highlight places in a process where work moves from one group or person to another and reveals how groups or individuals relate to one another throughout the process. The deployment flowchart is particularly useful when the goal is to optimize roles and functions within a process.

Deployment flowcharts are read both vertically and horizontally.

- The vertical dimension shows how the process is progressing.
- The horizontal dimension shows who does what and the handoffs between individuals or between groups.

What Are Some Tips for Creating a Deployment Flowchart?

Start by drawing a table with columns for the people, roles, or groups that the process flows through. Enter the name of a person, role, or group at the top of each column.

After you have created the table, insert the sequential flowchart steps to show which person, role, or group is responsible for which action. The horizontal lines define internal customer-supplier relationships. Correct identification of these

FIGURE 17.5. SECTION OF DEPLOYMENT FLOWCHART FOR ENROLLMENT IN OUTPATIENT CYSTIC FIBROSIS CLINIC.

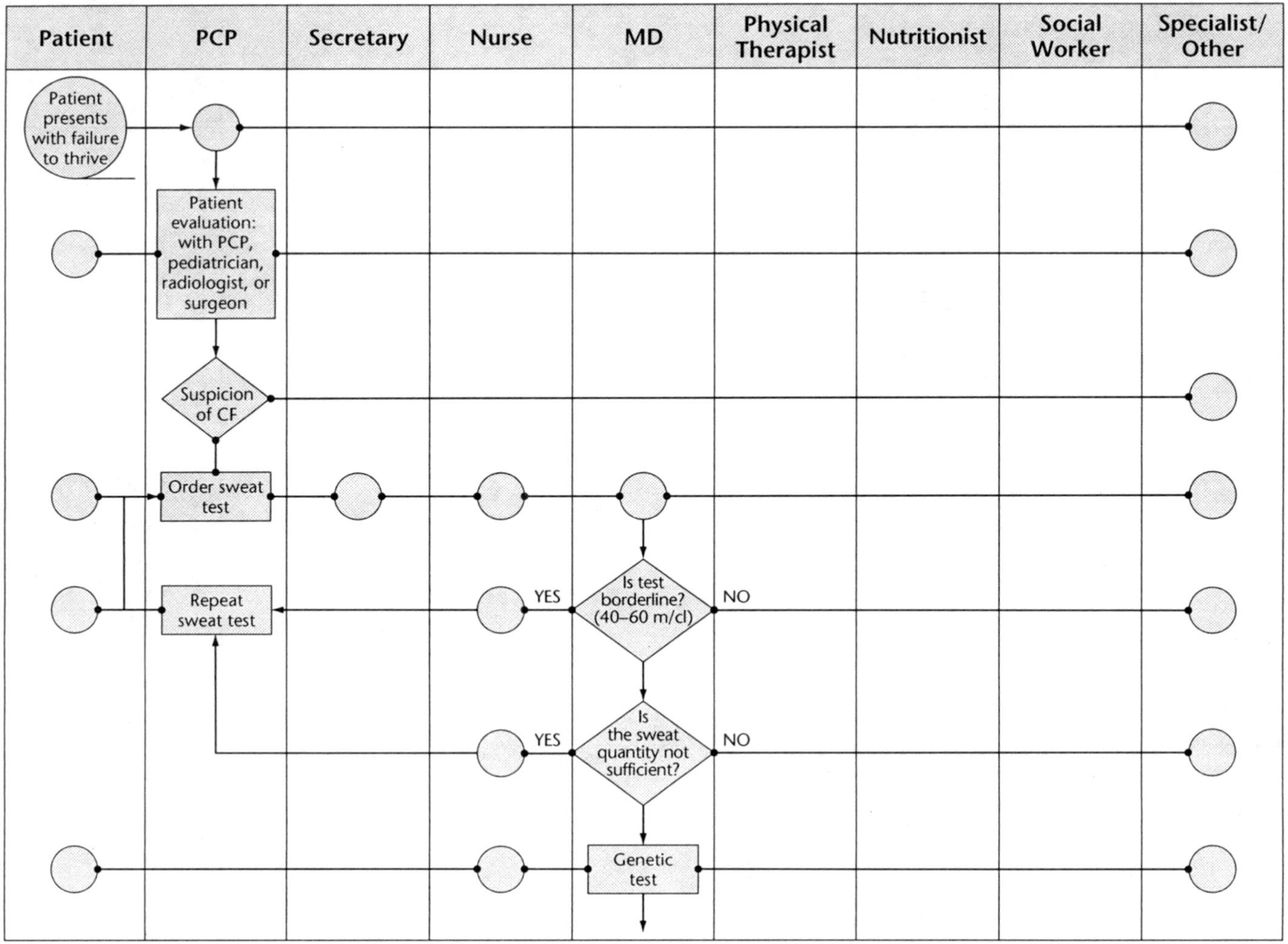

customer-supplier relationships is important if the handoffs are to become de-fect free. It is very useful to use a deployment flowchart when you are beginning to explore customer requirements within a process that must be actively designed to produce value-added activities and outcomes.

Case Studies

Intermediate Cardiac Care Unit (ICCU)

The ICCU lead improvement team members made a high-level flowchart of the process of admission to the ICCU. They used their global aim to identify the start point and end point of their work. Their high-level flowchart is shown in Figure 17.6.

FIGURE 17.6. HIGH-LEVEL FLOWCHART OF ICCU ADMISSION PROCESS.

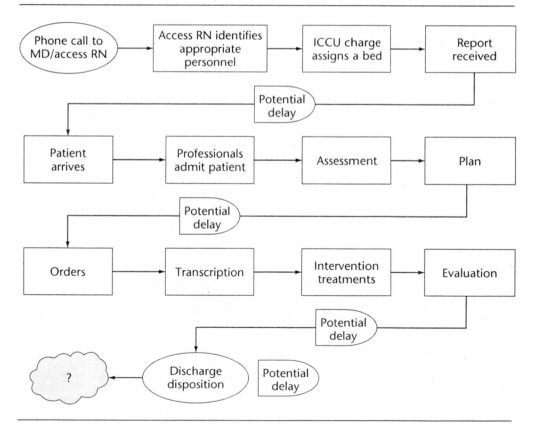

FIGURE 17.7. HIGH-LEVEL FLOWCHART FOR BEGINNING OF BREAST REDUCTION PROCESS.

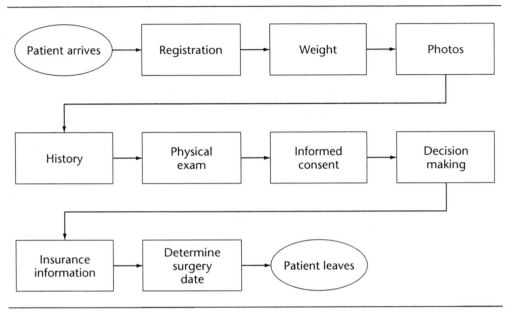

Plastic Surgery Section

To improve access to care, the Plastic Surgery Section lead improvement team members reviewed the current state of appointments for one subpopulation of patients. They chose the breast reduction procedure patients because the lead physician did that procedure with high frequency. It is usually wise to start with an interested physician who can test new ideas with the interdisciplinary team and then you can spread the improvement effort to other physicians and processes. The process shown in Figure 17.7 was completed one breast reduction patient at a time repeatedly throughout the workday. The lead improvement team started to think that there might be a better way to provide care to this special population that might improve access to care and overall quality, satisfaction, and efficiency.

Review Questions

1. What is process mapping?
2. What is the difference between high-level flowcharts and deployment flowcharts?

3. How does the global aim statement inform the flowchart process?
4. What are the common symbols used in flowcharts?
5. How would you create a high-level flowchart?
6. How would you create a deployment flowchart?
7. What does the horizontal dimension highlight in a deployment flowchart? What does the vertical dimension highlight?
8. Who should be involved in the flowcharting process?
9. How might you engage all members of your clinical setting in this process?

Between Sessions Work

1. Draft a flowchart of the process identified in your global aim statement.
2. Display the flowchart draft for all the staff to review and add to.
3. Modify the flowchart based on feedback.

Reference

Nelson, E. C. (2006). Teaching session delivered to Cincinnati Children's Hospital Learning Collaborative, Cincinnati, OH.

CHAPTER EIGHTEEN

SPECIFIC AIM

Chapter Purpose

Aim. To create a detailed, specific aim statement based on the selected theme and the global aim statement to further guide and focus improvement activities.

    Objectives. At the completion of this unit, you will be able to

- Define what a specific aim is.

- Describe the connections between specific aim, process flow, global aim selection, and theme.
- Use the specific aim template.
- Describe the improvement ramp that leads microsystem members to meet overall improvement aims.

This step in the microsystem improvement process follows your review of the process map (see Figure 18.1). After the current process is mapped, understood, and agreed upon, your next step, as described in this chapter, is to make a specific aim statement that provides a clear focus for the improvement.

What Is a Specific Aim?

The *specific aim* provides a detailed focus for improvement. It is based on the global aim statement, the flowchart, and an analysis of the overall process. It establishes the measurable outcomes you wish to achieve and a precise focus for tests of change.

FIGURE 18.1. IMPROVEMENT RAMP: SPECIFIC AIM.

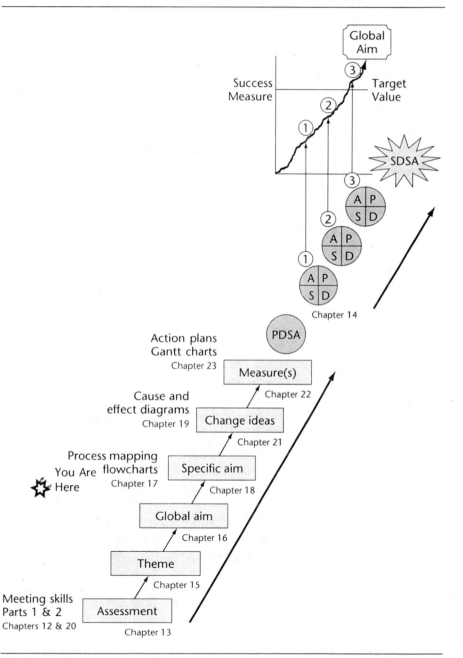

Why Use a Specific Aim?

A good specific aim offers detailed focus for your improvement work. A good specific aim has a sharp focus. It specifies what you can improve now, usually something within your "control" so that you do not require additional "permission" to test a change and make an improvement. It also describes the measurable outcomes that you wish to achieve. Specifying and measuring these outcomes can help you maintain improvement intention and focus.

Where Do Specific Aims Come From?

There are many good sources from which you can develop promising change ideas that can be adapted to your local context, using the specific aim approach, and then tested out, using the plan-do-study-act (PDSA) method. Change ideas and specific aims frequently come from these five areas:

- *Process analysis.* Mapping the current process "as is" will usually reveal several specific steps that do not work as well as they might, and ideas for changing them arise as this is realized.
- *Cause and effect analysis.* Constructing a fishbone diagram (Chapter Nineteen) to explore the web of causes involved in the effects you are trying to improve will often prompt ideas about what might be changed in order to improve a desired outcome.
- *Direct observation.* Directly observing the actual work process can reveal steps that could be eliminated or that might work better.
- *Change concepts.* A wide variety of general suggestions have been developed for improving any process. Applying these ideas as part of a process analysis can identify numerous specific ideas about designing change.
- *Evidence-based and best practices.* Increasingly, the scientific literature about improving care will offer evidence in support of specific ideas or will make possible a formal comparative exploration of a best practice—the process of benchmarking (Mohr, Mahoney, Nelson, Batalden, & Plume, 1998).

Where Does the Specific Aim Fit in the Overall Improvement Process?

A global aim and theme usually end up with multiple specific aims linked to them. Start with one specific aim, and use the PDSA method to begin testing changes. Often, multiple specific aims and PDSA cycles will be helpful in achieving the global aim identified. These tests of change can become progressively complex, as suggested by the *improvement ramp* diagram we are using throughout Part Two (see, for example, Figure 18.1). This idea was developed by Tom Nolan, Brian Joiner, and the Institute for Healthcare Improvement (Langley, Nolan, Norman, Provost, & Nolan, 1996) and has been adapted by the authors of this book. An improvement ramp offers an overview of the sequence of changes involved in the improvement of a specific process.

The first test of change is often a relatively simple one. In the execution of that test additional ideas usually emerge that seem worth testing and that require a bit more time and effort to test. By sequencing the tests so that the easiest come early in the process, you can learn more about the global aim that has been selected and accelerate its realization. Once it is realized, you can take steps to standardize the new level of performance, using the standardize-do-study-act (SDSA) approach.

How Do You Write a Specific Aim?

Figure 18.2 offers a template for writing a clear specific aim statement. You will note that it invites clear, measurable outcomes and a target date for completion.

What Are the Next Steps?

It is common at this point to have more insight and understanding about the process you wish to improve and to have many ideas worth testing for change and improvement.

FIGURE 18.2. TEMPLATE FOR WRITING A SPECIFIC AIM STATEMENT.

Specific Aim Statement

Create a specific aim statement that will keep your focus clear and your work productive.

Use numerical goals, specific dates, and specific measures

Specific Aim: _____

_____

Measures: _____

_____

Case Studies

Intermediate Cardiac Care Unit (ICCU)

Based on the ICCU's overall picture of communication and flow, the ICCU lead improvement team selected its first specific aim. This specific aim states:

> *We aim to improve communication of patient plans* of *care,* including discharge, through an *interdisciplinary morning round approach starting February 27, 2006.* We will have *100% participation of all roles, 100% accuracy of plans of action,* and detailed discharge plans to facilitate bed availability for new admissions.

Plastic Surgery Section

Informed by the 5 P's, the theme of access improvement, and the flowchart of the current process for patients wishing breast reduction, the Plastic Surgery lead improvement team wrote its specific aim statement. This specific aim states:

> *We aim to reduce the backlog of patients by 50%, improve patient satisfaction* with scheduling, and *improve staff satisfaction within 6 months.*

Review Questions

1. Where does the specific aim fit in the overall improvement process?
2. How do the global aim and the flowchart inform your specific aim?
3. What does the specific aim template ask you to do?

Between Sessions Work

1. Create your specific aim based on your flowchart.

References

Langley, G. J., Nolan, K. M., Norman, C. L., Provost, L. P., & Nolan, T. W. (1996). *The improvement guide: A practical approach to enhancing organizational performance.* San Francisco: Jossey-Bass.

Mohr, J., Mahoney, C. C., Nelson, E. C., Batalden, P. B., & Plume, S. K. (1998). Learning from the best: Clinical benchmarking for best patient care. In E. C. Nelson, P. B. Batalden, & J. C. Ryer (Eds.), *Clinical improvement action guide.* Oakbrook Terrace, IL: Joint Commission on Accreditation of Healthcare Organizations.

CHAPTER NINETEEN

CAUSE AND EFFECT DIAGRAMS

Chapter Purpose

Aim. To define cause and effect diagrams and the process of creating them to gain deeper knowledge of the factors that contribute to end results.

    Objectives. At the completion of this session, you will be able to

- Define cause and effect diagrams (fishbone diagrams).
- Describe the principle of the web of causation in relation to a fishbone diagram.

- Create a cause and effect diagram specific to the outcome you are studying.
- Describe the function of cause and effect diagrams in the big picture of improvement.
- Develop a process to engage all staff in the creation and modification of a fishbone diagram.

    Cause and effect diagrams give you yet more information about causal factors influencing your specific aim and related processes. As described in this chapter, constructing such a graphic can help microsystem members understand the forces that are contributing to a specific aim and thereby identify what might be changed to attain improvement goals. Figure 19.1 shows you where the cause and effect diagram fits in the improvement ramp.

FIGURE 19.1. IMPROVEMENT RAMP:
CAUSE AND EFFECT DIAGRAMS.

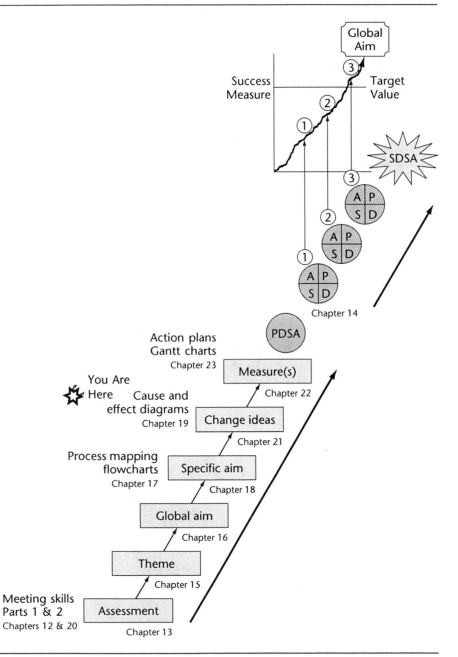

What Is a Cause and Effect Diagram?

A *cause and effect diagram* is an analysis tool that depicts the possible causes that contribute to a single effect. First described in 1968 by a committee of the Japanese Union of Scientists and Engineers (JUSE) led by Kaoru Ishikawa (1976), it has also been called an *Ishikawa diagram* and, because it resembles the skeleton of a fish, a *fishbone diagram*.

Brian MacMahon (MacMahon & Pugh, 1970) described exploring causes and effects as creating a *web of causation*. He noted that outcomes are almost always the result of many interrelated causes and rarely the result of a single cause. He suggested that we are best served when we think of results as being produced by such a causal network, that is, by a system of causes that combine to produce an effect (or effects). Graphically depicted, this concept more closely resembles a spider's web than a simplistic cause and effect, "*x* causes *y*" diagram (see Figure 19.2).

MacMahon would argue, for example, that the acorn does not *cause* the oak tree. The web of causation for the oak tree includes interactions of soil, water, temperature, sunshine, nightfall, nutrients, an acorn, and freedom from harm caused by predators, illness, and injury.

Although MacMahon's spider web model is a wonderful way to think about causes and effects in the real world, a cause and effect diagram in the

FIGURE 19.2. WEB OF CAUSATION.

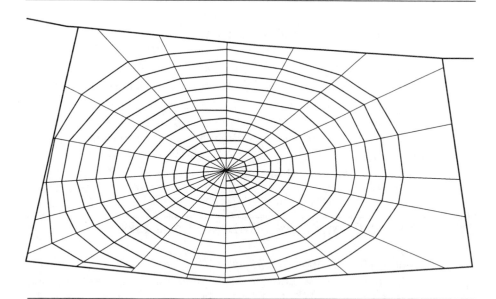

form of a fishbone diagram often provides a straightforward way to translate a web of interactions into an easy-to-construct and easy-to-understand visual display that helps people get started with designing and testing changes for improvement.

Why Use a Fishbone Diagram?

The fishbone diagram is an important scientific tool used to identify and clarify the causes of an effect of interest. When lead improvement team members construct such a diagram, it allows them to build a visual theory about potential causes and effects that can be used to guide improvement work. The fishbone diagram can stimulate the formation of *hunches* worth empirically testing, using plan-do-study-act (PDSA) cycles.

In addition, the fishbone diagram promotes a disciplined use of major categories of potential causes. As a result, rather than allowing people to focus on a few top-of-the-mind areas, it facilitates deeper thinking about possible causation. Finally, it can help the team answer the question of where to begin the process of improvement.

What Is the Structure of a Fishbone Diagram?

As we said earlier, the fishbone diagram looks like a fish skeleton consisting of a spine and attached bones, as shown in Figure 19.3. The big bones attached directly to the spine represent major categories of causation. Some examples of commonly used major categories are process, equipment, materials, people, and environment.

Once the major categories are defined, the discrete causal elements (specific causes and contributing factors) within each category are listed on the smaller bones attached to the big bones. With the diagram shown in Figure 19.3, asking the question Why is this a cause? five times will result in getting to the multiple causes of the outcome of interest.

What Does a Completed Fishbone Look Like?

Figure 19.4 is a fishbone diagram that shows many of the factors that contribute to the undesirable result of medical appointments that last much longer than needed. The main causal categories are people, equipment, materials, environment, and process. The details within each category reflect *why* the category is a

FIGURE 19.3. FISHBONE DIAGRAM.

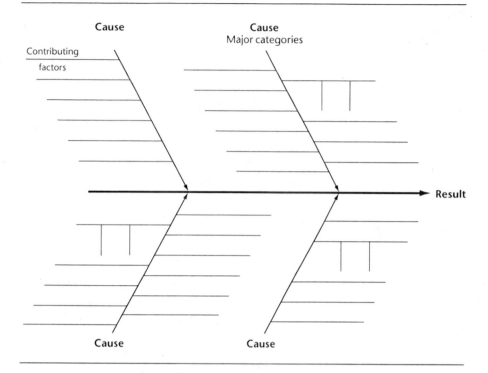

FIGURE 19.4. FISHBONE DIAGRAM SHOWING CAUSES OF LENGTHY APPOINTMENTS.

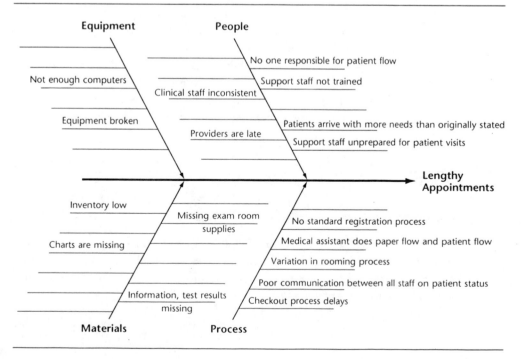

cause, illustrating the many waits, delays, and flow problems that are specific causes of this (undesired) effect.

What Are Some Tips for Creating a Fishbone Diagram?

- Review the specific aim that you want to work on.
- Clarify the effect. It is important that everyone involved is clear about the effect, or the outcome of interest, which can be stated as an *undesired* result (such as lengthy appointments) or as a *desired* result (such as a hypertensive patient whose blood pressure is under control) or as a *neutral* result (such as the amount of time it takes to place a patient ready to be discharged from the emergency department in an inpatient unit bed.)
- Determine the major categories of causation that contribute to the effect, and brainstorm to identify the detailed causes within these larger categories. Visual display of the categories can often stimulate broader thinking about potential detailed causes. However, sometimes it is easier for a team to work the other way—from the particular to the general categories. To do this, lead improvement team members hold a session in which they brainstorm causes leading to an identified result by writing possible causes on Post-it Notes, grouping the notes according to similarity of ideas, and then giving a category name to each major grouping. This is called *affinity grouping.*
- Refine the fishbone diagram. Once the process is completed, review the diagram, and consider whether causes should be re-sorted and whether categories should be split or aggregated to make the most sense.
- Share the fishbone diagram with others, and use their feedback to improve it. Once you have created a draft fishbone, post it in a place where all members of the microsystem can review it and add their comments. This can result in a more accurate cause and effect diagram and greater shared understanding of the findings.

Case Studies

Intermediate Cardiac Care Unit (ICCU)

Using the selected specific aim of the ICCU concerning the timeliness of assigning patients to beds, the lead improvement team created a fishbone to identify the reasons why the admissions department could not get a bed for a new admission within thirty minutes of the initial phone call (see Figure 19.5).

FIGURE 19.5. FISHBONE DIAGRAM FOR ICCU BED ASSIGNMENT.

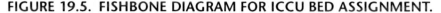

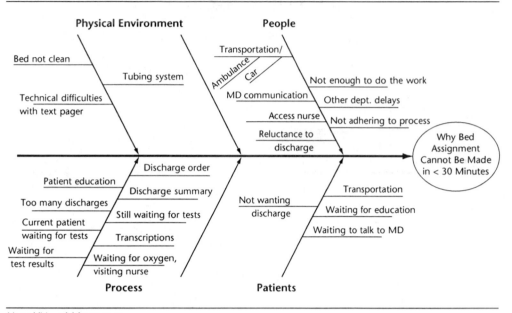

Note: VN = visiting nurse.

Plastic Surgery Section

The lead improvement team created a cause and effect diagram showing the causes of the backlog of appointments keeping patients from being seen in a timely manner (see Figure 19.6). The main categories included patients, processes, providers, and support staff.

Review Questions

1. What is a fishbone diagram?
2. How would you describe a web of causation?
3. What are the benefits of using cause and effect diagrams as an improvement tool?
4. What is a common structure used to draw cause and effect diagrams?
5. How do you make a fishbone diagram when you are in an improvement team?
6. How might you engage all members of your microsystem in creating and refining a fishbone diagram?

FIGURE 19.6. FISHBONE DIAGRAM FOR PLASTIC SURGERY APPOINTMENT BACKLOG.

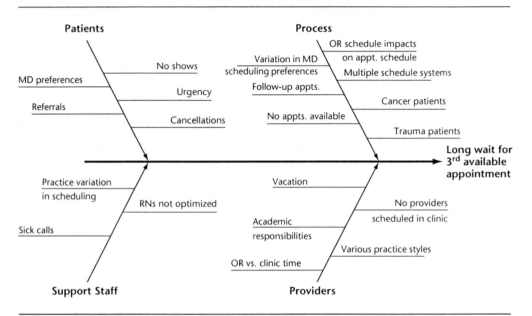

Note: OR = operating room.

Between Sessions Work

1. Create a fishbone diagram to show the causes that contribute to your specific aim.
2. Display the draft fishbone diagram for all to review and modify.
3. Make the modifications to the fishbone diagram based on feedback.

References

Ishikawa, K. (1976). *Guide to quality control.* Tokyo: Asian Productivity Organization.
MacMahon, B. T., & Pugh, T. F. (1970). *Epidemiology: Principles and methods.* Boston: Little, Brown.

CHAPTER TWENTY

EFFECTIVE MEETING SKILLS II

Brainstorming and Multi-Voting

Chapter Purpose

Aim. To define the process that a lead improvement team can use to develop a large list of ideas for improving a process and then to systematically reduce the number to the very best ideas.

    Objectives. At the completion of this unit, participants will be able to

- Define the methods and describe the steps in the process of brainstorming and multi-voting.

- Describe the differences between interactive brainstorming, silent brainstorming, and nominal group techniques.
- Apply brainstorming and multi-voting to a topic in order to select a specific change idea to test.
- Develop a process to engage all staff in the review and consideration of the results of the brainstorming and multi-voting session.

For lead improvement team members to work well together it is extremely helpful if they have good methods for surfacing creative ideas for improvement—the more ideas the better—and if they have a method for selecting the best idea(s) to work on next. Therefore a good time to use brainstorming (to generate ideas) and multi-voting (to select an idea to test) is when the team must decide on what the first or the next test of change will be. This chapter describes both methods (see Figure 20.1).

FIGURE 20.1. IMPROVEMENT RAMP: BRAINSTORMING AND MULTI-VOTING.

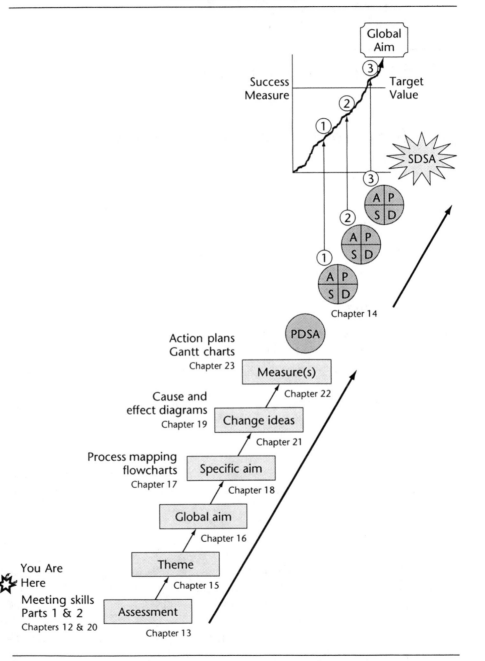

What Is Brainstorming?

Brainstorming is a method of provoking a group of people to generate creative ideas. Brainstorming can be used for many different purposes. Improvement teams often find it useful to use brainstorming to develop a long list of ideas for changing or improving a process or for doing something that is new to the organization.

What Are the Benefits of Brainstorming?

Successful brainstorming involves everyone in the team, encourages creative thinking, generates a great deal of energy and enthusiasm, and produces a long list of ideas.

More specifically, brainstorming

- Involves all members of the lead improvement team in idea generation—no idea is too small, too big, or out of the question.
- Increases the sense of camaraderie among those working on the improvement process.
- Increases team members' ability to listen carefully to others' ideas and to build on those ideas, which increases the team's creativity.
- Produces ideas that are new and different from those usually offered.

What Are Some Different Types of Brainstorming?

There are several ways to conduct brainstorming sessions. This section describes three of them. First, there is *group interactive brainstorming.* This approach can be loud and expressive. When group members think out loud, that stimulates ideas that build on each other, resulting in a list of many ideas. Ideas can be posted on a large flipchart as individuals call them out. It is important for the recorder to capture each individual's idea by writing his or her *exact words* on the flipchart and for others to refrain from commenting on or evaluating the ideas offered.

A second technique is *silent brainstorming.* Each person on the team first thinks about ideas during a silent period and then writes each idea on a Post-it Note and hands the batch of completed notes to the recorder, who reads each idea out loud before posting it on a flipchart. One form of this written, silent brainstorming is called the *nominal group technique.* In this method the team does not engage in a highly interactive form of conversation and idea building; it is literally a group in name only. Instead, each member of the group quietly writes down his or her ideas, one idea per Post-it Note, for a set period of time. When the idea generation time is finished, the recorder goes around the group eliciting ideas, one at a time, until all ideas are posted. This type of brainstorming works well for highly controversial topics.

It is possible to blend these different brainstorming methods. For example, a team could start with silent brainstorming, giving everyone a chance to think and get some ideas out, and then move to interactive brainstorming.

What Are Some Tips for Conducting Brainstorming?

- Clarify the objective before starting the brainstorming. If the team is not clear on the purpose of the brainstorming session, the outcome is likely to be less productive than desired. It is also helpful to clarify the ground rules about the process, defining what is desired and what behaviors are to be avoided, for example.
- Setting a target that expresses the number of fresh ideas expected (for example, "Let's generate forty ideas in the next ten minutes") can boost the number of ideas produced and encourage creative thinking within a limited time.
- It is usually best to take a few minutes to allow the team members to think quietly about their ideas before engaging in an interactive brainstorming session.
- Set some good practices for team members to follow:

  Listen to everyone's ideas and build on them. Listen carefully to what others are saying. This often results in more creative thinking than would otherwise be produced.

  Do not judge, criticize, or comment on other people's ideas. Try to verbalize ideas in rapid succession, and attempt to avoid a commentary after each idea—no facial grimaces or groans! (Multiple recorders who record suggestions alternately may increase or at least maintain the speed of the process.)

  Do not hold back your ideas, no matter how crazy they seem to you. In fact a far-out idea can open creative thinking in others. Your idea may stimulate someone else to be creative and to come up with a good idea. Feel free to suspend prior assumptions about the topic that you are brainstorming.

- After the ideas have been generated and posted on a flipchart, the leader of the meeting reads each idea out loud, and the team's understanding of the idea is clarified where necessary. The person who contributed an idea is the only person who should clarify that idea.

- Some teams find the use of Post-it Notes helpful in capturing brainstorming ideas. Each idea is written on one Post-it and then placed on a flipchart. The Post-its eliminate the need to erase or cross out ideas. When you review and consolidate similar ideas, you can move the Post-its and group them as needed. Other teams call out their ideas while the recorder for the meeting makes the list. Depending on the size and energy of the team, a second recorder may be helpful during a brainstorming session to keep up with the flow of ideas. It is important for the recorder to write the offered idea using the person's own words, to capture that person's meaning.
- Gathering ideas from the team in a methodical way, going around the team one by one, helps everyone participate. If a member does not have an idea, he or she can simply "pass" to the next person. The rounds continue until all ideas are exhausted.
- Gathering ideas by having all ideas called out, in no particular order, by the session participants has the benefit that ideas are often stimulated by hearing another's ideas. If this approach is used, it may be important for the facilitator to encourage everyone to participate.

What Is Multi-Voting?

Multi-voting is a method that engages all members of the team in agreeing on the best ideas to focus the improvement work on. It involves voting to reduce the idea list generated during a brainstorming session to the top choices. This is accomplished through a series of votes, each round of voting reducing the list and finally resulting in a consensus on a few top ideas to focus on next.

The word *consensus* comes from a Latin verb meaning "to share thoughts and feelings." Consensus does not mean that everyone is in total agreement but rather that everyone is reasonably comfortable with the decision from the team. The process of brainstorming and multi-voting provides an opportunity for all to be heard and for issues and concerns to be explored and discussed to the satisfaction of the team.

Do Teams Always Multi-Vote After a Brainstorming Session?

No. Brainstorming can be used for many different purposes: to stimulate thinking about causes and effects, to increase knowledge about a process, or to make a list of people to consider inviting for an improvement activity. If brainstorming is used to generate ideas for improvement work, the large list of ideas will need to be narrowed down and this can be accomplished through the multi-voting process.

How Do You Multi-Vote?

1. Review all the ideas generated by the team; the ideas should be read out loud for clarification. Once the ideas are clarified, similar ideas can be merged (with the permission of the people who contributed the ideas).
2. Letter the consolidated list of ideas: the first idea will be labeled A, the second B, the third C, and so on.
3. Each person should be asked to vote for about one-third of the total number of ideas on the list. For example, if the list generated by the brainstorming session contains fifteen ideas, then each person gets five votes to cast for the most promising ideas based on the selection criteria. Team members review the full list of ideas and quietly write their top five choices on a piece of paper.
4. It is important in this step to discuss selection criteria with the team members. When choosing their top choices, what selection criteria should they consider? Here are some criteria often used by teams selecting change ideas to test:
   - *Short lead time.* The test can be started fast.
   - *Low cost.* The change does not cost much if any additional money.
   - *High leverage.* The effort is small in relation to the impact on the process.
   - *Control.* The idea can be tested by the team without getting "permission" from others outside the team.
5. Count the votes. To tally the team's results, the leader of the meeting can use one of several methods:
   - Read each item and ask for a show of hands.
   - Ask each person to put a hash mark next to each of his or her top choices on the flip chart (several people can do this concurrently).
   - Give "sticky dots" to each member to place next to his or her top choices.
6. After each vote the leader can ask if anyone believes that an idea that did not get many votes should be kept under consideration for compelling reasons that should be stated. This is a good time to hold a brief discussion about the remaining items.
7. Once the group has narrowed the original long list by the first round of votes, the list is then shortened again by repeating the process, giving group members a number of votes corresponding to approximately one-third of the new number of items.

8. The voting process is repeated until group members reach general agreement on what they want to work on first (or next).

What Does a Brainstorming Session with a Multi-Voting Outcome Look Like?

Figure 20.2 shows an example of multi-voting. The lead improvement team started with six change ideas (1). Team members combined two ideas (2), they voted for their top-rated ideas (3), and they finished with two change ideas to test using the plan-do-study-act (PDSA) method (4).

Case Studies

Intermediate Cardiac Care Unit (ICCU)

The ICCU lead improvement team was gaining deeper knowledge of its clinical microsystem and becoming very good at employing effective meeting skills in its weekly meetings. Through practice, reminders to each other, and an improvement coach, the team members were making meeting skills a regular habit. An agenda was created during each meeting for the next meeting, and the roles of leading, recording, and keeping time were rotated. The team dynamics were changing, and the enthusiasm remained high. New meeting skills were now required for the tasks of reviewing all the data team members had collected and of coming to agreement on what to change and how "to improve communication of patient plans of care, including discharge, through an interdisciplinary morning round approach." They reviewed the rules for brainstorming and multi-voting to ensure that everyone was part of the solution and the decision making in selecting improvements to test. Their brainstorming session produced the following list of good ideas:

- Interdisciplinary morning rounds in the conference room
- Walking interdisciplinary rounds in the morning
- Resident and attending physicians walking rounds with charge nurses
- All physicians rounding with only the charge nurse

The multi-voting resulted in the team's selecting interdisciplinary morning rounds with all staff in the conference room. The discussion revealed how much the team valued having all staff involved and informed about patient plans of care and discharge plans.

FIGURE 20.2. BRAINSTORMING AND MULTI-VOTING EXAMPLE.

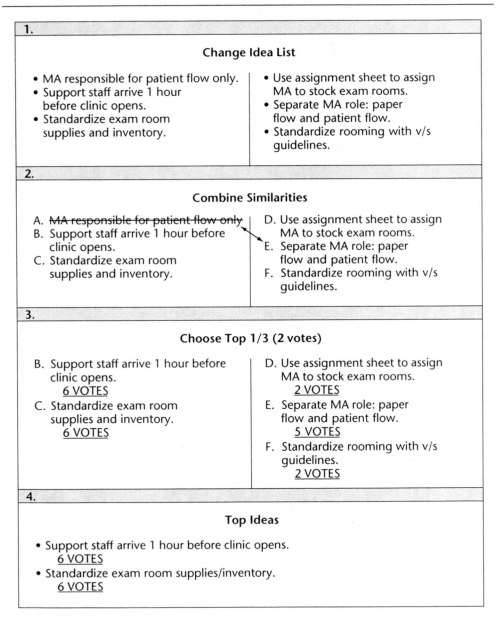

1.

Change Idea List

- MA responsible for patient flow only.
- Support staff arrive 1 hour before clinic opens.
- Standardize exam room supplies and inventory.

- Use assignment sheet to assign MA to stock exam rooms.
- Separate MA role: paper flow and patient flow.
- Standardize rooming with v/s guidelines.

2.

Combine Similarities

A. ~~MA responsible for patient flow only~~
B. Support staff arrive 1 hour before clinic opens.
C. Standardize exam room supplies and inventory.

D. Use assignment sheet to assign MA to stock exam rooms.
E. Separate MA role: paper flow and patient flow.
F. Standardize rooming with v/s guidelines.

3.

Choose Top 1/3 (2 votes)

B. Support staff arrive 1 hour before clinic opens.
   6 VOTES
C. Standardize exam room supplies and inventory.
   6 VOTES

D. Use assignment sheet to assign MA to stock exam rooms.
   2 VOTES
E. Separate MA role: paper flow and patient flow.
   5 VOTES
F. Standardize rooming with v/s guidelines.
   2 VOTES

4.

Top Ideas

- Support staff arrive 1 hour before clinic opens.
  6 VOTES
- Standardize exam room supplies/inventory.
  6 VOTES

Note: MA = medical assistant; v/s = vital signs.

Plastic Surgery Section

The lead improvement team brainstormed ideas for working down the backlog of appointments. Team members reviewed best practices and, through the Institute for Healthcare Improvement, turned to the access improvement work of Mark Murray and Catherine Tantau (2006). They reviewed the suggested list of steps to reduce the backlog to determine what would work best in their practice. The team's initial assessment showed that each physician tended to have a certain pattern of scheduling patients for follow-up visits, that these patterns varied for no apparent reason, and that these follow-up appointments could fill space needed for new patients. The list of brainstormed change ideas to improve appointment access included these approaches:

- Discuss with each physician the need to reduce follow-up appointment frequency.
- Measure demand for appointments.
- Shorten length of appointments.
- Limit the number of appointment types.
- Use shared medical appointments.

When discussion resulted in a deeper understanding of the lead physician's frustration with repeatedly saying the same thing to patients wishing to have breast reductions, the lead improvement team selected the idea of shared medical appointments. The team also realized that the backlog of patients waiting for a first appointment for breast reduction could be drastically reduced through seeing eight to twelve patients in a ninety-minute time period. Through brainstorming and multi-voting, team members determined that they would explore group visits to improve the appointment process and thereby improve access to appointments. They also decided to share the follow-up appointment scheduling variations with all the physicians to increase physician awareness of the variation and possibly encourage each physician to rethink her or his own pattern for scheduling follow-up appointments.

Review Questions

1. What is brainstorming?
2. What are three types of brainstorming?
3. What are the steps for conducting a brainstorming session?
4. When would you use multi-voting after a brainstorming session?
5. What is the difference between brainstorming and multi-voting?

Between Sessions Work

1. Brainstorm and multi-vote to choose a change idea to test that is related to your specific aim statement.
2. Develop a process to engage all staff in the review and consideration of the results of your brainstorming and multi-voting work.
3. Develop a clear plan to test a change idea.
4. Review the plan with all staff.
5. Determine dates and preparation needed to test the change idea quickly.
6. Use the PDSA ↔ SDSA worksheet (Figure A.15 in the Appendix) to guide actions.

Reference

Murray, M., & Tantau, C. (2006). *Shortening waiting times: Six principles for improved access.* Retrieved June 26, 2006, from http://www.ihi.org/IHI/Topics/OfficePractices/ Access/Literature/ShorteningWaitingTimesSixPrinciplesforImprovedAccess.htm.

CHAPTER TWENTY-ONE

CHANGE CONCEPTS

Chapter Purpose

Aim. To understand how change concepts can contribute to developing new change ideas for improvement.

    Objectives. At the completion of this unit, you will be able to

- Define a change concept.
- List common change concept categories.

- Identify when change concepts enter the overall improvement process.
- Describe how a change concept can lead to specific change ideas.
- Describe a clinical example of a change concept applied to a change idea.

C hange concepts help to stimulate change ideas for testing the process you hope to improve. The more good change ideas you have the better your prospects for successfully reaching your aim. This chapter describes how you can use a change concept to stimulate specific change ideas and thereby expand your options for redesigning processes and for improving care. A good time to employ change concepts is when you are considering possible changes that can be tested using the plan-do-study-act (PDSA) method (see Figure 21.1).

FIGURE 21.1. IMPROVEMENT RAMP: CHANGE IDEAS.

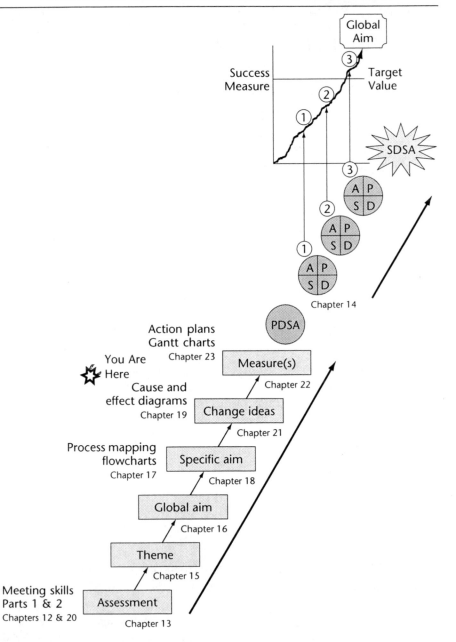

What Is a Change Concept?

Change concepts are stimulants for developing and designing detailed and specific tests of change. Combining change concepts with your deep knowledge of a process can lead you and your team to new thinking about the process and specific, high-yield change ideas to test. De Bono (1992) suggests that if you understand an underlying concept on which a specific idea is based, you can use that concept to develop numerous ideas and options.

It is important to note that a change concept cannot be used as a substitute for examining the process you aim to improve. Using change concepts is successful when coupled with your process knowledge.

Why Use Change Concepts?

Change concepts can help you clarify your thinking about where in a process a change can be made to result in substantive improvement. Change concepts are useful for jump-starting improvement ideas and offering new perspectives for change that you might not have considered previously. When you are ready to consider changes in a process, using change concepts can enrich your thinking and amplify idea generation.

Change concepts have been popularized in two books:—*The Improvement Action Guide: A Practical Approach to Enhancing Organizational Performance* (Langley, Nolan, Norman, Provost, & Nolan, 1996) and the *Clinical Improvement Action Guide* (Nelson, Batalden, & Ryer, 1998). Langley et al. list seventy change concepts, based in part on Deming's system of profound knowledge (Deming, 1986). These concepts and their categories are listed in Table 21.1.

How Can You Use Change Concepts in a Process?

Figure 21.2 provides a visual example of some ways that change concepts can be used to redesign care. This diagram is based on actual improvement work focusing on hip replacements. The interdisciplinary lead improvement team's aim was to achieve superior clinical and functional health status, satisfaction, and cost outcomes for this population. By first creating a flow diagram and studying the current process of care and then considering change concepts, the team was able to generate specific ideas for improving the hip replacement process.

TABLE 21.1. LANGLEY'S CHANGE CONCEPTS.

Category	Change Concepts
Eliminate waste	• Eliminate things that are not used • Eliminate multiple entry • Reduce or eliminate overkill • Reduce controls on the system • Recycle or reuse • Use substitution • Reduce classifications • Remove intermediaries • Match the amount to the need • Use sampling • Change targets or set points
Improve work flow	• Synchronize • Schedule into multiple processes • Minimize handoffs • Move steps in the process close together • Find and remove bottlenecks • Use automation • Smooth workflow • Do tasks in parallel • Consider people as in the same system • Use multiple processing units • Adjust to peak demand
Optimize inventory	• Match inventory to predicted demand • Use pull systems • Reduce choice of features • Reduce multiple brands of same item
Change the work environment	• Give people access to information • Use proper measurements • Take care of basics • Reduce demotivating aspects of pay system • Conduct training • Implement cross-training • Invest more resources in improvement • Focus on core processes and purpose • Share risks • Emphasize natural and logical consequences • Develop alliance/cooperative relationships
Enhance the producer/ customer relationship	• Listen to customers • Coach customers to use product/service • Focus on the outcome to a customer • Use a coordinator • Reach agreement on expectations • Outsource for "free" • Optimize level of inspection • Work with suppliers

TABLE 21.1. (*Continued*)

Category	Change Concepts
Manage time	• Reduce setup or startup time • Set up timing to use discounts • Optimize maintenance • Extend specialist's time • Reduce wait time
Manage variation	• Standardization (create a formal process) • Stop tampering • Develop operational definitions • Improve predictions • Develop contingency plans • Sort product into grades • Desensitize
Design systems to avoid mistakes	• Exploit variation • Use reminders • Use differentiation • Use constraints • Use affordances
Focus on the product or service	• Mass customize • Offer product/service anytime • Offer product/service anyplace • Emphasize intangibles • Influence or take advantage of fashion trends • Reduce the number of components • Disguise defects or problems • Differentiate product using quality dimensions

Source: Langley et al., 1996. Used with permission.

What Are the Next Steps?

After refining an idea for change—based on process knowledge and change concepts—you are ready to design a test of change using the PDSA method.

Case Studies

Intermediate Cardiac Care Unit (ICCU)

The ICCU's lead improvement team brainstormed ideas on *where* to focus improvement. Once the team members had all contributed their ideas, they multi-voted, which led them to a decision to focus on morning rounds. They learned

FIGURE 21.2. CHANGE CONCEPTS APPLIED
TO A CLINICAL PROCESS.

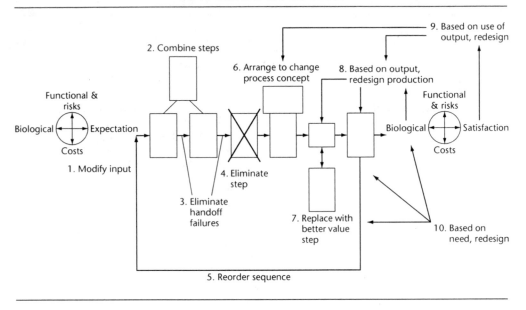

that morning rounds were not interdisciplinary and that the clinical team often did not know the specific care plans for each patient. This resulted in inconsistent communication to patients, families, and staff concerning the plan of the day, which in turn led to delays in discharges and transfers. After morning rounds were selected as a focus, the team brainstormed ideas for improvement. Walking rounds with all professionals—including patients and families—was suggested, as well as holding consolidated interdisciplinary rounds in the conference room, and "just forcing" people to communicate better. After the team members brainstormed all their ideas, they multi-voted and decided to test the approach of consolidated interdisciplinary rounds in the conference room. It was clear that the different clinical disciplines needed to learn to value each other's contributions to patient care and also to learn how to communicate differently.

The first PDSA cycle was conducted. This led to many subsequent PDSA cycles, each building on the lessons from the prior cycle (see Figure 14.7). The new insights about communication, professional relationships, and patient care plans were enormous. The medical director spoke frequently with the attending staff and house staff to coach and educate colleagues about the process changes that were being tested. To keep everyone up to date, the ICCU nursing director communicated frequently with all nursing staff using verbal communications, change of shift updates, and visual displays.

Plastic Surgery Section

With the specific aim to decrease the backlog for appointments by 50 percent (with a starting baseline measure of ninety-nine days), the Plastic Surgery Section lead improvement team designed tests of change for *shared medical appointments,* a type of medical care popularized by Noffsinger (Carlson, 2003).

The Plastic Surgery team reviewed its flowchart and fishbone diagram to see how shared medical appointments might improve patient satisfaction and clinical productivity while reducing the backlog of patients. The new model included the following elements:

- Patient knowledge: previsit mailing of comprehensive information
- Flowchart of new process: a detailed diagram of patient flow and provider actions
- Role redesign: changing the role of the registered nurses

Developing the detailed diagram of process flows was a key to success for the first shared medical appointment. The lead improvement team also identified the importance of a detailed plan of education and training to optimize the roles of the RNs. The team also believed that practice makes perfect, so conducting mock shared medical appointments—to simulate the patient and provider flows—was an important part of preparing for the first shared medical appointment.

Review Questions

1. How might you define change concepts?
2. What are eight categories of change concepts?
3. Where do change concepts fit in the overall improvement process?
4. How does a change concept lead to a change idea?
5. What are the next steps after you have selected a change concept?

Between Sessions Work

1. Review the change concept list, and use it to stimulate thinking about ways to redesign your process.
2. Research the best-known change ideas for the process you aim to improve.

References

Carlson, R. (2003). *Shared appointments improve efficiency in the clinic.* Retrieved June 26, 2006, from http://www.managedcaremag.com/archives/0305/0305.sharedappointments.html.

De Bono, E. (1992). *Serious creativity: Using the power of lateral thinking to create new ideas.* New York: HarperBusiness.

Deming, W. E. (1986). *Out of the crisis.* Cambridge, MA: MIT Center for Advanced Engineering Study.

Langley, G. J., Nolan, K. M., Norman, C. L., Provost, L. P., & Nolan, T. W. (1996). *The improvement guide: A practical approach to enhancing organizational performance.* San Francisco: Jossey-Bass.

Nelson, E. C., Batalden, P. B., & Ryer, J. C. (Eds.). (1998). *Clinical improvement action guide.* Oakbrook Terrace, IL: Joint Commission on Accreditation of Healthcare Organizations.

CHAPTER TWENTY-TWO

MEASUREMENT AND MONITORING

Chapter Purpose

Aim. To understand how to make and interpret run charts and control charts, two methods for measuring and displaying data trends over time.

    Objectives. At the completion of this unit, you will be able to

- Describe how plotting data over time and using run charts and control charts fit into the improvement process.
- Make and interpret a run chart.
- Make and interpret one type of control chart.

The focus in this chapter is planning measurement specific to PDSA ↔ SDSA cycles to determine whether change ideas are really improvements. A goal of the Dartmouth Microsystem Improvement Curriculum is to build the capability of microsystem staff to improve quality of care and their own worklives by becoming a community of scientists. Scientists reflect on the world around them, they make hypotheses about causes and effects (what causes what), they run experiments (tests of change) to test their hypotheses, and they collect data to provide evidence to support or reject their hypotheses.

    One way to look at the plan-do-study-act ↔ standardize-do-study-act (PDSA ↔ SDSA) process is to view it simply as putting the scientific method into a clinical microsystem's everyday work of finding better ways to do things. Clearly, the PDSA ↔ SDSA model represents the scientific method that we all learned in high school and college. The use of this model in health care organizations represents a way to popularize and localize the scientific method.

As you saw in our discussion of PDSA and SDSA in Chapter Fourteen, the improvement process includes gathering data related to your aim to determine whether a change is an improvement. The *plan* step involves planning data collection, the *do* step involves collecting data, and the *study* step involves evaluating the data to determine the pilot test's effect on specific aim-related measures.

Also, as you learned in our earlier discussion about the improvement ramp, the overall idea is to define your microsystem's global aim and to find a measure that can be tracked over time to determine whether all the changes you make as you ascend the ramp are helping your system to approach the target value that represents success.

In general you will want to use trend charts, such as run charts and control charts, to determine whether you are making measurable progress on reaching your aim. Once you have achieved your aim, you will want to use trend charts to monitor performance over time so you can avoid slipping back into a worse performance zone without quickly knowing it (see Figure 22.1).

As your clinical microsystem progresses to become increasingly performance driven and process minded, you will build out your data wall and graphical displays that will feature trend charts for showing changes in critical measures over time and for monitoring performance to make sure that the microsystem is maintaining consistent, high-level performance.

What Are Measures, What Makes Measures Good, and How Do They Relate to Aims?

In general you can think of *measures* (or *variables*) as things to be counted so you can evaluate the amount (or the status) of a thing of interest. People in clinical microsystems use many different types of measures to evaluate such interesting and important things as quality, safety, costs, satisfaction, productivity, reliability, and so forth.

Good measures have several important characteristics.

- Good measures can provide an answer to a critical question. For example, an emergency department might ask, "Have we reached our specific aim of doing an ECG and drawing cardiac enzymes on every appropriate patient within fifteen minutes of arrival?" and the appropriate measures would answer that question.

FIGURE 22.1. IMPROVEMENT RAMP: MEASUREMENT.

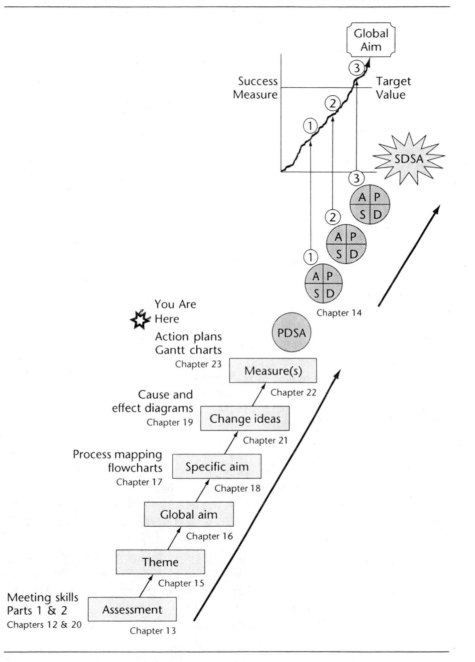

- Good measures are sufficiently accurate (reliable and valid) for the purpose at hand, such as having your own local, relevant evidence on your microsystem's level of performance.
- Good measures have such basic working parts as
    A descriptive name
    A conceptual definition describing the measure
    An operational definition describing the method to be used to score or categorize the measure
    Graphical (or tabular) data displays that can be used to answer the critical question

It takes good measures to determine whether your global aim and specific aims are being met.

Recall that the basic model for improvement begins with three questions (see Chapter Fourteen).

1. *Aim.* What are we trying to accomplish?
2. *Measures.* How will we know that a change is an improvement?
3. *Changes.* What changes can we make that will result in an improvement?

Look again at the improvement ramp, and you will see how all of this fits together—aims, measures, use of the scientific method in the form of PDSA to make changes to reach a targeted level of performance, and use of SDSA to maintain the needed level of performance.

What Is a Run Chart?

A *run chart* is a graphical data display that shows trends in a measure of interest; trends reveal what is occurring over time. Run charts are the most common type of trend chart, and we all are accustomed to seeing them in newspapers, financial reports, reference books, and particularly in modern improvement work.

A run chart shows data points in time order. The value of the measure of interest is shown on the vertical dimension and the value of the measure at each point, *running* over time, is shown on the horizontal dimension. You will often see run charts used to show trends related to patients or organizations or clinical units. You might make or see run charts for many different measures, for example:

- Fasting blood sugar. Blood sugar levels for a person with diabetes might be plotted daily for a month (see Figure 22.2).

FIGURE 22.2. RUN CHART DISPLAYING FASTING BLOOD SUGAR LEVELS.

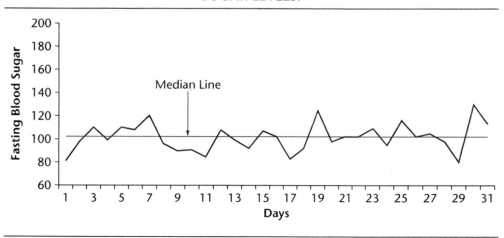

FIGURE 22.3. RUN CHART DISPLAYING NO SHOWS.

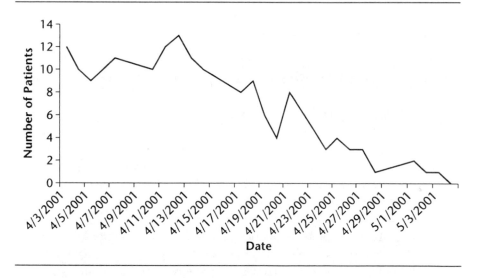

- No shows. The number of patients who do not arrive for an appointment at a clinic might be plotted daily for a month (see Figure 22.3).
- Appointment access. The number of days to the third next available appointment might be plotted over a two-year time period as changes are made to improve access to care (see Figure 22.4).

FIGURE 22.4. RUN CHART DISPLAYING DAYS TO THIRD NEXT AVAILABLE APPOINTMENT.

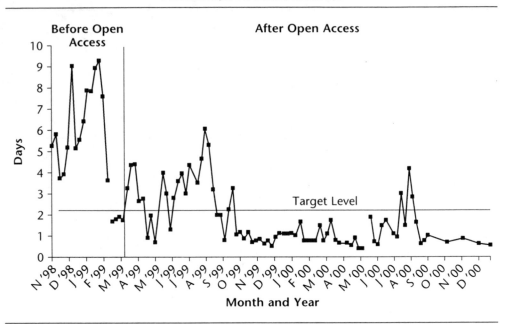

What Are the Benefits of Using a Run Chart?

There are many advantages to using run charts:

- They are easy to make and easy to interpret.
- They provide a "picture" that reveals how the process is performing, communicating more information more clearly than a table that contains the same information.
- They can be used for several important purposes:
    To detect problems that might otherwise go unnoticed
    To see if your microsystem is performing at the targeted level
    To determine if a change (or all the changes being made) is associated with movement of an aim-related measure in the right direction
    To show how much variation there is in the process you are working to improve, which may give you a hint about the underlying system of causes influencing the process

How Do Run Charts Fit in the Overall Improvement Process?

As represented in the improvement ramp (Figure 22.1), one place that run charts fit into the overall improvement process is to show if the changes being made are causing an aim-related outcome measure to move into the targeted zone of success. Consequently, as soon as a general aim is established it is important to find a way to measure current performance of a measure related to that aim and to track movement in this measure over time as changes are planned and executed. What you want to do is to make the most powerful changes possible in the least amount of time to attain the desired level of performance as measured by run chart (time-trended) results.

Run charts also fit into the overall improvement process when your lead improvement team is conducting individual tests of change using PDSA cycles. Each cycle may involve using run charts to see if specific changes are being made in upstream processes (doing something "this way each time") or in *downstream* results (getting certain outcomes as a result of doing it "this way each time").

What Do Run Charts Tell You About Your Performance Level and Variation?

Run charts show the amount of the measure on the vertical axis, and they show the time when this value occurred on the horizontal axis. As the number of data points builds up, and as you start connecting the data points, you see some important things:

- First, you see whether or not the measure is "running" in the targeted or desired zone. Measures related to aims should, in general, have a specified target value that can be used to determine if performance is adequate or inadequate.
- Second, you see how much variation there is point to point and over time. In general you want to have results that stay in the targeted performance zone, or at the desired level, with only a small amount of variation. When this state of affairs is achieved, you have a reliable process that is producing consistent results that are at the desired level.

What Are Special Cause and Common Cause Variation?

It should be noted here that as you gain knowledge about causes and effects you will also gain knowledge about sources of variation. Deming popularized the idea of two types of variation: special cause and common cause.

- *Common cause variation* occurs when the system of causes, or the web of causation, is relatively consistent and the variation in outcomes is being produced by *chance causes,* by random variation in the causal system.
- *Special cause variation* occurs when the system of causes, or the web of causation, experiences a *new* or *special* or *assignable* cause(s) that enters the causal system for either a short or extended period of time and that has an effect on outcomes beyond what can be accounted for by random variation.

All causal systems have common cause—that is, chance or random—variation. Sometimes causal systems have both common cause and special cause variation embedded in them.

Common causes typically take the form of a large number of small and ongoing sources of variation. For example, random variation in arrival times of patients to a clinic might be due to such things as weather, vehicle problems, parking issues, traffic volume, and so forth. Special causes are not part of the process all of the time. They arise from less ordinary circumstances. For example, patients arriving late to a clinic due to a strike by bus drivers are being affected by a special cause.

For another example, imagine that you are on a track team and run the 100-meter dash in twenty track meets. If you stay in about the same physical condition, then your times will vary by a few tenths of a second up or down depending on such common causes as the direction of the wind, how quickly you react to the starting gun, the condition of the track, and so forth. However, if you are injured one day, if you pull a muscle in your leg and have severe pain, your time for the 100-meter dash that day will be several seconds slower, because of the special leg problem. Once your muscle pull heals, and you are back to normal, your times will return to their prior performance zone. This is a simple example of a system that has both common cause and special cause sources of variation.

When making improvements, it is important to know if the system you are seeking to make better is subject to only common cause, or random, variation or if it is subject to both common cause and special cause variation.

- If it has special cause variation—and this variation causes extraordinarily poor results,—then you will want to identify the special cause and find a way to remove it (or design it out of) the system. For example, if access to care is poor every

February because many staff take a vacation during a school holiday, then you might wish to set up a policy that rations time off during the choicest time periods.

- If it has special cause variation and if this variation causes extraordinarily good results,—then you will want to identify the special cause and try to find a way to reproduce it (or design it into) the system. For example, if one physician's patients with newly diagnosed hypertension do much better at rapidly reducing their blood pressure and keeping it in a safe zone than the patients of all the other clinicians in the practice do, then it might be helpful to determine what process that one clinician uses to educate newly diagnosed patients with hypertension, and to encourage the other clinicians to try adapting that process to their patients. This is the practice of process benchmarking, whereby you identify the best process, the one that produces consistently superior results, and attempt to incorporate this best process's features into your own process.
- If it has common cause variation only and yet the performance level is not adequate or is too highly variable, then the best way to improve the process is to use disciplined improvement work or to make innovations in the way the process works.

The reason you need to understand common cause and special cause variation is that part of the value of trend charts—both run charts and control charts—is that they provide your microsystem with a method for determining whether or not its processes are subject only to common cause variation or if they are subject to both common and special cause variation. As you will see, the rules for interpreting run chart and control chart results give you a way of judging the likelihood that your outcomes are subject to special cause as well as common cause variation.

How Do You Make a Run Chart?

You may find it helpful to use a data collection tool for making run charts and control charts (see Figure 22.5).

Here are some general steps for making a run chart.

1. Select a measure that can answer a critical question.
2. Document your operational definition to explain the details of how you will collect data on the measure.
3. Make a plan (who does what, when, in following which process) to collect data on the measure at set intervals, such as hourly, daily, weekly, or monthly.
4. Collect data on the measure, and record them on a measurement worksheet.
5. Make your run chart.
   a. Plot your data points in a time-ordered sequence. Use the vertical dimension to show the value of the measure and the horizontal dimension to show variation over time.

FIGURE 22.5. WORKSHEET FOR COLLECTING DATA TO MEASURE A KEY VARIABLE.

MEASUREMENT OF KEY VARIABLE

Variable: _____ Unit of Measure: _____ Method of Measurement: _____

1. Enter your data

	1	2	3	4	5	6	7	8	9	10	11	12	13	14	15	16	17	18	19	20	21	22	23	24	25	26	27	28	29	30	31	32
Date																																
Time																																
Measures (X)																																
Moving range (R)																																

2. Do these calculations

Average = $\bar{X}$ = _____ Sum of X's / # of X's

Moving Range = $R = (X_2 - X_1)$ Absolute #'s only

Average Range = $\bar{R}$ = _____ Sum of R's / # of R's

Upper Natural Process Limit = $\bar{X} + (2.66 \times \bar{R})$ = _____

Lower Natural Process Limit = $\bar{X} - (2.66 \times \bar{R})$ = _____

Upper Control Limit for Range Limit = $3.27 \times \bar{R}$ = _____

3. Plot limits, data, averages

Measurements (X)

1	2	3	4	5	6	7	8	9	10	11	12	13	14	15	16	17	18	19	20	21	22	23	24	25	26	27	28	29	30	31	32

Moving range (R)

1	2	3	4	5	6	7	8	9	10	11	12	13	14	15	16	17	18	19	20	21	22	23	24	25	26	27	28	29	30	31	32

   b. Name your run chart. A good way to do this is to write the question that
      the run chart answers above the run chart. For example:
      - Are the fasting blood sugar levels of this patient in a safe zone?
      - Do our diabetic patients have HbA1c levels under 7?
      - How long do patients need to wait for an appointment?
6. Connect the data points to make it easy to see the pattern they represent.
7. Calculate the mean or the median to show where the distribution is centered.
8. Make sense out of the results by studying them and understanding their pattern, following the common rules for interpreting run charts.
9. Overlay the target value for the measure that you have set as a performance goal and determine whether the process being measured has or has not yet reached the desired level, or whether it is approaching the target level.

As a rule of thumb, you should seek to have about twenty-five or more data points to determine the pattern of results that your process is producing. Wheeler (1993) recommends this number as a minimum for process analysis but states that you can begin to make provisional assessments with as few as twelve data points.

How Do You Interpret Run Chart Results?

Use these questions to interpret the pattern of results represented in your run chart.

1. Is the measure running at or above the target level?
   - If the measure is at or above the target level, what actions might you take to maintain the process? Consider using SDSA.
   - If the measure is below the target level, what actions might you take to improve or innovate? Consider using PDSA.
2. How much variation is there in the measure?
   - Do the levels of the measure's high points or low points mean that the process is unreliable?
3. Are there any special cause signals? Here are some of these signals:
   - Eight data points in a row are above or below the center line (the mean or the median value).
   - Six data points in a row are going up.
   - Six data points in a row are going down.

A word of caution about point 3. There are many different guidelines for detecting special cause patterns in process performance data plotted on run charts. The three special cause rules we have listed are often used to interpret run chart results, but they are not perfect rules. It is possible to get a pattern of points that matches one of these rules and for this signal to be a false alarm. The odds of the alarm's being false are relatively small, but the more rules that are used, the more likely it is to get a false alarm (Wheeler, 1995, chap. 1, "Shewhart's Control Charts").

What Is a Control Chart?

Run charts and control charts are similar in that they both use time-ordered data. The difference is that control charts provide limits within which observed variation can be characterized as random and expected, and outside which you can recognize variation as extraordinary. With control charts you have more ways than run charts provide to detect special cause signals.

As mentioned earlier there are three common rules for detecting special cause signals in run charts. These same rules apply to control charts but additional rules can be used with control charts because they have an added feature, calculated upper and lower *control limits*, or upper and lower *natural process limits*, that can be used to detect special causes in your process.

We illustrate the essential difference between these two types of trend charts in Figures 22.6 and 22.7.

Figure 22.6 shows the gross anatomy of a run chart. It has a variable, X, whose value is measured on the vertical dimension and is shown at each point in a time-ordered sequence on the horizontal dimension. The run chart also has a center line based on either the calculated average value or the median value of the points.

Figure 22.7 shows the gross anatomy of a control chart. It has all the features of the run chart but in addition has upper and lower *calculated limits*. These calculated limits are shown, by convention, as dotted lines and are called the *upper control limit* (UCL) and *lower control limit* (LCL), respectively. Another set of terms for these calculated limits, one that Wheeler prefers (1993, 1995), is *upper natural process limit* and *lower*

FIGURE 22.6. GROSS ANATOMY OF A RUN CHART.

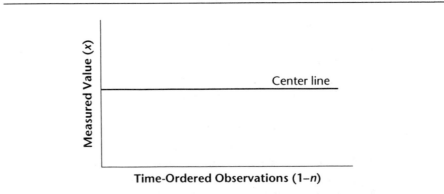

FIGURE 22.7. GROSS ANATOMY OF A CONTROL CHART.

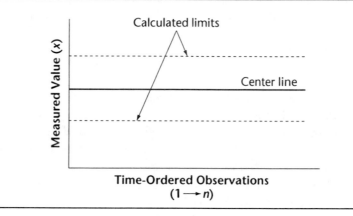

FIGURE 22.8. CONTROL CHART FOR INDIVIDUALS WITH DIABETES IN A GENERAL MEDICINE PRACTICE.

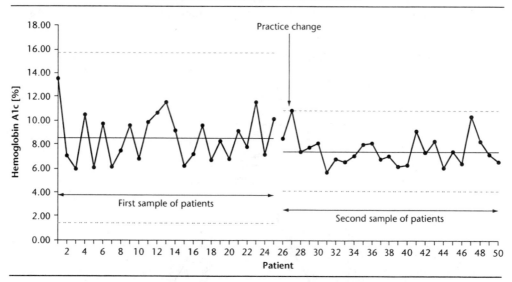

natural process limit. Wheeler prefers this terminology because it is a better reflection of the principle of special cause and common cause variation, described earlier.

In general you can interpret the results of a run chart by looking for data points above the upper limit or below the lower limit. If a data point falls *outside* these calculated upper or lower limits, it is a special cause signal, because the likelihood that a point will fall outside these limits due to a common cause is very low (less than 1 out of 100).

Figure 22.8 provides a real-life example of a control chart, one that a physician colleague of ours (Mark Splaine) used to measure progress in managing blood sugar levels in his patients with diabetes. This figure shows that after Splaine made changes in his practice, the average level of blood sugar control improved and the variation over time was reduced.

What Is the Theory Behind Control Charts?

The term *control* chart is short for *statistical process control* (SPC) chart. What control charts reveal is whether observed variation in a process is consistent with random variation due to innumerable common causes. When variation occurs within control limits, the process is said to be in *statistical control*, free from special cause effects or assignable cause variation. The process is subject only to chance factors or random cause variation.

As mentioned earlier, calculated upper and lower control limits (or, more correctly labeled, statistical process control limits) are added to a run chart to make it into a control chart. Control limits are calculated on the basis of statistical theory describing distribution of values within any population of data.

Figure 22.9 shows a typical normal distribution (called *normal* because it applies to so much of the data that we all typically encounter). It is also known as a Gaussian

FIGURE 22.9. NORMAL DISTRIBUTION, AKA THE BELL CURVE.

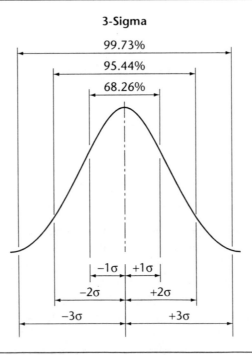

(after Gauss, the person who first described it) or bell (for the obvious reason) curve. The normal distribution is formed by showing graphically the spread of results from observing a variety of samples (a sample might be, for example, a group of patients) drawn from a universe of possible samples. What the normal distribution shows is that samples tend to have average values that center on the true average value but that most samples are either above or below the true average value by a little bit, by a medium amount, or by a large amount. The likelihood that a sample's value will be close to the true average value is greater than the likelihood that it will be far away. The mathematics for normal distributions uses the concept of *standard deviations* of values from the true center value of the distribution. The way this works is that about 68 percent of sample values will fall within 1 standard deviation (1 SD, or 1 sigma) and that about 95 percent of sample values will fall within 2 SD, or 2 sigma, and that more than 99 percent will fall within 3 SD, or 3 sigma.

Upper and lower control limits are generally calculated so that values that fall outside 3 SD are displayed as falling outside the control limit. Those data points that fall outside 3 SD, or 3 sigma, are very unlikely to happen by chance. The normal distribution tells us that the vast majority of data points (99.73 percent) will fall within the upper and lower range (within 3 SD) and thus it is likely that the process is experiencing special causes when a point falls outside these calculated statistical process control limits. Figure 22.10 illustrates this concept by juxtaposing a control chart and the normal distribution. The reason for setting your limits

FIGURE 22.10. CONTROL CHART IN RELATION TO NORMAL DISTRIBUTION.

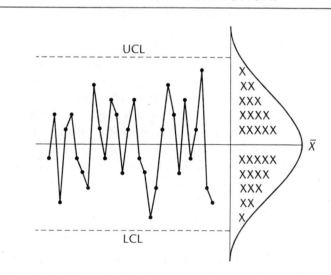

at 3 standard deviations rather than 2, as is customary in much scientific writing, is based on Walter Shewhart's observation that it is generally more effective, from a practical, economic point of view, to restrict investigation for special causes to situations in which the data are quite different from what one would expect, not just somewhat different (Shewhart, 1931/1980, 1939/1986).

What Are the Benefits of Using a Control Chart Instead of a Run Chart?

The primary benefit of using a control chart is that it provides another guideline for identifying special cause signals. When you see a run chart, you will often see a point that looks extremely high or extremely low relative to the other points. You might be tempted to say that something special is happening. But absent calculated control limits, it is not possible to know from the chart itself whether this apparently very high or very low point is likely to be due to chance variation or likely to signal a special cause event or pattern.

What Are the Different Kinds of Control Charts?

Because there are different types of measures (that is, different kinds of variables), there are different types of control charts. What they all have in common is the mathematics of probability theory. The basic idea is that your choice of control chart depends on the type of measure that you are using.

Measures can be made using various methods for counting or classifying data. Here are two common types of measures:

- *Variables* data are measures of such things as times, blood glucose levels, dollars, or other types of counts or measures that can conceivably take any value (that are *continuous*). A good control chart for variables data is the XmR chart.
- *Attributes* data are measures of such conditions as infected/not infected, defective/not defective, error/no error, and other types of classifications that indicate whether a characteristic is present or absent in each case examined. Attributes data for a series of cases are often summarized as a proportion: for example, the proportion infected or the proportion defective or the proportion with error. A good control chart for attributes data is the P-chart.

What Is an XmR Control Chart?

Because the most common types of measures involve variables data we will discuss the XmR control chart in this chapter.

FIGURE 22.11. GROSS ANATOMY OF AN XMR CHART.

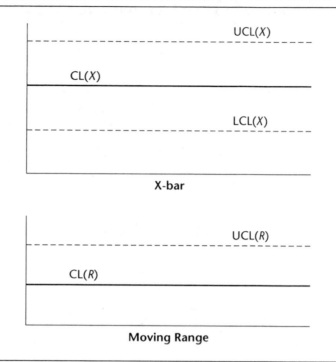

The XmR chart is both versatile and relatively easy to make. The calculated control limits use simple formulas that require only basic arithmetic (adding, subtracting, multiplying, and dividing) and nothing more. An excellent book that introduces both control chart thinking and the use of the XmR chart is *Understanding Variation,* by Donald Wheeler (1993); it is a good book for novices to read to gain insight and practical knowledge on the topic of control charts.

Figure 22.11 shows the basic anatomy of an XmR control chart. It is made by using a pair of trend charts. The upper chart (the *X*-bar display) shows each value and its average over time. The lower chart (the moving range display) shows the amount of difference between successive points and their average difference, each from its predecessor, over time. An example of an actual XmR chart for fasting blood glucose levels in an individual patient is shown in Figure 22.12.

How Do You Make an XmR Control Chart?

You can use the data collection worksheet (Figure 22.5) to turn your run chart into an XmR control chart. Instructions are summarized on the worksheet and discussed in more detail here:

FIGURE 22.12. XMR CHART SHOWING FASTING BLOOD SUGAR VARIANCE IN ONE PATIENT OVER ONE MONTH.

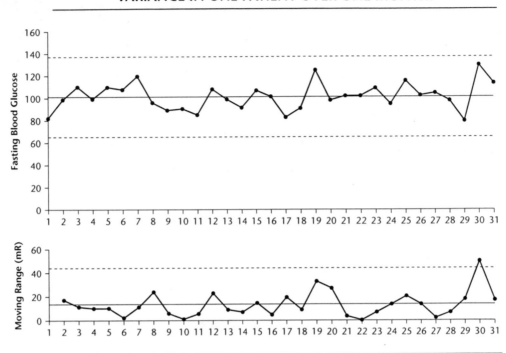

1. Specify the name of your measure (variable, for example, systolic blood pressure), the unit of measure (for example, mm) and the method of measurement.
2. Enter your data:
   a. The first two rows provide space for entering the data and the time of data collection and can be used when helpful.
   b. Row 3 provides space for entering the value of each measurement that you take.
3. Do these calculations:
   a. Moving range. Row 4 provides space to enter the moving range. This is done by calculating the absolute value of the difference between each two time-ordered points: that is, the difference between Points 1 and 2, then the difference between Points 2 and 3, then the difference between Points 3 and 4, and so forth.
   b. Average $= X$ bar. The sum of the measures in Row 3 divided by the number of measures listed in Row 3 (the sum of the X's divided by the total number of X's).

    c. Average range = R bar. The sum of the measures in Row 4 divided by the number of moving ranges in Row 4 (the sum of the R's divided by the total number of R's).

    d. Upper natural process control limit (UCL) = X bar + (2.66 × R bar).

    e. Lower natural process control limit (LCL) = X bar − (2.66 × R bar).

    f. Upper control limit for moving range = UCL_R.

4. Plot your data for the upper chart showing the time trend for your measures (values of X), keeping in mind that the upper and lower control limits must fit onto the chart:

    a. Plot the data for each point in time order (all the X's), and connect the dots.

    b. Draw the center line, using the average value of all the X's (X bar).

    c. Draw in the upper control limit for X, using a dotted line.

    d. Draw in the lower control limit for X, using a dotted line.

5. Plot your data for the lower chart, showing the time trend for the moving range between your measures (values of R):

    a. Plot the data for each point in time order (all the R's), and connect the dots, keeping in mind that the upper control limit must fit onto the chart.

    b. Draw in the center line using the average value of all the R's (R bar).

    c. Draw in the upper control limit for R (UCL_R), using a dotted line; there is no lower control limit for the moving range because absolute values are used to show point-to-point variation.

6. Interpret the results by studying them and understanding the patterns; use the common rules for interpreting control charts.

7. Overlay the target value (on the upper chart) for the measure that you have set as a performance goal and determine whether your system has or has not yet reached the desired level or whether you are approaching the target level.

How Do You Interpret Control Chart Results?

As we mentioned earlier, you can interpret your control chart results using the same approach used for run charts except that now you have another way to identify possible special cause signals in your data. You will know you have a likely special cause signal when one or more points fall outside the upper or lower control limits.

    Figures 22.13, 22.14, and 22.15 illustrate special cause signals occurring in control charts.

FIGURE 22.13. SPECIAL CAUSE SIGNAL: EIGHT CONSECUTIVE POINTS ON SAME SIDE OF CENTER LINE.

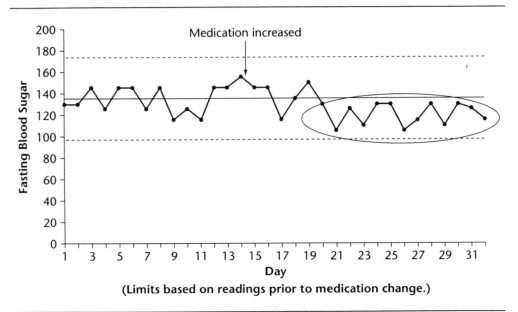

(Limits based on readings prior to medication change.)

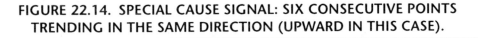

FIGURE 22.14. SPECIAL CAUSE SIGNAL: SIX CONSECUTIVE POINTS TRENDING IN THE SAME DIRECTION (UPWARD IN THIS CASE).

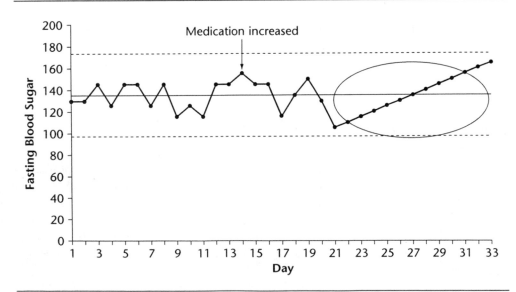

FIGURE 22.15. SPECIAL CAUSE SIGNAL: A POINT OUTSIDE A CONTROL LIMIT.

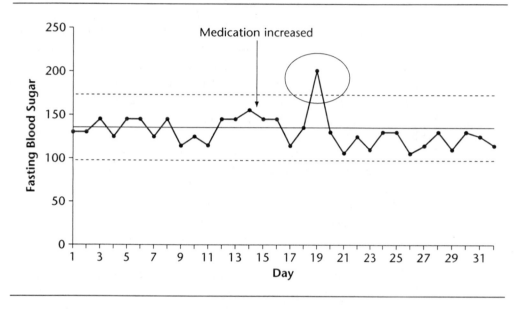

When Do You Recalculate Control Chart Values?

As you start using control charts and run charts in your microsystem—and as you measure processes and make changes that lead to improvement—you will also need to know when to recalculate the values (the average value and the upper and lower control limits) on your control charts.

For example, once you have ascended the improvement ramp and your microsystem has achieved a new level of performance, you should consider recalculating the center line and the control limits, using the new pattern of data that your process is producing. To do this, you will accumulate twelve to twenty-five new observations, made after the level of performance changed, and use this new series of data points to calculate the center line and the control limits. You may wish to make provisional calculations based on twelve points and then make further calculations—ones that you expect to be "fixed" for a time—after reaching twenty-five data points.

In general it is smart to consider recalculating your control chart's average value and control limits when you see any substantial change in the process (in a positive or a negative direction) signaled by a consistent shift in the data (such as consistently running eight or more points above or below the center line).

What Are Some Tips for Using Run Charts and Control Charts?

- *Take intelligent action.* Remember that the purpose of measuring and monitoring is to gain information that helps you answer critical questions and then to take intelligent action. The more you use your data to answer good questions and to guide action, the more successful you will be at improving processes and in taking some of the *chaos* out of your microsystem's worklife.
- *Make a data wall.* Display a data wall that has run charts and control charts, and use it to discuss everyone's work.
- *Hold daily huddles.* Hold your daily huddles by your data wall so you can make use of that information to monitor your work and to stay close to improvements being tested.
- *Have a data captain.* Ask one of the numbers-oriented staff in your microsystem to serve as the data captain for a period of time and to take responsibility for making and posting trend charts. Alternatively, develop a *data squad* so that several members of the microsystem share this responsibility.
- *Stay close to the data.* When you are running tests of change, draw the run charts (or control charts) on large flipchart pages, and post new values as close to real time as possible (such as hourly, at the end of each shift, or at the end of the workday).
- *Take advantage of technology.* Use electronic spread sheets with control chart *macros* embedded in them to make it easy to enter data and to have your control charts "automatically" produced by the software. This is easy to do in standard spreadsheet programs, such as Microsoft Excel. Alternatively, use special statistical packages that have control charts and run charts included as options.
- *Compile trend reports.* Develop routine reports (daily, monthly, quarterly, and yearly) that make use of the power of showing trends in data over time and are based on run-chart and control-chart methods.

Case Studies

Intermediate Cardiac Care Unit (ICCU)

The measurements the ICCU lead improvement team tracked during the system's PDSA cycles included the following:

- Number of patients discharged before noon
- Portion of newly admitted patients who receive a bed assignment within thirty minutes of staff notifying the ICCU

- Patient satisfaction with the discharge and admission processes
- Staff ratings of interdisciplinary communication and ease of discharge and admission processes

Plastic Surgery Section

Several measures were used during the lead improvement team's PDSA cycles to evaluate the impact of shared medical appointments. Patient satisfaction was measured through qualitative and quantitative measures. An important measure was whether or not the patients felt all their questions were answered. This patient-reported measure showed the greatest gain from the shared medical appointment process for patients considering breast reduction.

The primary success measure was access to care. The initial access backlog measure changed over time after shared medical appointments were launched. The baseline value for the third next available appointment was ninety-nine days and it improved to thirty days over a one-year period.

Review Questions

1. How do control charts differ from run charts?
2. What is the importance of having a data wall for visually displaying measures?
3. How can you establish responsibility for data collection and analysis?

Between Sessions Work

1. Create a run or control chart specific to your PDSA cycle.
2. Display the chart on a data wall for all staff to see real-time progress.
3. Build measurement into every microsystem member's activities.

References

Shewhart, W. A. (1980). *Economic control of quality of manufactured product.* Milwaukee, WI: American Society for Quality Control. (Original work published 1931)

Shewhart, W. A., with Deming, W. E. (1986). *Statistical method from the viewpoint of quality control.* New York: Dover. (Original work published 1939)

Wheeler, D. J. (1993). *Understanding variation: The key to managing chaos.* Knoxville, TN: SPC Press.

Wheeler, D. J. (1995). *Advanced topics in statistical process control.* Knoxville, TN: SPC Press.

CHAPTER TWENTY-THREE

ACTION PLANS AND GANTT CHARTS

Chapter Purpose

Aim. To create a clear action plan of next steps for planning and monitoring improvement activities and progress made.

    Objectives. At the completion of this unit, you will be able to

- Describe the importance of an action plan.
- Differentiate between an action plan and a Gantt chart.

- Explain the connections among the action plan, the Gantt chart, and your improvement work.
- Describe how to manage improvement activities over time.
- Write an action plan or Gantt chart, or both.

A s your microsystem members begin to blend Job 1—doing the work—with Job 2—improving the way they do the work—it will be smart to look ahead to the future and to devise a plan to follow over time. A good time to make a first draft plan is when you begin making tests of change (see Figure 23.1). By this time you will have started to get a sense of pace, rhythm, and discipline; these can be reinforced by using time-planning tools. As described in this chapter, action plans keep immediate activities on track, and Gantt charts keep the big picture and major steps in the overall journey on track.

FIGURE 23.1. IMPROVEMENT RAMP: ACTION PLANS AND GANTT CHARTS.

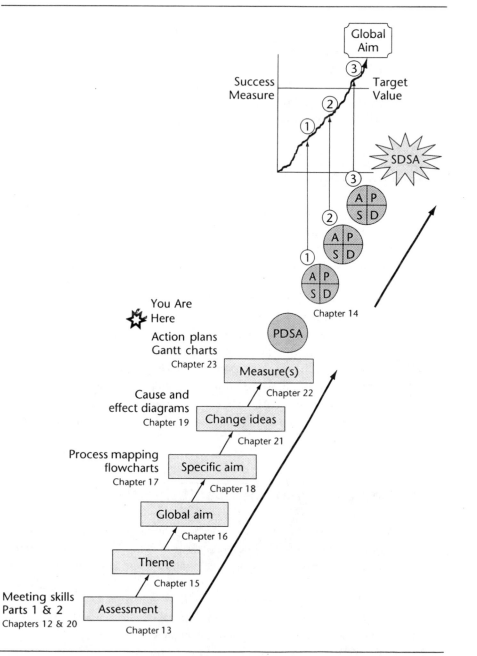

What Is an Action Plan?

An *action plan* is a list of tasks specific to the next steps that need to be completed to achieve your stated improvement goals. The action plan is a simple, helpful organizing tool to keep improvement activities on track over time. It is often created at the end of the weekly improvement meeting to ensure that all the steps that need to be completed before the next meeting are achieved and to document additional action steps and timelines. The action plan changes weekly and is updated as tasks are completed.

What Is a Gantt Chart?

A *Gantt chart* is a horizontal bar chart developed by Henry L. Gantt (1910), an American engineer and social scientist. Gantt charts are useful tools that are frequently used to manage overall improvement work. A Gantt chart provides a graphical illustration of the improvement activity schedule; it helps you to plan, coordinate, and track specific tasks. It allows you to show how long an improvement initiative is expected to take, to determine the resources needed, and to lay out the order in which tasks will be carried out.

A Gantt chart may be used to plan the entire improvement initiative. These charts may be simple displays drawn by hand on graph paper or complex diagrams made with computer programs such as Microsoft Project or Excel.

When improvement activities are under way, Gantt charts help you to monitor whether the activities are on schedule. If they are not on schedule, these charts allow you to pinpoint the remedial action necessary to put them back on schedule.

Why Use Action Plans and Gantt Charts?

Action plans and Gantt charts help busy clinical teams stay on track with intended improvement activities. They also serve to record who is to do what, and when, and to track progress over time. Action plans and Gantt charts

- Help you lay out the tasks that need to be completed.
- Provide a basis for scheduling when tasks will be carried out.
- Specify the resources needed to complete the tasks.
- Clarify the critical path for an improvement activity.

How Do You Write an Action Plan?

At the end of each weekly improvement meeting, an action plan should be completed to maintain the momentum and rhythm of improvement. To create an action plan, first, list the tasks that need to be carried out to achieve the goal. Second, list who will complete each task by a certain date. It is helpful to list the actual completion dates and the actual names of the individuals responsible for completing each task.

How Do You Create a Gantt Chart?

A Gantt chart tracks the progress of the improvement journey over time. List the steps or tasks in the overall improvement process on the left-hand side of the chart and then create horizontal bars on the right to show when each phase of the improvement process is scheduled to occur (see Figure 23.2). When improvements are begun, it helps to strategize about the improvement activities over the upcoming months. This will help you and your team maintain the pace of improvement.

FIGURE 23.2. EXAMPLE OF A GANTT CHART.

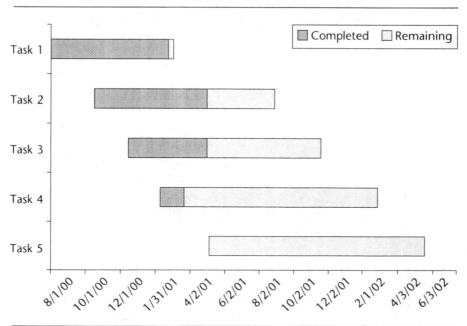

What Are the Next Steps?

Once you have created your action plan, it is smart to track the completion of the listed tasks between weekly meetings. Follow up with individuals who have been assigned to each task to determine their progress and to offer assistance as needed.

Sometimes, due to competing interests and limited time, a task may not be completed by the next scheduled meeting. Adjustments to the agenda and timeline may need to be made if the deadline is not met.

The Gantt chart can be reviewed to monitor progress over time; it can be modified based on actual experience. To keep everyone's energy high, it is helpful to periodically review what has been accomplished.

Case Studies

Intermediate Cardiac Care Unit (ICCU)

Each weekly meeting of the ICCU lead improvement team produces action plans to follow up between meetings. An example of an action plan detailing next steps follows:

- Stay with PDSA 7.
- Give the attending physician's beeper to the nurse practitioner to decrease interruptions during rounds.
- Post a sign on the conference room door to decrease interruptions during rounds.
- Adjust "scripts" for each role during morning rounds to accurately reflect what the roles are reporting and to keep everyone on track; repost the scripts on the wall for all to see during rounds.
- Use the charge nurse beeper to alert each RN when it is time for that RN to come to the conference room to report on her or his patients.

The ICCU team members created a Gantt chart to provide a road map for their long-term improvement activities and to help them to stay on track (Figure 23.3).

Plastic Surgery Section

Since 2003, the Plastic Surgery Section lead improvement team has continued to meet weekly and improve processes and roles. The weekly meetings have changed

Action Item	Responsible	Jan. '06				Feb. '06				March '06				April '06				May '06				June '06				July '06			
Month / Week		1	2	3	4	1	2	3	4	1	2	3	4	1	2	3	4	1	2	3	4	1	2	3	4	1	2	3	4
Organize and conduct weekly meetings	Jean/Ed																												
Create PDSA for A.M. rounds in conference room	Lead Improvement Team																												
Interdisciplinary morning walking rounds	Jean & Ed																												
Optimization of roles with standardization of function	Jean & Shelly																												
New care model design	Jean & Pilot Group																												

over time. Team members now use laptop computers to research data during the meeting, and they have an LCD projector to display findings for all to see during the meeting. They continue to work through their list of changes and to engage new members of the Plastic Surgery Section to learn about improvement and apply the concepts in daily practice. Both leaders and microsystem members realize improvement is a continuous journey. Not only are there weekly improvement meetings but the section also holds monthly all-staff meetings to ensure that everyone is aware of improvements and to provide opportunities to discuss progress and new initiatives. Annual retreats are part of the microsystem culture; they are held to review progress and to set goals for the coming year.

The improvement activity has moved beyond just the section's outpatient practice. Active discussions and applications of improvement knowledge and tools are occurring with the operating room staff and other specialty groups who share patient populations with the Plastic Surgery Section. Improvement science is the foundation for all their activities. They have developed the habit of comingling, doing their work (Job 1) along with improving their work (Job 2).

Review Questions

1. What is the difference between an action plan and a Gantt chart?
2. What are the benefits of action plans and Gantt charts?
3. How might a Gantt chart boost morale?

Between Sessions Work

1. Write a Gantt chart specific to your long-term improvement plan.
2. Each week, write an action plan to promote between-meeting completion of tasks.

Reference

Gantt, H. L. (1910). *Work, wages, and profits: Their influence on the cost of living.* New York: Engineering Magazine.

CHAPTER TWENTY-FOUR

FOLLOW THROUGH ON IMPROVEMENT

Storyboards, Data Walls, and Playbooks

Chapter Purpose

Aim. To make plans to tell the improvement story, measure progress over time, and sustain improvement using standard processes.

    Objectives. At the completion of this unit, you will be able to

- Describe the improvement fundamentals needed to maintain and sustain improvement.
- Identify where improvement data can be posted for viewing by all microsystem members to increase their knowledge about purpose, progress, and priorities.
- Design a microsystem playbook that documents standard ways of performing processes and that can be used in orientation, performance appraisals, and daily improvement work.
- Develop a storyboard to document your microsystem's improvement journey and progress made over time.

It is essential to anchor new ways of thinking, behaving, and communicating in the daily environment of the microsystem. This chapter discusses three tangible products that are extremely valuable for fostering microsystem cultural transformation—storyboards, data walls, and playbooks. Each of these products helps you create a visual environment; they are viewable artifacts that reinforce the microsystem's aspiration to be a high-performing unit.

What Is the Importance of Follow Through?

Well-intended efforts to make meaningful improvements are at risk of not being sustained over time after early aims are achieved. Systems and processes are constantly under pressure, professionals come and go, processes morph as time passes, and unless someone is actively doing the *follow-through*, improvements can be lost. Intentional planning to hold the gains, through monitoring processes and reviewing data, is essential to prevent old habits from encroaching on the new and improved ways.

What Can You Do to Follow Through?

The key follow-through activities for microsystem leaders are following the fundamentals of improvement, creating a data wall to display ongoing performance measures, creating and updating a microsystem playbook, and maintaining a storyboard of the system's improvement journey.

What Are the Fundamentals of Improvement?

Practicing the fundamentals of microsystem improvement is important to ensure that the right things consistently happen in your microsystem. These fundamentals include

- *Leadership.* Ensure that the microsystem has an effective leadership team—often a physician and a nurse or an administrative person—that communicates and reinforces the microsystem's vision in words and action.
- *Discipline.* Consistently use improvement science methods when change is required. Using the improvement model and the techniques embodied in the Dartmouth Microsystem Improvement Curriculum will foster continued learning, new habits, and ongoing growth.
- *Rhythm.* Maintain the weekly or biweekly lead improvement team meetings and use effective meeting skills. Holding daily huddles to review clinical care and improvement progress helps to remind everyone of the imperative for ongoing improvement. Monthly all-staff meetings should have improvement on every

agenda to promote the vitality of the process. Reporting of data specific to new improvements and conducting process monitoring keep metrics that matter on everyone's radar screen.

- *Pace.* Clinical care has its ups and downs. Continuing to maintain the rhythm just described, even during peak periods of clinical activity, is important. Be sensitive to high-volume, high-acuity times; avoid launching work on new improvement themes when it will compete with clinical demands.

What Is a Data Wall?

A data wall is a clearly defined physical space where vital measures of performance can be posted on the wall for all members of the microsystem to review. The posted measures can reflect not only the microsystem's improvement work and performance metrics but also the work and metrics of the larger organization. Chapter Twenty-Two recommends identifying a *data captain* and building measurement into daily work. It is important to know who will *own* the data wall and keep it up to date and relevant. The data captain can own the data wall, review the metrics on a regular basis, and determine, with the lead improvement team, when data no longer need to be posted and which subset of data will be needed for monitoring.

Data come from many sources; they can be provided by the macrosystem or the microsystem may collect its own data. Secretaries, nurses, physicians, assistive personnel, patients, and families in the microsystem can all contribute vital information to the data wall. Using run charts and control charts to display data over time reinforces the idea that processes and outcomes vary as time passes and that a basic goal is to increase reliability. The data displays do not necessarily need to come from a software program; they can be simple pieces of graph paper showing daily, weekly, and monthly measures and can be posted manually by someone who is close to the process.

Many high-performing microsystems review their data walls at monthly all-staff meetings to (1) ensure that all members are informed of the gains being made, and (2) draw attention to early warning signs of poor results that require attention.

What Is a Playbook?

A playbook is a collection of core and supporting processes used routinely by your microsystem. It includes flowcharts and diagrams of processes that have been tested using improvement science and that represent "the way we want this process done." The aim of a playbook is to provide a place to collect standard processes of care.

How Is the Playbook Used?

The playbook is used to maintain high performance and to promote safety, efficacy, and efficiency. This can be accomplished in many ways:

- *Interviewing job candidates.* Review of the playbook offers clear communication about how the microsystem functions and how it expects members of the microsystem to interact with each other.
- *Orienting a new staff member.* The playbook is an efficient way to teach new staff about the way the microsystem work is done. Because playbooks use flowcharts and diagrams, the steps in each process are easy to understand. Flowcharts provide an easy way for new staff to learn and remember process steps.
- *Conducting performance reviews.* The playbook can be used for performance evaluation, enabling staff to review expected performance vis-à-vis actual performance. It can be used periodically to check whether everyone who uses a specific process is using the standard version of that process.
- *Orienting temporary staff.* Temporary staff—such as per diems, floats, and travelers—may become part of your microsystem for a period of time. The playbook is a helpful resource for them, helping them do their work the right way.

How Do You Create a Playbook?

Once you have completed testing changes to a process, you can create the *final* (SDSA) version of how that process should be executed all the time. It is usually best to use a deployment flowchart to show what actions should be taken by whom and in what order.

In addition to flowchart(s), the playbook can include tools that support the process, such as

- Data collection forms
- Blank forms such as huddle sheets and report forms
- Pictures of how to complete a process

There are three basic steps to making a playbook:

1. *Table of contents.* Create a table of contents listing the individual processes included. A notebook is a convenient place to store the materials and to make

it easy to copy and update the flowcharts. You may wish to create an electronic playbook to provide better access and to simplify updates.

2. *Checklist templates.* Complete a playbook checklist for each process (see Figure 24.1) to outline what is included in each section and when updates are scheduled.

3. *Flowcharts.* Following each checklist, insert the appropriate process flowchart(s) and additional information. Repeat this for each process listed in the table of contents. If you are using a notebook, consider using clear *sleeves* to store the flowcharts and forms, in order to protect the pages and to make extra copies readily available.

How Do You Maintain Your Playbook?

Playbooks evolve over time as you test processes and identify new best practices. It is important to *refresh* your playbook at predetermined intervals and when improvement cycles are done. Not only should the playbook be refreshed but critical review of the SDSA processes over time will often identify the need to move from SDSA back to PDSA, because of new knowledge, new equipment, or new technology. A key principle of the PDSA $\leftrightarrow$ SDSA method is the notion that ongoing improvement work shifts back and forth between experimentation and standardization.

Use the checklist to identify who will be responsible for reviewing and updating and when the process will be kept current. In general, people who are part of the process should be the ones responsible for keeping the playbook current.

A good method to ensure that the recommended steps in a process are being completed as planned is to identify someone to observe the current process, step by step, and make notes when the steps are not performed as documented.

Performance lapses may occur for assorted reasons:

- The individuals were not aware of the best practice.
- The process has changed but the playbook has not been updated.
- Some people have decided to execute the process using their own style.
- Changes have occurred in equipment or materials or supplies.
- A physical space has changed.

All of these reasons reveal why playbooks, education, and reminders are important. Staying close to the process helps you to identify when the playbook needs to change and when new flowcharts need to be completed.

FIGURE 24.1. PLAYBOOK CHECKLIST TEMPLATE.

PLAYBOOK CHECKLIST

Name of Process _____

Contact Person _____

Which of the following are included in this section?

☐   Flowcharts

        ☐ _____

        ☐ _____

        ☐ _____

        ☐ _____

☐   Forms

        ☐ _____

        ☐ _____

        ☐ _____

        ☐ _____

☐   Data collection sheets: Include measures that will be monitored to ensure
standardized process specifications are being followed.

        ☐ _____

        ☐ _____

        ☐ _____

        ☐ _____

☐   Pictures

        ☐ _____

        ☐ _____

        ☐ _____

        ☐ _____

WHO will observe, review & update? _____
                                         Name

                _____
                           Frequency of Review

DATE of review _____
                               Date

DATE to report findings of review to lead improvement team _____
                                                              Date

What Is a Storyboard?

Storyboards can communicate the highlights of your work to others in a way that is easy to follow and graphically interesting. The storyboard communicates more in graphs and pictures than in words. The format is easy to use, maintain, and read, and it memorializes achievements. Someone new to the work should be able to understand what was done and why by following the logic of the storyboard's graphical displays, data analyses, and conclusions.

How Do You Make a Storyboard?

There are many ways to construct a storyboard. You can make one the old-fashioned way, using boards and graphics and pictures on paper. Increasingly, however, people are choosing to use Microsoft PowerPoint to create a storyboard as a PowerPoint slide, and then to print that slide as a poster, using a large format printer. This method allows you to import data and other graphics directly into PowerPoint and to create the poster without rework.

Materials often used for a storyboard include

- Foam core board for a freestanding display
- Colored poster board
- Pictures
- Graphics, data, flowcharts, and fishbone diagrams
- Spray glue

A general format for a storyboard follows. Start your story in the upper-left-hand corner.

1. List your facility's name, microsystem name, and lead improvement team's name. In addition:
   - Supply the location of the facility.
   - List the names or roles of the team members involved in improvement efforts.
   - Give the dates of interaction and a timeline.
2. Document your AIM statement:
   - State what you and your team were trying to accomplish.
   - Include the area worked in and the scope of the aim. If applicable, also mention the extent of the spread of improvement beyond the initial area and scope.
3. List the diagnostic tools used to identify the need to improve.
4. List the measures monitored during the improvement cycles.

5. List the change ideas implemented. Also list the change ideas tested.
6. Display qualitative and quantitative results.
7. Summarize the effort, and indicate the next steps.

Discussion

The improvement journey is hard work and never ends. Even harder is ensuring that the improvement gains and successes you have made are sustained and continuously improved on. High-performing microsystems continue to achieve success and reach new levels of performance when they stay true to the fundamentals of improvement, when they follow through—using data walls, playbooks, and storyboards—and when they keep improvement omnipresent in busy clinical settings. The follow-through tools presented here will help you keep the visual environment vibrant with improvement knowledge and outcomes and serve as reminders to celebrate improvement progress by the members of the microsystem. The habits of improvement need to be woven into the fabric of everyday work and reinforced using (1) visual reminders, (2) meeting skills, and (3) active engagement from everyone.

Case Studies

Intermediate Cardiac Care Unit (ICCU)

The ICCU lead improvement team maintains a dynamic storyboard for all ICCU staff to review (see Figure 24.2). This storyboard serves as an educational source for staff to communicate progress and as a talking point for leaders and others who visit the ICCU. The conference room walls chronicle the history of ICCU's improvement journey because meeting notes are recorded on flipcharts along with graphics and diagrams.

The data wall continues to grow, blending organizational measures with relevant ICCU data. The data portray real-time progress and help keep the ICCU team alert to progress and trends that might trigger investigation.

The ICCU playbook is under construction. The lead improvement team's initial work resulted in a clear, uniform process for interdisciplinary morning rounds participation with defined roles, defined content for reports, and action items.

Plastic Surgery Section

A visual display of improvement activities and the 5 P's provide constant reminders of the focus and goals of improvement for the Plastic Surgery Section (see Figure 24.3). The data wall keeps staff current on performance and shows when certain processes

FIGURE 24.2. STORYBOARD DISPLAY OF THE ICCU IMPROVEMENT JOURNEY.

Case Study: Intermediate Cardiac Care Unit
Dartmouth-Hitchcock Medical Center, Lebanon, New Hampshire

PURPOSE
The ICCU will create an environment in which cardiac patients and their families can receive excellent, comprehensive, specialized state of the art quality care.

TEAM

Jean R.N.	Joanne
Shelly	Dara
Melanie	Laurie
Edward M.D.	Dhaval
Kate	Mary
Jessica	Lucia
Shelby	Tiffany
Nancy	Marcia (cardiac patient)

TIMELINE
January '06
Attended Coach the Coach (educational session)
Established regular team meetings with effective meeting skills
Review 5P's
February '06
Begin interdisciplinary rounds
March '06
Interdisciplinary rounds clarification of roles in rounds
Creation of script for each role
Order of reporting modified
Discharge ticket initiated
April '06
Continued testing of rounding report process
Discharge planning ticket revised

DIAGNOSIS
THEME: Communication
Global Aim
  We aim to improve the process of communication in our ICCU. The process begins with the initial notification of the need for patient admission. The process ends with the appropriate discharge disposition of the patient. By working on this process we expect: Improved patient care and efficiency; improved flow of consistent information between patients, providers and families, improved communication along the health care continuum; a reduction in readmissions; a reduction in stress. It is important to work on this process now because we have identified the need to improve: satisfaction of patients, families, and care professionals. We need to eliminate near misses and errors due to poor communication and have clearer plans of care.

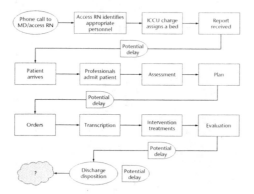

Specific Aim Statement
We aim to assign and communicate assigned bed for patients within 30 minutes of request for admission.

  Measures
  1. Time from phone call to time of admit bed communicated
  2. # of admissions/day
  3. % of discharges before noon (to open beds for admits)

Figure 19.5 Fishbone Diagram: ICCU Bed Assignment*

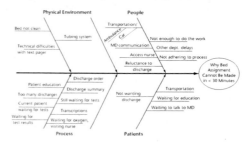

*Note. This figure shows the factors that contribute to the delays in bed assignment that prevent achievement of the specific aim: assign and communicate bed assignment for needed admission in 30 minutes

PDSA CYCLES

PDSA Ramp of Tests*

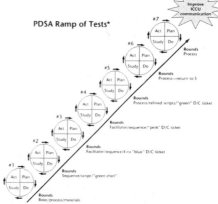

*Note. The ICCU team used repeated rapid tests of change, based on stringing together PDSA cycles, to attain the aim regarding improving the communication process of morning rounds.

NEXT STEPS
1. Continue to test interdisciplinary morning rounds.
2. Prepare scripts and process to move interdisciplinary morning rounds to the bedside to include patients and families.
3. Review and post data on data wall.
4. Review roles and functions to ensure optimized roles.
5. Consider redesign of "care teams" to improve continuity and reliability of patient care.

FIGURE 24.3. PLASTIC SURGERY SECTION DATA WALL.

Ambulatory Clinical Practice Committee

Surgery

Plastic Surgery

Technical Excellence

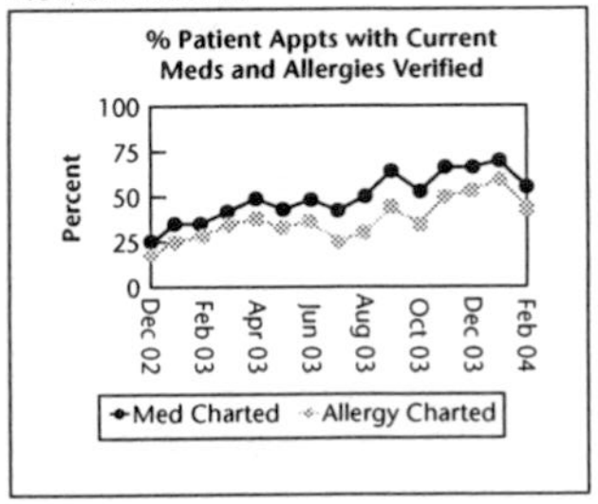
% Patient Appts with Current Meds and Allergies Verified
Percent
100
75
50
25
0
Dec 02
Feb 03
Apr 03
Jun 03
Aug 03
Oct 03
Dec 03
Feb 04
Med Charted
Allergy Charted

Service Excellence

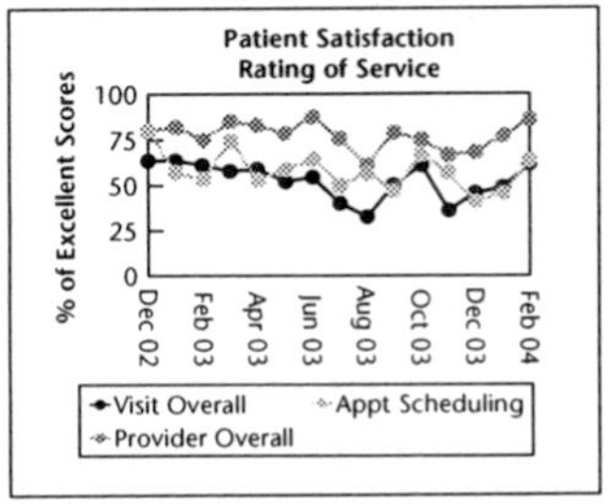
Patient Satisfaction Rating of Service
% of Excellent Scores
100
75
50
25
0
Dec 02
Feb 03
Apr 03
Jun 03
Aug 03
Oct 03
Dec 03
Feb 04
Visit Overall
Appt Scheduling
Provider Overall

Patient Characteristics

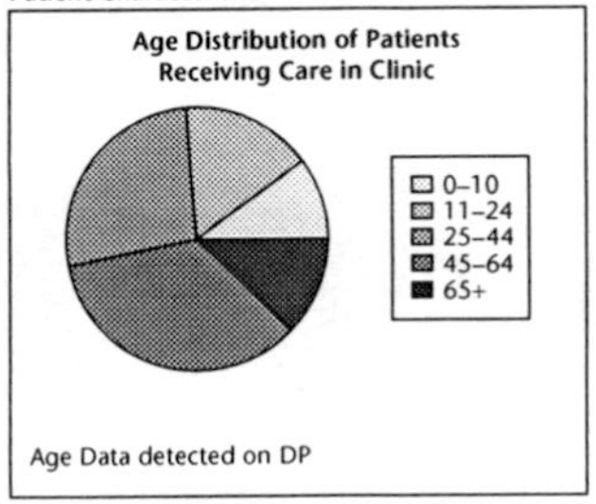
Age Distribution of Patients Receiving Care in Clinic
0–10
11–24
25–44
45–64
65+
Age Data detected on DP

Cost Excellence

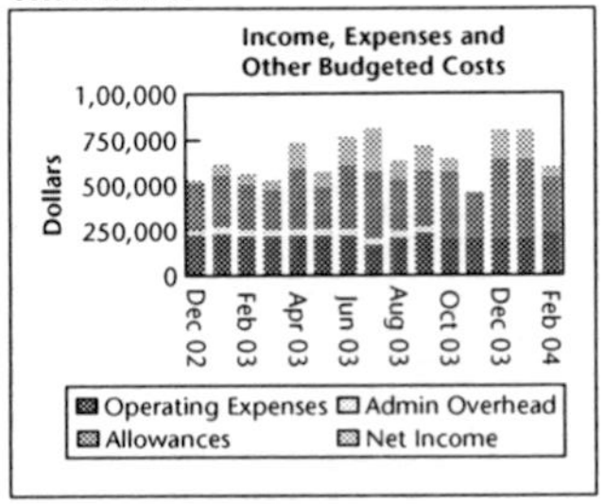
Income, Expenses and Other Budgeted Costs
Dollars
1,00,000
750,000
500,000
250,000
0
Dec 02
Feb 03
Apr 03
Jun 03
Aug 03
Oct 03
Dec 03
Feb 04
Operating Expenses
Admin Overhead
Allowances
Net Income

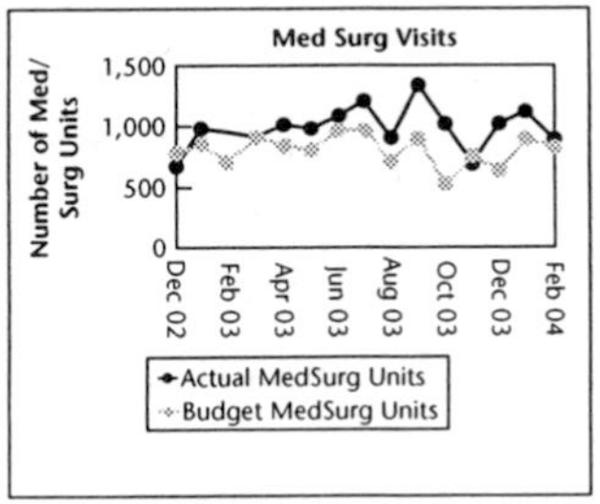
Med Surg Visits
Number of Med/ Surg Units
1,500
1,000
500
0
Dec 02
Feb 03
Apr 03
Jun 03
Aug 03
Oct 03
Dec 03
Feb 04
Actual MedSurg Units
Budget MedSurg Units

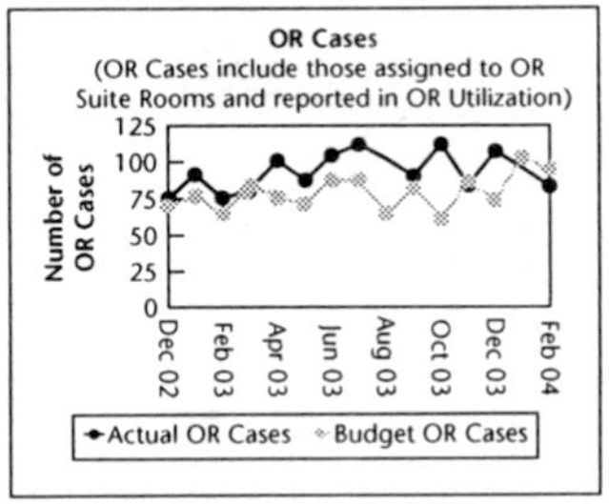
OR Cases
(OR Cases include those assigned to OR Suite Rooms and reported in OR Utilization)
Number of OR Cases
125
100
75
50
25
0
Dec 02
Feb 03
Apr 03
Jun 03
Aug 03
Oct 03
Dec 03
Feb 04
Actual OR Cases
Budget OR Cases

Ambulatory Clinical Practice Committee

Surgery

Plastic Surgery

Cost Excellence: Volume and Efficiency

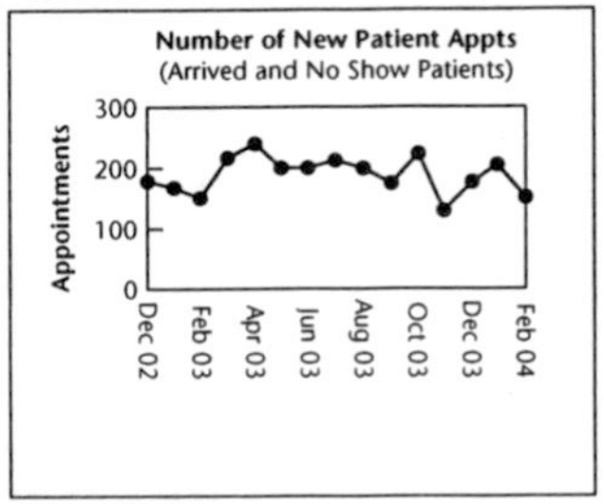
Number of New Patient Appts
(Arrived and No Show Patients)
Appointments
300
200
100
0
Dec 02
Feb 03
Apr 03
Jun 03
Aug 03
Oct 03
Dec 03
Feb 04

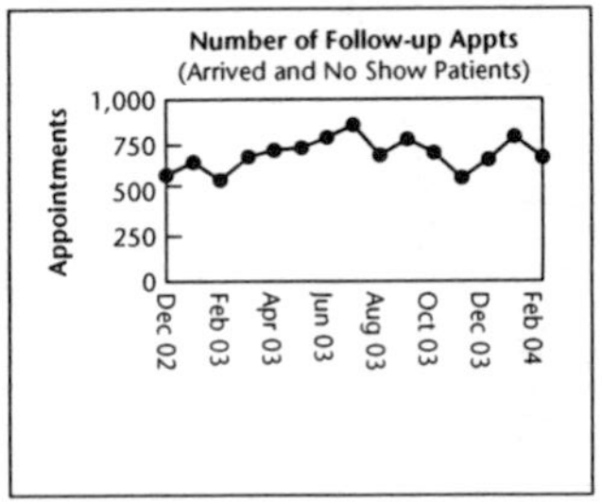
Number of Follow-up Appts
(Arrived and No Show Patients)
Appointments
1,000
750
500
250
0
Dec 02
Feb 03
Apr 03
Jun 03
Aug 03
Oct 03
Dec 03
Feb 04

Service Excellence: Access

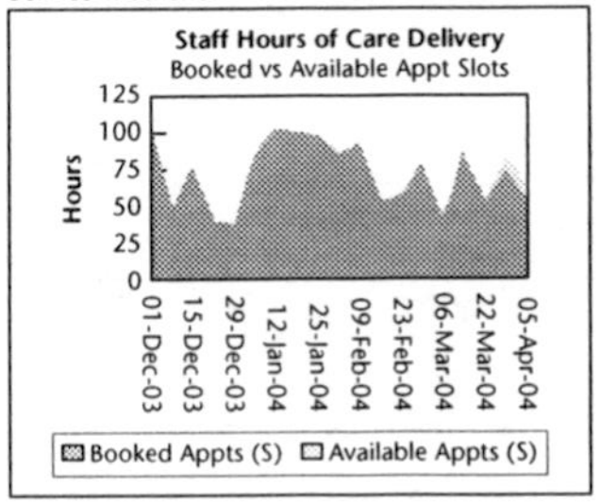
Staff Hours of Care Delivery
Booked vs Available Appt Slots
Hours
125
100
75
50
25
0
01-Dec-03
15-Dec-03
29-Dec-03
12-Jan-04
25-Jan-04
09-Feb-04
23-Feb-04
06-Mar-04
22-Mar-04
05-Apr-04
Booked Appts (S)
Available Appts (S)

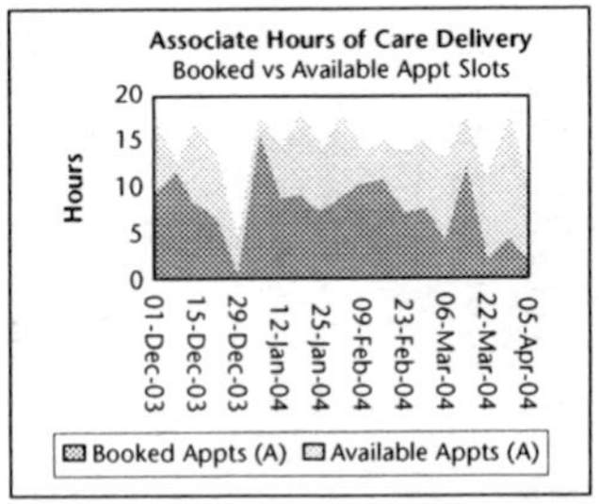
Associate Hours of Care Delivery
Booked vs Available Appt Slots
Hours
20
15
10
5
0
01-Dec-03
15-Dec-03
29-Dec-03
12-Jan-04
25-Jan-04
09-Feb-04
23-Feb-04
06-Mar-04
22-Mar-04
05-Apr-04
Booked Appts (A)
Available Appts (A)

Top 10 Conditions/Diagnoses	% of All OP Dxs
Other aftercare	32.2
Other skin disorders	9.9
Open wounds of head, neck, and trunk	5.5
Residual codes, unclassified	5.3
Nonmalignant breast conditions	4.7
Other congenital anomalis	4.4
Chronic ulcer of skin	4.3
Other nervous system disorders	3.9
Other and unspecified design necalism	3.6
Other connective tissues disease	3.1

Referring Provider Distribution	% of All OP Referrals
ALL OTHER	42.0
INTERNAL-LEBANON	29.3
DOCTOR NOT ENTERED	25.4
INTERNAL-NORTHERN REGIONAL OFFICE	3.3
INTERNAL-SOUTHERN REGION	0.0
INTERNAL-NO LONGER ACTIVE	0.0
DOCTOR NONE/SELF/UNKNOWN	0.0

may need attention to avoid backsliding. The Plastic Surgery playbook continues to grow. Scheduling methods, contingency plans, daily huddles, and shared medical appointments are some of the activities contained in this microsystem's playbook.

Review Questions

1. What are the essential follow-through practices that sustain and monitor improvement gains?
2. What fundamentals of improvement maintain the momentum of improvement?
3. How do data walls, storyboards, and playbooks compare and contrast?
4. What playbook functions can be used in a microsystem?

Between Sessions Work

1. Create a storyboard showing your microsystem's current state.
2. Start and maintain a data wall of results, achievements, and processes to be monitored.
3. Create and actively manage your microsystem playbook.

CHAPTER TWENTY-FIVE

CONCLUSION

Continuing on the Path to Excellence

In this, the final chapter, we will take a quick look back to recap what has been covered and then we will provide a quick glimpse of the future and offer an invitation to you to get started on using microsystem thinking to make a difference in your part of the world.

Looking Back

We set out to write this book to provide health care system leaders with a good start for improving care from the inside out, beginning with microsystems—the places where patients and families and care teams meet. We have explained how microsystems are the natural building blocks that come together to form all health systems—both small ones and large ones. If you keep your eye on the patient, you will find professionals and support staff forming a system around that patient to attempt to ease the burden of illness. The first main message is that health care professionals, patients, and families can have successful health care systems if, and only if, those systems have successful microsystems that *perfect* their own processes and *perfect* the handoffs of patients, services, and information between and across microsystems.

In Part One of this book we provided case studies from the real world to highlight high-performing microsystems and the principles and methods on which their achievements are based. We explored many critical facets of microsystems—leading and leadership, measuring and measurement, designing care and services for discrete populations, building staff capability and morale, and designing safety and reliability into the fabric of the microsystem. And most important, we began to show how microsystem thinking can be used strategically and operationally to enable senior and midlevel leaders to create the conditions in their organizations for genuine empowerment of staff and for ongoing improvement and innovation at the frontlines of care. We believe strongly that the greater the focus of the front office on what happens at the front line, the greater the chance for the organization's health mission to be more than nice words that have only limited carryover into daily operations.

In Part Two of this book we provided a way to get started, or as Donald Berwick is fond of saying, *a path forward*. The path that we point out is open to anyone who cares about building improvement efforts into the daily work of health care professionals. The first and most important message behind Part Two is the concept that in today's world every health care professional really has two jobs—doing the work and improving the work. This is easy to say, and many people are beginning to see the need for this but have not yet found a way to translate the need into action with traction. We offered the Dartmouth Microsystem Improvement Curriculum (DMIC) as a step-by-step guide for getting started along the path to improving care as part of everyone's daily work.

By starting with teams hailing from intact, naturally occurring clinical microsystems and their supporting macrosystems, we have seen that it is possible to begin to make cultural transformations in frontline clinical units. Real people have made real improvements in important outcomes measures, in worklife, and in organizational performance by using this learn-and-take-action method. Therefore, over time, we developed a powerful learning program—one that can be adapted to virtually any clinical setting and that can provide the knowledge, methods, and value-based rationale for making improvement integral to the daily work of frontline teams.

In Chapters Ten to Twenty-Four we traced out proven methods and techniques for diagnosing the strengths and weaknesses of microsystems, and we showed how this information can be used to test changes iteratively, to redesign care systems, and to make measured improvements that can be sustained. We firmly believe that absent the creation of process mindedness, systems thinking, and a penchant for experimenting with ways to improve quality and value, there is little hope for positive changes that are deep and lasting. Learning new ways of thinking, doing, and acting (and unlearning old behaviors and sentiments) is the only sure pathway that we know of to transform health care.

By the way, if you have been wondering about what the Dartmouth Microsystem Improvement Curriculum led to in the cases cited in Part Two—the

Intermediate Cardiac Care Unit and the Plastic Surgery Section—you will be most interested in the following short answers.

Intermediate Cardiac Care Unit (ICCU)

This case study occurred over a brief, sixteen-week period, beginning in January 2006. The ICCU made significant headway using the DMIC approach. ICCU staff are learning to see new things in their microsystem and are learning to work together in new ways based on a common purpose. The unit's nursing director and medical director, who share the ICCU leadership, are also leading the way to clarify the vision and to set the rhythm, pace, and discipline of improvement. Their genuine commitment and role modeling have been critical to making these early efforts to improve the ICCU successful and visible. (For further information contact Jean.Tenhaken@hitchcock.org.)

Plastic Surgery Section

This case extended over a two-year period. After one leading physician in the Plastic Surgery Section began studying and applying microsystem thinking in her clinical unit, a lead improvement team was formed, and it has made great strides. First, team members have fine-tuned and popularized the shared medical appointment method and have applied it to several different clinical populations at the Dartmouth-Hitchcock Medical Center (DHMC). This in turn led to other clinical programs at DHMC adopting this innovative way of seeing patients, and now the approach has become a subject of evaluative research. In addition, the Plastic Surgery Section has had dramatic measured improvements in patient satisfaction, staff satisfaction, access to care, and clinical productivity. In fact this microsystem is now the leading clinical program for achieving productivity rates exceeding national benchmarks (its productivity is 125 percent of the relevant national benchmark value; the next most productive clinical program is 118 percent of the national norm). The motto of this microsystem is "work smarter not harder," and staff practice what they preach every day. (For further information contact Barb.Rieseberg@hitchcock.org.)

Looking Forward and an Invitation: Make It Personal and Make It Happen

We invite you to take microsystem thinking into all the nooks and crannies of your health system. Make a line-of-sight plan for going from statements of vision and mission and values and strategy all the way to the front line of care where these statements either become actions—for the benefit of patients and the community—or they do not. Make it possible for your health system to have the characteristics of a hologram. By this we mean that the smallest units embody all of the elements of the largest units with respect to the ends (vision) and the means (strategy) and the worthy aims (values) that inspire people to put forth their best effort and feel good about their work, rather than feeling worn down by the grind.

These images of taking improvement into all the nooks and crannies and of becoming holographic are based on a few principles that we have covered before and that are hard to deny:

- Systems thinking will be needed to improve the health care system.
- Smaller systems are embedded in bigger systems and function together to produce the results enjoyed or deplored by the larger systems.
- The best hope for making health systems ever better is for the members of these systems, at all levels, to work intelligently and consistently to improve results for patients and to improve their own worklife.

In light of these principles we would like to offer every reader an invitation. It is simple and has just four parts.

1. Read this book and think about what it says.
2. Try using the ideas and methods contained in this book. Start here and start now. Do what makes sense to you.
3. Master the ideas and methods. Refine and improve upon them based on your good judgment, your hard work, and your intelligent adaptation to the conditions that shape your world.
4. Celebrate your successes and share what you have learned with others and invite them to do what you have done.

We would like to hear from you about what you do and what you learn. Visit www.clinicalmicrosystem.org frequently and send us your results and stories.

We wish you good luck in turning your aspirations for achieving better outcomes and better working conditions into tangible results that you, your patients, and their families can be proud of.

APPENDIX A:
PRIMARY CARE WORKBOOK

Clinical Microsystems
The Place Where Patients, Families and Careteams Meet
Assessing, Diagnosing and Treating
Your Outpatient Primary Care Practice

> Purpose
> Patients
> Professionals
> Processes
> Patterns

www.clinicalmicrosystem.org

Strategies for Improving the Place Where Patients, Families, and Careteams Meet

Clinical microsystems are the frontline units that provide most health care to most people. They are the places where patients, families, and careteams meet. Microsystems also include support staff, processes, technology, and recurring patterns of information, behavior, and results. Central to every clinical microsystem is the patient.

The microsystem is the place where

- Care is made
- Quality, safety, reliability, efficiency, and innovation are made
- Staff morale and patient satisfaction are made

Microsystems are the building blocks that form practices. The quality of care can be no better than the quality produced by the small systems that come together to provide care. Here is the quality equation:

$$\text{Health System Quality} = \text{Quality of Microsystem 1} + \text{Quality of Microsystem 2} + \text{Quality of Microsystem 3} - n.$$

All health care professionals—and we believe all frontline clinical and support staff are professionals—have two jobs. Job 1 is to provide care. Job 2 is to improve care.

Finding time to improve care can be difficult, but the only way to improve and maintain quality, safety, efficiency, and flexibility is by blending analysis, change, measuring, and redesigning into the regular patterns and the daily habits of frontline clinicians and staff. Absent intelligent and dedicated improvement work by all staff in all units, quality, efficiency, and pride in work will not be made nor sustained.

This workbook provides tools and methods that busy careteams can use to improve the quality and value of patient care as well as the worklife of all staff who contribute to patient care. These methods can be adapted to a wide variety of clinical settings, large and small, urban and rural, community-based and academic. This workbook has been adapted from its original form to better integrate with the materials already provided in the chapters of this book.

This workbook provides a guide for making a *path forward* toward higher performance. Just as you can assess, diagnose, and treat patients, you can assess, diagnose, and treat your clinical microsystem. This workbook is designed to guide your clinical microsystem on a journey to develop better performance. There are many good ways to improve performance; research shows that this is one of those good ways.

You can access more examples, tools, talleysheets, and blank forms to customize at www.clinicalmicrosystem.org.

The Path Forward

Step 1: Organize a Lead Improvement Team

Successful, sustainable cultural change requires the commitment and active involvement of all members of the clinical microsystem. To keep the microsystem on track and focused, a lead improvement team, made up of representatives of all roles in the microsystem, should be formed.

Step 2: Do the Assessment

Assess your microsystem using the 5 P's as your guide. Review your current performance metrics.

- *Purpose*
- *Patients*
- *Professionals*
- *Processes*
- *Patterns*
- Metrics that matter

Step 3: Make a Diagnosis

Using the information you gathered in Step 2, review your 5 P's assessment and your metrics that matter to make your diagnosis. You should select a *theme* and *aims* for improvement that reflect this diagnosis and your organization's strategic priorities.

Step 4: Treat Your Microsystem

Use scientific improvement methods and tools.

Step 5: Follow Up

Design and execute monitoring processes, outcomes, and results. Once you have achieved success with your first improvement theme, move to your next improvement theme.

Step 1: Organize a Lead Improvement Team

Assemble a lead improvement team to represent all disciplines and roles in your practice. Include MDs, RNs, NPs, clinical support staff, clerical staff, and patients and their families, along with any other professionals who are regularly in your practice providing care and service.

Must Do's

- Have the lead team meet weekly to maintain focus, make plans, and oversee improvement work.
- Use effective meeting skills in the weekly meetings.
- Hold monthly *all*-staff meetings to engage and inform all members of the practice.
- Explore creative ways to communicate and stay engaged with all staff on all shifts and all days of the week. Use e-mail, newsletters, listservs, messages on paper, verbal messages, visual displays, communication boards, conference calls, and buddy systems.
- Remember, true innovation is achieved through active engagement of the patient and his or her family with the lead team.

Step 2: Assess Your Primary Care Practice

Complete the "5 P's" assessment. This process needs to be completed by the interdisciplinary lead improvement team. Building common knowledge and insight into the microsystem among all members of the practice will create a sense that everyone has equal value and ability to contribute to the improvement activities.

Start with purpose. Why does your practice exist?
Raise this question with *everyone* in your practice to create the best statement of purpose, one that everyone can buy into.

Assess your patients, professionals, processes, and patterns using the tools provided here and in the chapters. The aim is to create the *big picture* of your system, to see beyond one patient at a time. Assessing the 5 P's and then reflecting on their connections and interdependence often reveals new improvement and redesign opportunities.

Create a timeline for the assessment process. Some microsystems have the capacity and resources to move quickly through the materials in this book and this workbook appendix. Many microsystems, however, need to pace themselves, completing the worksheets and assessment on a longer timeline. Some microsystems may need to start an important improvement immediately, even as they are starting the assessment process. If this is your situation, the ongoing assessment will give you needed context and will help you make better improvements.

Remember, however you choose to progress through these materials, it *must* be done within the context of your interdisciplinary team.

Use the data review sheet (Figure A.1) to outline and track which data and information will be retrieved from current systems and which data and information will be measured through a worksheet. Review the worksheets in this workbook. Determine which worksheets you will copy and use to collect new data and information. Determine which worksheets you will not use because you have systems that can provide useful, timely data for you without a special effort.

Microsystem Assessment of Data Sources and Data Collection Actions

With your interdisciplinary team, use Figures A.1 and A.2 to determine which measures you can obtain from your organization and which you will need worksheets for. Be sure the data you collect are current and not months old.

Once you determine which worksheets will be used, plan who will complete each worksheet and when and how.

Also decide who will oversee the compilation of each worksheet or alternative data source.

FIGURE A.1. MICROSYSTEM ASSESSMENT OF DATA SOURCES AND DATA COLLECTION ACTIONS.

Type of Data	Data Source or Data Collection Action	Date and Owner
Know your patients (Figure A.2)		
Estimated age distribution of patients (Figure A.2)		
Estimated number of unique patients in practice (Figure A.2)		
Disease-specific health outcomes (Figure A.2)		
Top diagnoses and conditions (Figure A.2)		
Top referrals (Figure A.2)		
Patients who frequent practice (Figure A.2)		
Clinical microsystems (Figure A.2)		
Patient satisfaction scores (Figures A.2)		
Patient point of service survey (Figure A.3)		
Patient viewpoint survey (Figure A.4)		
Care for chronic conditions survey (Figure A.6)		
Patient population census (Figure A.2)		
"Through the eyes of your patients" survey (Figure A.5)		
Out-of-practice visits (Figure A.2)		
Know your professionals (Figure A.2)		
Current staff (Figure A.2)		
Float pool (Figure A.2)		
On-call (Figure A.2)		
Third next appointment available (Figure A.2)		
Days of operation (Figure A.2)		
Hours of operation (Figure A.2)		
Appointment type (Figure A.2)		
Appointment duration (Figure A.2)		
Staff satisfaction scores (Figures A.2)		
Staff satisfaction survey (Figure A.7)		

(continued)

FIGURE A.1. MICROSYSTEM ASSESSMENT OF DATA SOURCES AND DATA COLLECTION ACTIONS. (*Continued*)

Type of Data	Data Source or Data Collection Action	Date and Owner
Personal skills assessment (Figure A.8)		
Activity survey (Figure A.9)		
Know your processes (Figure A.2)		
Flowcharts of routine processes		
Patient cycle time tool (Figure A.10)		
Core and supporting processes (Figure A.11)		
High-level flowchart		
Know your patterns (Figure A.2)		
Most significant pattern (Figure A.2)		
Successful change (Figure A.2)		
Most proud of (Figure A.2)		
Financial picture (Figure A.2)		
Unplanned activity tracking card (Figure A.12)		
Telephone tracking log (Figure A.13)		

FIGURE A.2. PRIMARY CARE PRACTICE PROFILE.

A. Purpose: Why does your practice exist?

Site Name:	Site Contact:	Date:
Practice Manager:	MD Lead:	Nurse Lead:

B. Know your patients. Take a close look into your practice; create a high-level picture of the *patient population* that you serve. Who are they? What resources do they use? How do the patients view the care they receive?

Est. Age Distribution of Patients	%
Birth–10 years	
11–18 years	
19–45 years	
46–64 years	
65–79 years	
80 + years	
% Females	
Est. # (unique) pts. in practice	
Disease-specific health outcomes (Fig. A.17)	
Diabetes HbA1c =	
Hypertension B/P =	
LDL <100 =	

List Your Top 10 Diagnoses/Conditions

1.	6.
2.	7.
3.	8.
4.	9.
5.	10.

Top Referrals (for example, GI, Cardiology)

Patients who are frequent users of your practice and their reasons for seeking frequent interactions and visits

Other clinical microsystems you interact with regularly as you provide care for patients (for example, OR, VNA)

Patient Satisfaction Scores	% Excellent
Experience via phone	
Length of time to get your appointment	
Saw whom you wanted to see	
Satisfaction with personal manner	
Time spent with person today	

Pt. population census: Do these numbers change by season? (Y/N)	#	Y/N
Patients seen in a day		
Patients seen in last week		
New patients in last month		
Disenrolling patients in last month		
Encounters per provider per year		
Out-of-practice visits		
Condition-sensitive hospital rate		
Emergency room visit rate		

(continued)

FIGURE A.2. PRIMARY CARE PRACTICE PROFILE. (Continued)

Complete "Through the Eyes of Your Patient" (Fig. A.5).

C. *Know your professionals.* Use the following template to create a comprehensive picture of your practice. Who does what and when? Is the right person doing the right activity? Are roles being optimized? Are all roles that contribute to the patient experience listed? What hours is your practice open for business? How many appointment types do you have, and what is the duration of each type? How many exam rooms do you currently have? What is the morale of your staff?

Current Staff	FTEs	Comment/Function	3rd Next Available		Cycle Time
			PE	Follow-Up	Range
Enter names below totals. Use a separate sheet if needed.					
MD total					
NPs/PAs total					
RNs total					
LPNs total					
LNAs/MAs total					
Secretaries total					
Others:					
Do you use float pool?	Yes _____	No _____			
Do you use on-call?	Yes _____	No _____			

Days of Operation	Hours
Monday	
Tuesday	
Wednesday	
Thursday	
Friday	
Saturday	
Sunday	

Do you offer the following? Check all that apply.

- ☐ Group visit
- ☐ E-mail
- ☐ Web site
- ☐ RN clinics
- ☐ Phone follow-up
- ☐ Phone care management
- ☐ Disease registries
- ☐ Protocols/guidelines

Appoint. Type	Duration	Comment

Staff Satisfaction Scores	%
How stressful is the practice?	% Not stressful
Would you recommend it as a good place to work?	% Strongly agree

Each staff member should complete the Personal Skills Assessment (Fig. A.8) and Activity Survey (Fig A.9).

D. **Know your processes.** How do things get done in the microsystem? Who does what? What are the step-by-step processes? How long does the care process take? Where are the delays? What are the handoffs between microsystems?	
1. Track cycle time for patients from the time they check in until they leave the office, using the **Patient Cycle Time worksheet (Fig. A.10). Also list ranges of time per provider on this worksheet.**	
2. Complete the Core and Supporting Process worksheet (Fig. A.11)	
E. **Know your patterns.** What patterns are present but not acknowledged in your microsystem? What is the leadership and social pattern? How often does the microsystem meet to discuss patient care? Are patients and families involved? What are your results and outcomes?	
• Does every member of the practice meet regularly as part of a team?	• Do the members of the practice regularly review and discuss safety and reliability issues?
• How frequently?	• What have you successfully changed?
• What is the most significant pattern of variation?	• What are you most proud of?
	• What is your financial picture?
	Complete the Metrics That Matter worksheet (Fig. A. 14).

Patients

Patients have valuable insight into the quality and process of care health professionals provide. Real-time feedback can pave the way for rapid responses and quick tests of change. Patients or their family members can be asked to complete the following survey (Figure A.3) at the time of their visit to provide real-time measurement of satisfaction.

FIGURE A.3. POINT OF SERVICE SURVEY: PATIENT/FAMILY SATISFACTION WITH PRIMARY CARE PRACTICE ACCESS.

Date: _____

Think about this visit.

1. How would you rate your satisfaction with getting through to the office by phone?

   ❑ Excellent   ❑ Very good   ❑ Good   ❑ Fair   ❑ Poor

2. How would you rate your satisfaction with the length of time you waited to get your appointment today?

   ❑ Excellent   ❑ Very good   ❑ Good   ❑ Fair   ❑ Poor

3. Did you see the clinician or staff member that you wanted to see today?

   ❑ Yes   ❑ No   ❑ Did not matter who I saw today

4. How would you rate your satisfaction with the personal manner of the person you saw today (courtesy, respect, sensitivity, friendliness)?

   ❑ Excellent   ❑ Very good   ❑ Good   ❑ Fair   ❑ Poor

5. How would you rate your satisfaction with the time spent with the person you saw today?

   ❑ Excellent   ❑ Very good   ❑ Good   ❑ Fair   ❑ Poor

Comments:

Thank You for Completing This Survey

Review Section B (Know Your Patients) of the Primary Care Profile (Figure A.2). Determine if there is information you need to collect or if you can obtain this data within your organization. Remember, the aim is to collect and review data and information about your patients and families that might lead to a new design of process and services.

Conduct the Point of Service Survey (Figure A.3) for two weeks with patients and families if you currently *do not* have a method to survey patients and families. If you *do* have a method, be sure the data are up to date and reflect the current state of your practice.

The Patient Viewpoint Survey is a validated survey tool created from the Medical Outcomes Study (MOS) Visit-Specific Questionnaire in 1993 (see Figure A.4). This survey evaluates from the patient perspective the operations of the practice and explores what actions have delighted patients and resulted in loyalty to the practice.

FIGURE A.4. PRIMARY CARE PRACTICE PATIENT VIEWPOINT SURVEY.

Today's Office Visit

Please rate the following questions about the visit you just made to this office.

	Excellent	Very good	Good	Fair	Poor
1. The amount of time you waited to get an appointment.	❏	❏	❏	❏	❏
2. Convenience of the location of the office.	❏	❏	❏	❏	❏
3. Getting through to the office by phone.	❏	❏	❏	❏	❏
4. Length of time waiting at the office.	❏	❏	❏	❏	❏
5. Time spent with the person you saw.	❏	❏	❏	❏	❏
6. Explanation of what was done for you.	❏	❏	❏	❏	❏
7. The technical skills (thoroughness, carefulness, competence) of the person you saw.	❏	❏	❏	❏	❏
8. The personal manner (courtesy, respect, sensitivity, friendliness) of the person you saw.	❏	❏	❏	❏	❏
9. The clinician's sensitivity to your special needs or concerns.	❏	❏	❏	❏	❏
10. Your satisfaction with getting the help that you needed.	❏	❏	❏	❏	❏
11. Your feeling about the overall quality of the visit.	❏	❏	❏	❏	❏

(continued)

FIGURE A.4. PRIMARY CARE PRACTICE PATIENT VIEWPOINT SURVEY. (*Continued*)

General Questions

Please answer these general questions about your satisfaction with this practice.

12. If you could go anywhere to get health care, would you choose this practice or would you prefer to go someplace else?

  ❑ Would choose   ❑ Might prefer   ❑ Not sure
      this practice   someplace else

13. I am delighted with everything about this practice because my expectations for service and quality of care are exceeded.

  ❑ Agree   ❑ Disagree   ❑ Not sure

14. In the last 12 months, how many times have you gone to the emergency room for your care?

  ❑ None   ❑ One time   ❑ Two times   ❑ Three or more times

15. In the last 12 months was it always easy to get a referral to a specialist when you felt like you needed one?

  ❑ Yes   ❑ No   ❑ Does not apply to me

16. In the last 12 months how often did you have to see someone else when you wanted to see your personal doctor or nurse?

  ❑ Never   ❑ Sometimes   ❑ Frequently

17. Are you able to get to your appointments when you choose?

  ❑ Never   ❑ Sometimes   ❑ Always

18. Is there anything our practice can do to improve the care and services for you?

  ❑ No, I'm satisfied   ❑ Yes, some things   ❑ Yes, many things
      with everything   can be improved   can be improved

  Please specify improvement: _____

19. Did you have any good or bad surprises while receiving your care?

  ❑ Good   ❑ Bad   ❑ No surprises

  Please describe: _____

About You

20. In general, how would you rate your overall health?

  ❑ Excellent   ❑ Very good   ❑ Good   ❑ Fair   ❑ Poor

21. What is your age?

  ❑ Under 25 years ❑ 25–44 years   ❑ 45–64 years   ❑ 65 years or older

22. What is your gender?

  ❑ Female   ❑ Male

Sources: Medical Outcomes Study (MOS) Visit-Specific Questionnaire, 1993; Rubin et al., 1993.

Gain insight into how your patients experience your practice. One simple way to understand the patient experience is to experience the care. Members of the staff should do a *walk through* in your practice. Try to make this experience as real as possible. The form in Figure A.5 can be used to document the experience. You can also capture the patient experience by making an audio- or videotape.

FIGURE A.5. THROUGH THE EYES OF YOUR PATIENTS.

Tips for making your "walk through" most productive:

1. Determine with your staff where the starting point and ending point should be, taking into consideration making the appointment, the actual office visit process, follow-up, and other processes.
2. Two members of the staff should role-play these two roles: patient and patient's partner or family member.
3. Set aside a reasonable amount of time to experience the patient journey. Consider walking through the multiple experiences along the patient journey at different times.
4. Make it real. Include the time spent on registration, lab tests, new patient procedures, follow-up, and physicals. Sit where the patient sits. Wear what the patient wears. Make a realistic paper trail, including chart, lab reports, and follow-up materials.
5. During the experience note both positive and negative experiences, as well as any surprises. What was frustrating? What was gratifying? What was confusing? Again, making an audio- or videotape can be helpful.
6. Debrief your staff on what you did and what you learned.

Date:_____ Staff Members:_____

Walk Through Begins When:_____ Ends When:_____

Positives	Negatives	Surprises	Frustrating/Confusing	Gratifying

Obtaining deeper information about your patients can be difficult. One method is to use the HowsYourHealth Web site (www.howsyourhealth. org). On the home page choose "For Health Professionals." This will tell you about the features of the program and how to customize the survey on this site for your practice setting. A beginning step is to have all the practice staff complete the survey to gain insight into survey process for patients and to see how aggregate data about a group might be used in developing plans of care. You might also administer the following survey (Figure A.6).

FIGURE A.6. ASSESSMENT OF CARE FOR CHRONIC CONDITIONS.

Staying healthy can be difficult when you have a chronic condition. We would like to learn about the type of help you get from your health care team regarding your condition. This might include your regular doctor, the nurse, or the physician's assistant who treats your illness.

Over the past 6 months, when I received care for my chronic conditions, I was

	None of the Time	A Little of the Time	Some of the Time	Most of the Time	Always
1. Asked for my ideas when we made a treatment plan.	$\square_1$	$\square_2$	$\square_3$	$\square_4$	$\square_5$
2. Given choices about treatment to think about.	$\square_1$	$\square_2$	$\square_3$	$\square_4$	$\square_5$
3. Asked to talk about any problems with my medicines or their effects.	$\square_1$	$\square_2$	$\square_3$	$\square_4$	$\square_5$
4. Given a written list of things I should do to improve my health.	$\square_1$	$\square_2$	$\square_3$	$\square_4$	$\square_5$
5. Satisfied that my care was well organized.	$\square_1$	$\square_2$	$\square_3$	$\square_4$	$\square_5$
6. Shown how what I did to take care of myself influenced my condition.	$\square_1$	$\square_2$	$\square_3$	$\square_4$	$\square_5$
7. Asked to talk about my goals in caring for my condition.	$\square_1$	$\square_2$	$\square_3$	$\square_4$	$\square_5$
8. Helped to set specific goals to improve my eating or exercise.	$\square_1$	$\square_2$	$\square_3$	$\square_4$	$\square_5$

FIGURE A.6. ASSESSMENT OF CARE FOR CHRONIC CONDITIONS. (*Continued*)

	None of the Time	A Little of the Time	Some of the Time	Most of the Time	Always
9. Given a copy of my treatment plan.	❑₁	❑₂	❑₃	❑₄	❑₅
10. Encouraged to go to a specific group or class to help me cope with my chronic condition.	❑₁	❑₂	❑₃	❑₄	❑₅
11. Asked questions, either directly or on a survey, about my health habits.	❑₁	❑₂	❑₃	❑₄	❑₅
12. Sure that my doctor or nurse thought about my values, beliefs, and traditions when they recommended treatments to me.	❑₁	❑₂	❑₃	❑₄	❑₅
13. Helped to make a treatment plan that I could carry out in my daily life.	❑₁	❑₂	❑₃	❑₄	❑₅
14. Helped to plan ahead so I could take care of my condition even in hard times.	❑₁	❑₂	❑₃	❑₄	❑₅
15. Asked how my chronic condition affects my life.	❑₁	❑₂	❑₃	❑₄	❑₅
16. Contacted after a visit to see how things were going.	❑₁	❑₂	❑₃	❑₄	❑₅
17. Encouraged to attend programs in the community that could help me.	❑₁	❑₂	❑₃	❑₄	❑₅
18. Referred to a dietitian, health educator, or counselor.	❑₁	❑₂	❑₃	❑₄	❑₅
19. Told how my visits with other types of doctors, like an eye doctor or surgeon, helped my treatment.	❑₁	❑₂	❑₃	❑₄	❑₅
20. Asked how my visits with other doctors were going.	❑₁	❑₂	❑₃	❑₄	❑₅

Professionals

Creating a joyful work environment starts with a basic understanding of staff perceptions of the practice. Staff members should complete the Staff Satisfaction Survey in Figure A.7. Use a tally sheet to summarize results.

Ask *all* practice staff to complete this survey. Often you can distribute this survey to any professional who spends time in your practice. Set a deadline of one week, and designate a place where the survey is to be dropped off. You may have an organization-wide survey in place that you can use to replace this survey, but be sure the measures you get from it are *current* data, not months old, and that you are able to use it to capture the needed data from all professionals specific to your workplace.

FIGURE A.7. PRIMARY CARE STAFF SATISFACTION SURVEY.

1. I am treated with respect every day by everyone that works in this practice.
   - ❏ Strongly agree ❏ Agree ❏ Disagree ❏ Strongly disagree

2. I am given everything I need—tools, equipment, and encouragement—to make my work meaningful to my life.
   - ❏ Strongly agree ❏ Agree ❏ Disagree ❏ Strongly disagree

3. When I do good work, someone in this practice notices that I did it.
   - ❏ Strongly agree ❏ Agree ❏ Disagree ❏ Strongly disagree

4. How stressful would you say it is to work in this practice?
   - ❏ Very stressful ❏ Somewhat stressful ❏ A little stressful ❏ Not stressful

5. How easy is it to ask anyone a question about the way we care for patients?
   - ❏ Very easy ❏ Easy ❏ Difficult ❏ Very difficult

6. How would you rate other people's morale and their attitudes about working here?
   - ❏ Excellent ❏ Very good ❏ Good ❏ Fair ❏ Poor

7. This practice is a better place to work than it was 12 months ago.
   - ❏ Strongly agree ❏ Agree ❏ Disagree ❏ Strongly disagree

8. I would recommend this practice as a great place to work.
   - ❏ Strongly agree ❏ Agree ❏ Disagree ❏ Strongly disagree

9. What would make this practice better for patients?

10. What would make this practice better for those who work here?

Development of each member in the practice is a key to success for staff and the microsystem. The Personal Skills Assessment tool (Figure A.8) helps determine the education and training needs of staff. All staff members should complete this survey and then discuss the action plan with leaders and other staff. The action plan is developed to help members achieve goals so they can become the best they can be.

This tool provides guidance for individual development plans and also assesses group needs so that you can plan larger learning and training sessions effectively.

FIGURE A.8. PRIMARY CARE STAFF PERSONAL SKILLS ASSESSMENT.

Name:_____ Unit:_____

Role:_____ Date:_____

Clinical Competencies

Please create your list of clinical competencies and evaluate.	Want to Learn	Never Use			Occasionally				Frequently		
	❏	1	2	3	4	5	6	7	8	9	10

Clinical Information Systems (CIS)

What features and functions do you use?	Want to Learn	Never Use			Occasionally				Frequently		
Provider/on-call schedule	❏	1	2	3	4	5	6	7	8	9	10
Patient demographics	❏	1	2	3	4	5	6	7	8	9	10
Lab results	❏	1	2	3	4	5	6	7	8	9	10
Pathology	❏	1	2	3	4	5	6	7	8	9	10
Problem list	❏	1	2	3	4	5	6	7	8	9	10
Electronic health record (EHR)	❏	1	2	3	4	5	6	7	8	9	10
Review reports/notes	❏	1	2	3	4	5	6	7	8	9	10
Documentation	❏	1	2	3	4	5	6	7	8	9	10
Direct entry	❏	1	2	3	4	5	6	7	8	9	10
Note templates	❏	1	2	3	4	5	6	7	8	9	10
Medication lists	❏	1	2	3	4	5	6	7	8	9	10
Medication ordering	❏	1	2	3	4	5	6	7	8	9	10
Action taken on surgical pathology	❏	1	2	3	4	5	6	7	8	9	10
Insurance status	❏	1	2	3	4	5	6	7	8	9	10
Durable power of attorney	❏	1	2	3	4	5	6	7	8	9	10
Radiology	❏	1	2	3	4	5	6	7	8	9	10
OR schedules	❏	1	2	3	4	5	6	7	8	9	10

Note: CIS refers to hospital- or clinic-based systems used for such functions as checking in patients, maintaining electronic medical records, and accessing lab and X-ray information. Customize your list of CIS features to reflect skills needed by your various staff members to optimize their roles.

(*continued*)

FIGURE A.8. PRIMARY CARE STAFF PERSONAL SKILLS ASSESSMENT. (*Continued*)

Technical Skills

Please rate the following on how often you use them.	Want to Learn	Never Use			Occasionally				Frequently		
CIS	❏	1	2	3	4	5	6	7	8	9	10
E-mail	❏	1	2	3	4	5	6	7	8	9	10
PDA (such as Palm Pilot)	❏	1	2	3	4	5	6	7	8	9	10
Digital dictation link	❏	1	2	3	4	5	6	7	8	9	10
Central dictation	❏	1	2	3	4	5	6	7	8	9	10
Word processing (such as MS Word)	❏	1	2	3	4	5	6	7	8	9	10
Spreadsheet (such as Excel)	❏	1	2	3	4	5	6	7	8	9	10
Presentation (such as PowerPoint)	❏	1	2	3	4	5	6	7	8	9	10
Database (such as Access or FileMaker Pro)	❏	1	2	3	4	5	6	7	8	9	10
Patient database/statistics	❏	1	2	3	4	5	6	7	8	9	10
Internet/intranet	❏	1	2	3	4	5	6	7	8	9	10
Printer access	❏	1	2	3	4	5	6	7	8	9	10
Fax	❏	1	2	3	4	5	6	7	8	9	10
Copier	❏	1	2	3	4	5	6	7	8	9	10
Telephone system	❏	1	2	3	4	5	6	7	8	9	10
Voice mail	❏	1	2	3	4	5	6	7	8	9	10
Pagers	❏	1	2	3	4	5	6	7	8	9	10
Tube system	❏	1	2	3	4	5	6	7	8	9	10

Meeting and Interpersonal Skills

What skills do you currently use?	Want to Learn	Never Use			Occasionally				Frequently		
Effective meeting skills (brainstorming/multi-voting)	❏	1	2	3	4	5	6	7	8	9	10
Timed agendas	❏	1	2	3	4	5	6	7	8	9	10
Role assignments during meetings	❏	1	2	3	4	5	6	7	8	9	10
Delegation	❏	1	2	3	4	5	6	7	8	9	10
Problem solving	❏	1	2	3	4	5	6	7	8	9	10
Patient advocacy process	❏	1	2	3	4	5	6	7	8	9	10
Open and effective communication	❏	1	2	3	4	5	6	7	8	9	10

FIGURE A.8. (*Continued*).

What skills do you currently use?	Want to Learn	Never Use			Occasionally				Frequently		
Feedback—provide and receive	❏	1	2	3	4	5	6	7	8	9	10
Managing conflict/negotiation	❏	1	2	3	4	5	6	7	8	9	10
Emotional/spiritual support	❏	1	2	3	4	5	6	7	8	9	10
Improvement Skills and Knowledge											
What improvement tools do you currently use?	Want to Learn	Never Use			Occasionally				Frequently		
Flowcharts/process mapping	❏	1	2	3	4	5	6	7	8	9	10
Trend charts	❏	1	2	3	4	5	6	7	8	9	10
Control charts	❏	1	2	3	4	5	6	7	8	9	10
PDSA = SDSA improvement model	❏	1	2	3	4	5	6	7	8	9	10
Aim statements	❏	1	2	3	4	5	6	7	8	9	10
Fishbone diagrams	❏	1	2	3	4	5	6	7	8	9	10
Measurement and monitoring	❏	1	2	3	4	5	6	7	8	9	10
Surveys—patient and staff	❏	1	2	3	4	5	6	7	8	9	10
STAR relationship mapping	❏	1	2	3	4	5	6	7	8	9	10

What do you spend *your* time doing? What is your best estimation of how much time you spend doing it? The goal is to have the right person doing the right thing at the right time. The group can discuss which activities are or are not appropriate for different people's level of education, training, and licensure.

You can start with one group of professionals, such as MDs, NPs, RNs, or clerical staff, assessing their activities using an activity survey along the lines of the examples shown in Figure A.9. These examples show surveys for an MD and an RN. This estimate of who does what is intended to reveal, at a high level, where there might be mismatches between education, training, licensure, and actual activities. It is good to eventually have all roles and functions complete this survey for review and consideration. Be sure to create the same categories for each functional role. People in some roles may hesitate to make time estimates; if this happens, just ask them to list their activities for the first review.

FIGURE A.9. PRIMARY CARE STAFF ACTIVITY SURVEY SHEETS.

Position: MD	% of Time
Activity: *See patients in clinic* Specific items involved: • Review chart history • Assess and diagnose patient • Determine treatment plan	
Activity: *Minor procedures*	
Activity: *See patients in hospital*	
Activity: *Follow-up phone calls* Specific items involved: • Answer patient messages and requests	
Activity: *Dictate or document patient encounter* Specific items involved: • Dictate encounter • Review transcriptions and sign off	
Activity: *Complete forms* Specific items involved: • Referrals • Camp or school physicals	
Activity: *Write prescriptions* Specific items involved: • Review chart/write prescriptions	

Position: RN	% of Time
Activity: *Triage patient issues and concerns* Specific items involved: • Phone • Face to face • Internet	15%
Activity: *Patient and family education* Specific items involved: • First time Diabetes	3%
Activity: *Direct patient care* Specific items involved: • See patients in clinic • Injections • Assist provider with patients • Review medication list	30%
Activity: *Follow-up phone calls* Specific items involved: • Call HTN pts/review plan of care	22%
Activity: *Review and notify patients of lab results* Specific items involved: • Normal with follow-up • Drug adjustments	5%

FIGURE A.9. PRIMARY CARE STAFF ACTIVITY SURVEY SHEETS. (*Continued*)

Position: MD | **% of Time**

Activity	%
Activity: *Manage charts*	
Activity: *Evaluate test results* Specific items involved: • Review results and determine next actions	
Activity: *See patients in nursing home*	
Activity: *Miscellaneous* Specific items involved: • CME; attend seminars; attend meetings	
Total	100%

Position: RN | **% of Time**

Activity	%
Activity: *Complete forms* Specific items involved: • Referrals • Camp or school physicals	18%
Activity: *Call in prescriptions* Specific items involved: • Fax prescription	5%
Activity: *Miscellaneous* Specific items involved: • CME; attend seminars; attend meetings	2%
Total	100%

Activity Occurrence Example

What's the next step? Insert the activities from the Activity Survey here.
Activities are combined by role from the data collected above. This creates a master list of activities by role. Fill-in *the number of times per session* (A.M. and P.M.) *that you perform the activity.* Make a tally mark (I) by the activity each time it happens, per session. Use one sheet for each day of the week. Once the frequency of activities is collected, the practice should review the volumes and variations by session, by day of week, and by month of year. This evaluation increases knowledge of predictable variation and supports improved matching of resources to need, based on demand.

Role: RN _____	Date: _____	Day of Week: _____	
	A.M.	P.M.	Total
Visit activities			
Triage patient concerns			
Family and patient education			
Direct patient care			
Nonvisit activities			
Follow-up phone calls			
Complete forms			
Call in prescriptions			
Miscellaneous			
Total			

Processes

Beginning to have all staff understand the processes of care and services in your practice is a key to developing a common understanding and focus for improvement. Start with the high-level process of a patient entering your practice by using the Patient Cycle Time tool in Figure A.10. You can assign someone to track all visits for a week with this tool to get a sample, or the tool can be initiated for all visits in a one-week period, with many people contributing to its collection and completion.

Typically, other processes needing to be measured will be uncovered, and you can create time-tracking worksheets like this one to measure other cycle times.

FIGURE A.10. PRIMARY CARE PRACTICE PATIENT CYCLE TIME.

Day: _____ Date: _____

Scheduled Appointment Time: _____   Provider You Are Seeing Today: _____

Time

_____   1. Time you checked in.

_____   2. Time you sat in the waiting room.

_____   3. Time staff came to get you.

_____   4. Time staff member left you in the exam room.

_____   5. Time provider came into the room.

_____   6. Time provider left the room.

_____   7. Time you left the exam room.

_____   8. Time you arrived at checkout.

_____   9. Time you left the practice.

Comments:

Review, adapt and distribute the following Core and Supporting Processes evaluation form (Figure A.11) to *all* practice staff. Be sure the processes list on the form is accurate for your practice and then ask staff to evaluate the *current* state of these processes. Rate each process by putting a tally mark under the column heading that most closely matches your overall understanding of the process. Also mark the final column if the process is a source of patient complaints. Other options to consider when obtaining staff input are to use an Internet-based survey tool to electronically have staff rate the processes or enlarge this survey tool to poster size, give each role a specific colored marker to use, and rate the processes in a public way. This process results with a large scatter plot display of microsystem member evaluations of the microsystem processes.

Tally the results to give the lead improvement team an idea of where to begin to focus improvement from the staff perspective.

Explore improvements for each microsystem process based on the outcomes of this assessment tool. Each of the processes listed on Figure A.11 should be *flowcharted* to reveal its current state. Once you have flowcharted the current state of your processes and determined your change ideas, use the PDSA ◄─► SDSA Worksheet (Figure A.15) to run tests of change and to measure.

FIGURE A.11. PRIMARY CARE PRACTICE CORE AND SUPPORTING PROCESSES.

Processes	Works Well	Small Problem	Real Problem	Totally Broken	Cannot Rate	We're Working on It	Source of Patient Complaint
Answering phones							
Appointment system							
Messaging							
Scheduling procedures							
Ordering diagnostic testing							
Reporting diagnostic test results							
Prescription renewal							
Making referrals							
Preauthorization for services							
Billing and coding							
Phone advice							
Assignment of patients to your practice							
Orientation of patients to your practice							
New patient workups							
Minor procedures							
Education for patients and families							
Prevention assessment and activities							
Chronic disease management							
Palliative care							

Deming (1982) has said, If you can't draw a picture of your process you can't improve anything. He is referring to the improvement tool of process mapping. With your interdisciplinary team, create a high-level flowchart of your microsystem's appointment process or the entire visit experience. Use the instructions, information, and examples in Chapter Seventeen.

Start with just *one* flowchart. Eventually you will wish to create flowcharts for many different processes in your practice and between your practice and other practices. Keep the symbols simple (see Figure 17.2 in Chapter Seventeen)!

Review your first flowchart to identify unnecessary rework, delays, and opportunities to streamline and improve.

Patterns

Patterns are present in our daily work and we may or may not be aware of them. Patterns can offer hints and clues to our work that inform us of possible improvement ideas. The Unplanned Activity Tracking Card (Figure A.12) is a tool you can ask staff to carry to track patterns of interruptions, waits, and delays in the process of providing smooth and uninterrupted patient care. Start with any group among the staff. Give each person a card to carry during a shift and to mark each time an interruption or other event occurs that means direct patient care is delayed or interrupted. The marks on the tracking cards should then be tallied for each person and for each group to review possible process and system redesign opportunities. Noticing patterns of unplanned activities can alert staff to possible improvements.

This collection tool can be adapted to the work of any role in the primary care practice in order to discover interruptions in work flow. Processes to further evaluate for possible improvements might be marked by circling them.

FIGURE A.12. PRIMARY CARE PRACTICE UNPLANNED ACTIVITY TRACKING CARD.

Name:	
Date: _____ Time: _____	
Place a tally mark (I) for each occurrence of an unplanned activity	**Total**
Interruptions	
• Phone	
• Secretary	
• RN	
• Provider	
Hospital admissions	
Patient phone calls	
Pages	
Missing equipment	
Missing supplies	
Missing chart: Same-day patient	
Missing chart: Patient	
Missing test results	
Other	

Name:	
Date: _____ Time: _____	
Place a tally mark (I) for each occurrence of an unplanned activity	**Total**
Interruptions	
• Phone HHH HHH HHH	15
• Secretary	
• RN HHH HHH	10
• Provider	
Hospital admissions HHH HHH II	12
Patient phone calls	
Pages HHH HHH HHH HHH	20
Missing equipment	
Missing supplies HHH	5
Missing chart: Same-day patient	
Missing chart: Patient HHH HHH	10
Missing test results	
Other	

Patterns can be found through tracking the volumes and types of telephone calls. Review the categories on the telephone tracking log (see Figure A.13); adapt them if necessary to ensure they reflect the general categories of calls your practice receives. Then ask clerical staff to track the telephone calls over the course of a week to find the patterns for each type of call and the volume peaks and valleys.

Put a tally mark (|) each time one of the phone calls is for one of the listed categories. Total the calls for each day, and then total the calls in each category for the week. Note the changes in volume by day of the week and by A.M. and P.M.

FIGURE A.13. PRIMARY CARE PRACTICE TELEPHONE TRACKING LOG.

Week of ___	Monday		Tuesday		Wednesday		Thursday		Friday		Saturday		Sunday		Week Total
	AM	PM	AM	PM	AM	PM	AM	PM	AM	PM	AM	PM	AM	PM	
Appointment for today															
Total															
Appointment for tomorrow															
Total															
Appointment for future															
Total															
Test results															
Total															
Nurse care															
Total															
Prescription refill															
Total															
Referral information															
Total															
Need information															
Total															
Message for provider															
Total															
Talk with provider															
Total															
Day total															

Metrics That Matter

Measures are essential if microsystems are to make and sustain improvements and to attain high performance. All clinical microsystems are awash in data, but relatively few have the rich information environments that allow the daily, weekly, and monthly use of *metrics that matter* (MTM). The key to having all the data that you actually need is to get started in a practical, doable way and to build out your metrics that matter and their vital use over time. Some guidelines for your consideration are listed here. Remember, these are just guidelines, and your microsystem should do what makes sense for its purpose, patients, professionals, processes, and patterns in the way it collects, displays, and uses metrics that matter.

Primary Care Metrics That Matter Guidelines

1. *What?* Every microsystem has vital performance characteristics, things that must happen for successful operations. Metrics that matter (MTMs) should reflect your microsystem's vital performance characteristics.
2. *Why?* The reason to identify, measure, and track MTMs is to ensure that you are not flying blind. Safe, high-quality, and efficient performance will give you specific, balanced, and timely metrics that show
   * When improvements are needed
   * Whether improvements are successful
   * Whether improvements are sustained over time
   * The amount of variation in results over time
3. *How?* Here are steps you can carry out to take advantage of MTMs.
   * *Lead improvement team.* Work with your lead team to establish the microsystem's *need* for metrics and their *routine* use. Quality begins with the intention to achieve measured excellence.
   * *Balanced metrics.* Build a *balanced* set of metrics, one that will give everyone insight into what's working and what's not working. Some data categories to consider are process flow, clinical, safety, patient perceptions, staff perceptions, operations, and finance and costs. Do not start with too many measures. Each of your metrics should have an operational definition, data owner, target value, and action plan. Strongly consider using the Joint Commission on Accreditation of Healthcare Organizations (JCAHO) and Centers for Medicare and Medicaid Services (CMS) metrics—ones that are already widely used by health care organizations across the nation— whenever they are relevant to your microsystem. Your own experience and strategic initiatives may suggest additional "vital" metrics for your system. Also consider what "gold standard" sets—such as measures from the National Quality Foundation (NQF) and from some professional organizations, such

as the American Society of Thoracic Surgeons (ASTS)—have to offer your practice.

- *Data owners or captains.* Start small. Identify one or more data owners for each metric. These data owners will be guided by the lead team. Each owner will be responsible for getting his or her measure and reporting it to the lead team. Seek sources of data from organization-wide systems. If the needed data are not available, use manual methods to get the required measures. Strive to build data collection into the flow of daily work.
- *Data wall displays.* Build a data wall, and use it daily, weekly, monthly, and annually. Gather data for each metric and display them on the data wall. For each process being tracked or worked on, report on the

    Current value or outcome

    Target value or outcome

    Action plan to improve or sustain value or outcome

    Display metrics as soon as possible—daily, weekly, and monthly metrics are the most useful—using visual displays such as time trend charts and bar charts.
- *Review and use.* Review your set of metrics on a regular basis—daily, weekly, monthly, quarterly, and annually. Use metrics in identifying and carrying out needed improvements whenever possible. Make metrics a fun, useful, and lively part of your microsystem development process. Discuss metrics that matter frequently with all staff and take action on these measures as needed.

Review the currently determined metrics that your practice should be monitoring, your *best metrics*.

Revise the worksheet in Figure A.14 so that it names and defines your best metrics. Use notes to identify measures sources if you wish.

Then use the worksheet to list your microsystem's current performance in these metrics and also the target values.

FIGURE A.14. PRIMARY CARE PRACTICE METRICS THAT MATTER.

Name of Measure	Definition and Data Owner	Current and Target Values	Action Plan and Process Owner
General Metrics			
Access			
3rd next available appointment**			
Staff morale			
Staff satisfaction**			
Voluntary turnover**			
Workdays lost per employee per year*			
Safety and reliability			
Identification of high-risk patient diagnosis and associated medications that put patient at risk (such as Coumadin and insulin), and related tests you must track			
Patient satisfaction			
Overall**			
Access**			
Finance			

FIGURE A.14. (*Continued*).

Name of Measure	Definition and Data Owner	Current and Target Values	Action Plan and Process Owner
Patient-Centered Outcome Measures*			
Assessment of Care for Chronic Conditions**			
Visit www.doqit.org for Data Submission Process information			
Coronary artery disease (CAD)			
Antiplatelet therapy			
Lipid profile			
Drug therapy for lowering LDL chol.			
LDL cholesterol level			
Beta-blocker therapy— prior MI			
ACE inhibitor therapy			
Blood pressure			
Heart failure (HF)			
Left ventricular function (LVF) assess			
Left ventricular function (LVF) testing			
Patient education			
Beta-blocker therapy			
ACE inhibitor therapy			
Weight measurement			

(*continued*)

FIGURE A.14. PRIMARY CARE PRACTICE METRICS THAT MATTER. (*Continued*)

Heart failure (HF)			
Blood pressure screening			
Warfarin therapy for pts. with atrial fib.			
Diabetes mellitus (DM)			
HbA1c management			
Lipid measurement			
HbA1c management control			
LDL cholesterol level			
Blood pressure management			
Urine protein testing			
Eye exam, foot exam			
Preventive care (PC)			
Influenza vaccination			
Pneumonia vaccination			
Blood pressure measurement			
Lipid measurement			
LDL cholesterol level			
Colorectal cancer screening			
Breast cancer screening			
Tobacco use			
Tobacco cessation			
Hypertension (HTN)			
Blood pressure screening			
Blood pressure control			
Plan of care			

*OSHA (Occupational Safety and Health Administration) Safety Log measure.
**IHI (Institute for Healthcare Improvement) Whole System Measures (2004).
***Measures from CMS (Center for Medicare and Medicaid Services); American Medical Association (AMA) Physician Consortium for Performance Improvement; National Diabetes Quality Improvement Alliance; National Committee for Quality Assurance (NCQA).

Step 3: Diagnose

With the interdisciplinary lead team review the microsystem's 5 P's assessment and metrics that matter. Also consider your organization's strategic plan. Then select a first theme, (for example, access, safety, flow, reliability, patient satisfaction, communication, prevention, or supply and demand) for improvement.

The purpose of assessing is to make an informed and correct overall diagnosis of your microsystem.

First, identify and celebrate the strengths of your system.

Second, identify and consider opportunities to improve your system:

- The opportunities to improve may come from your own microsystem. They might arise from the assessment, staff suggestions, or patient and family needs and complaints.
- The opportunities to improve may come from outside your microsystem. They might arise from a strategic project or from external performance or quality measures.
- In addition to looking at the detailed data from each assessment tool, you should also synthesize the findings of all the assessments and metrics that matter to get the *big picture* of your microsystem. Identify linkages within the data and information. Consider

    Waste and delays in the process steps. Look for processes that might be re-designed to result in better functions for roles and better outcomes for patients.

    Patterns of variation in the microsystem. Be mindful of smoothing the variations or matching resources with the variation in demand.

    Patterns of outcomes you wish to improve.

It is usually smart to pick out or focus on one important *theme* to improve at a time. Then you can work with all the "players" in your system to make a big improvement in the area selected.

Finally, write out your theme for improvement and a global aim statement. Follow the information and examples in Chapters Fifteen and Sixteen. Use the global aim template in Figure 16.2.

Step 4: Treat Your Primary Care Practice

Draft a specific aim statement and a way to measure that aim using improvement models—PDSA (plan-do-study-act) and SDSA (standardize-do-study-act).

Now that you've made your diagnosis and selected a theme worthy of improving, you are ready to begin using powerful change ideas, improvement tools, and the scientific method to change your microsystem.

This change begins with clearly identifying a *specific* aim and using the plan-do-study-act (PDSA) method, which is known as the *model for improvement*. After you have run your tests of change and have reached the target value for your specific aim, the challenge is to maintain the gains that you have made. This can be done using the standardize-do-study-act (SDSA) method, which is the other half of making improvement that has *staying power*.

To identify your specific aim, follow the information and examples in Chapter Eighteen. Use the specific aim template in Figure 18.2.

With your theme, global aim, and specific aim in hand, you are almost ready to begin testing change ideas with PSDA cycles. However, before you and your team brainstorm your own change ideas, you will be smart to avoid totally reinventing the wheel by first taking into consideration the best-known practices and the change ideas that other clinical teams have found really work. Also be aware that good change ideas will continue to be developed as more field testing is done and more colleagues design improvements (visit www.ihi.org and www. clinicalmicrosystem.org for the latest ideas).

A list of some of the best change ideas that might be adapted and tested in your practice follows. This list also offers Web resources for additional support and tools.

Primary Care Practice Change Ideas to Consider

1. Change ideas to improve access to care (http://www.clinicalmicrosystem.org/access.htm)
   - Shape demand.
   - Match supply and demand.
   - Redesign the system.
2. Change ideas to improve interaction
   - Design group visits or shared medical appointments (http://www.clinicalmicrosystem.org/sma.htm).
   - Use e-mail care.
   - Create a practice Web site.
   - Optimize professional roles for subpopulation care management.
3. Change ideas to improve reliability
   - Use a chronic care model, such as the Improving Chronic Illness Care (ICIC) model (http://www.improvingchroniccare.org).

4. Change ideas to improve vitality
   - Engage all staff in continuous improvement and research.
   - Develop strategies to actively develop individual staff.
   - Create a favorable financial status, which supports investments in the practice.
   - Begin holding a daily huddle with MDs, RNs, and clerical staff to review yesterday and plan for today, tomorrow, and the coming week (use the worksheet in Figure A.16 on page 430).

Also consider the change concepts discussed by Langley, Nolan, Norman, Provost, and Nolan (1996, p. 295). Here are Langley's main change categories:

- Eliminate waste
- Improve work flow
- Optimize inventory
- Change the work environment
- Enhance the producer/customer relationship
- Manage time
- Manage variation
- Design systems to avoid mistakes
- Focus on the product or service

Now you are ready to complete the PDSA ←—→ SDSA Worksheet (Figure A.15) to execute your chosen change idea in a disciplined measured manner, to reach the specific aim. This worksheet offers preparation steps as well as specific PDSA and SDSA steps. Steps 1 to 3 remind you to focus on your theme and specific aim for improvement. They involve big-picture, from 30,000-feet kinds of questions. Then Steps 4 to 7 take you through the PDSA method to improve your process. Steps 8 to 11 help you prepare to standardize your improved process. Then Steps 12 to 15 take you through the SDSA method to standardize the process.

FIGURE A.15. PDSA ←—→ SDSA WORKSHEET.

Name of Group: _____   **Start Date:** _____

TEAM MEMBERS:

1. Leader: _____   5. _____

2. Facilitator: _____   6. _____

3. _____   7. _____

4. _____   8. _____

Coach: _____   Meeting Day/Time: _____

Data Support: _____   Place: _____

1. *Aim* ——→ What are we trying to accomplish?

2. *Measures* ——→ How will we know that a change is an improvement?

3. *Current process* ——→ What is the process for giving care to this type of patient?

FIGURE A.15. (*Continued*).

4. ***Plan*** ⟶ How shall we *plan* the pilot? Who does what and when? With what tools or training? Are baseline data to be collected? How will we know if a change is an improvement?

Tasks to be completed to run test of change	Who	When	Tools or Training Needed	Measures

5. ***Do*** ⟶ What are we learning as we *do* the pilot? What happened when we ran the test? Any problems encountered? Any surprises?

6. ***Study*** ⟶ As we *study* what happened, what have we learned? What do the measures show?

7. ***Act*** ⟶ As we *act* to hold the gains or abandon our pilot efforts, what needs to be done? Will we modify the change? Make a *plan* for the next cycle of change.

(*continued*)

FIGURE A.15. PDSA ◄───► SDSA WORKSHEET (*Continued*).

8. *Standardize* ───► Once you have determined this PDSA result to be the current *best practice,* take action to standardize, do, study, act (SDSA). You will create the conditions to ensure this best practice in daily activities until a *new* change is identified and then the SDSA moves back to the PDSA cycle to test the idea to then standardize again.

9. *Trade-offs* ───► What are you *not* going to do anymore to support this new habit?

What has helped you in the past to change behavior and help you do the "right thing?"

What type of environment has supported standardization?

How do you design the new best practice to be the default step in the process?

Consider professional behaviors, attitudes, values, and assumptions when designing how to embed this new best practice.

FIGURE A.15. (*Continued*).

10. *Measures* ———➤ How will we know that this process continues to be an improvement?

What measures will inform us if standardization is in practice?

How will we know if old behaviors have appeared again?

How will we measure? How often? Who will measure?

11. *Possible changes* ———➤ Are there identified needs for change or new information or a tested best practice to test? What is the change idea? Who will oversee the new PDSA? Go to PDSA, Steps 4 to 7 on this worksheet.

(*continued*)

FIGURE A.15. PDSA ⟷ SDSA WORKSHEET (*Continued*).

12. *Standardize* ⟶ How shall we *standardize* the process and embed it into daily practice? Who? Does what? When? With what tools?

What needs to be *unlearned* to allow this new habit?

What data will inform us if this process is being standardized daily?

Tasks to be completed to embed standardization and monitor process to run test of change	Who	When	Tools or Training Needed	Measures
Note: Create a standard process map to be inserted in your playbook.

13. *Do* ⟶ What are we learning as we *do* the standardization? Any problems encountered? Any surprises? Any new insights to lead to another PDSA cycle?

14. *Study* ⟶ As we *study* the standardization, what have we learned? What do the measures show? Are there identified needs for change or new information or a tested best practice to adapt?

15. *Act* ⟶ As we *act* to hold the gains or modify the standardization efforts, what needs to be done? Will we modify the standardization? What is the change idea? Who will oversee the new PDSA? Design a new PDSA cycle. Make a *plan* for the next cycle of change. Go to PDSA, Steps 4 to 7 on this worksheet.

Step 5: Follow Up

Monitor the new patterns of results and select new themes for improvement. Embed new habits into daily work, using daily huddles, weekly lead team meetings, monthly "town hall" meetings, data walls, and storyboards.

Improvement in health care is a continuous journey.

New patterns need to be monitored to ensure improvements are sustained. Embedding new habits into daily work through the use of huddles to review and remind staff as well as weekly lead team meetings keeps everyone focused on improvements and results that can lead to sustained and continuous improvements.

Data walls, storyboards, and monthly all-staff meetings are also methods that should be used to embed new habits and thinking for improvement.

Finally, the lead team should continually repeat the improvement process described here for newly recognized themes and needed improvements that are identified by the microsystem's ongoing assessments and metrics that matter.

FIGURE A.16. HUDDLE WORKSHEET.

What can we proactively anticipate and plan for in our workday or workweek? At the beginning of the day, hold a review of the day, review of the coming week, and review of the next week. Frequency of daily review is dependent on the situation, but a midday review is also helpful. This worksheet can be modified to add more detail to the content and purpose of the huddles.

Practice: _____   Date: _____

Aim: To enable the practice to proactively anticipate and plan actions based on patient need and available resources and do contingency planning.

Follow-ups from yesterday

"Heads-up" information for today (special patient needs, sick calls, staff flexibility, contingency plans, and so forth)

Meetings

Review of tomorrow and proactive planning

Meetings

References

Deming, W. E. (1982). *Out of the crisis.* Cambridge, MA: MIT Center for Advanced Engineering Study.

Langley, G. J., Nolan, K. M., Norman, C. L., Provost, L. P., & Nolan, T. W. (1996). *The improvement guide: A practical approach to enhancing organizational performance.* San Francisco: Jossey-Bass.

Rubin H. R, Gandek, B., Rogers, W. H., Kosinski, M., McHorney, C. A., & Ware Jr., J. E. (1993). Patients' ratings of outpatient visits in different practice settings. *Journal of the American Medical Association, 270*(7), 835–840.

NAME INDEX

A

Abraham, M. R., 41, 50
Alexander, J., 192, 196
Amalberti, R., 86, 102
Argyris, C., 90, 93, 102
Arrow, H., 13, 32
Ashling, K., 51
Auroy, Y., 86, 102
Ayto, J., 52, 67

B

Baker, G. R., 102
Baker, L. S., 50
Barach, P., 86, 102, 165
Baribeau, P., 164
Barker, R. G., 94, 102
Barnes, B. A., 176
Barnhart, R., 52, 67
Barry, M., 151, 163
Batalden, P. B., 3, *11*, 12, 32, 33,
    34, 36, 44, 46, 49, 50, 51, 54,
    67, 69, *75*, 92, 93, 94, 95, 101,
    102, 104, 106, 107, 119, 123,
    124, 128, 131, 134, 146, 147,
    148, 164, 165, 166, 176, 178,

191, 196, 205, *209*, 227, 228,
    229, *231*, 232, 242, 261, 270,
    310, 312, 333, 338
Bate, P., 211, 229
Bates, D., 166, 176
Beckham, V., 164
Beer, M., 82, 102
Bennis, W. G., 73, 103
Bensimon, E. M., 93, 102
Berdahl, J., 13, 32
Berwick, D., 6, 32, 86, 87, 102,
    176, 205, 215, 235, 299, 381
Birnbaum, R., 93, 102
Bisognano, M., 102
Bladyka, K., 4, 7, 8, 9, 10
Blake, R. R., 65, 67
Blanchard, K. H., 121, 123
Blike, G., 165, 171, 176
Bodenheimer, T., 149, 152,
    163, 164
Bohlen, C., 107, 123
Böjestig, M., *73*, *212*, *213*, *214*
Bolman, L. G., 65, 67, 78, 80, *81*,
    93, 94, 95, 102
Bonomi, A. E., 164
Bossidy, L., xxxii, xxxvii, 77, 78,
    79, 100, 102

Box, G., 45, 49
Braddock, C. R., III, 157, 164
Brasel, K. J., 176
Brennan, T., 166, 176
Brown, P. W., 180, 196
Bruner, J. S., 216, 217, 218, 229
Bubolz, T., 131, 147
Buckingham, M., 121, 122, 123,
    210, 229
Burck, C., xxxii, xxxvii, 90, 102
Burdick, E., 176

C

Campbell, C., 50, 106, 147, 178
Capra, F., 12, 32
Carlson, R., 337, 338
Carthey, J., 166, 177
Charan, R., xxxii, xxxvii, 77, 78,
    79, 100, 102
Christenson, P., 121, 123
Cisneros-Moore, K. A., 41, 49
Clifton, D. O., 210, 229
Codman, E. A., 131, 146
Coffman, C., 121, 122, 123
Cohen, D. S., 82, 103, 210, 229
Coker, K., 41, 49

433

SUBJECT INDEX

A

Accelerating Improvement in CF CareCollaborative program, 5

Acceptance, importance of, *83*

Access to care: brainstorming and multi-voting to address, 329; change ideas to improve, 422; fishbone diagram of, *320*, 337; as the improvement global aim, 295; measured improvement in, reaching, 382; measuring and monitoring, 361; as a metric that matters, *418*; patterns of, assessing, case study involving, 268, *269*; run chart displaying, 343, *344*; specific aim statement addressing, 312; as a theme for improvement, 287, *288*, 289

Access to information, 173, 185

Accountability: fostering, 54, 98; for generating results, method for establishing, 194

Act step: in the PDSA cycle, *275*, 277, 425; in the SDSA cycle, 280, 428

Action guide. *See* M3 Matrix

Action learning, idea of, 216

Action planning, to improve the workplace and its staff, importance of, 119, 121–122

Action plans: case studies involving, 366, 368; clarification of, 277; defining, 364; developing, guide for, 205; distinguishing, from Gantt charts, 362; for education and training, developing, 403; good time to make, 362; how to write, 365; in the improvement ramp, *240*, *363*; organizational, alignment of staff development with, 107; reason for using, 364; reporting on, 417

Action steps, in leading macrosystems, 96–99

Action strategies: formulating more effective, 95; to improve patient safety, *175*

Action taking: being prepared for, 53; and empowerment, *84*; flexible approach to, importance of, 80; as a fundamental

process of leading, 54, 58, *59–62*; intelligent, 360; recommended, to address common oversights and wastes, *142–143*; time frame for, 205, *206–207*

Action-learning activity: creating conditions for, 98; embarking on, example of, 36

Action-learning program: model providing, 47; sponsoring an, 35; topics covered in, xxxv–xxxvi; using toolkits to guide, 227

Actions taken, to know the 5 P's, *140–141*

Activating, 159

Active involvement, as requisite, 388

Activities, assessing: reason for, 406; worksheets for, *406–407*

Activity occurrence example, *407*

Adaptive responses, to cost-cutting imperatives, example of, 38–39

Admission process, high-level flowchart of, *305*

Advanced information systems, myth about, 152, *153*, 154, 158